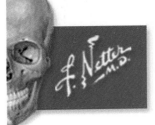
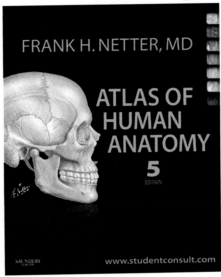

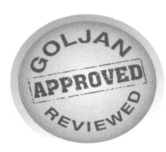

NETTER'S INTRODUCTION TO IMAGING

Larry R. Cochard, PhD
Assistant Professor of Medical Education
Augusta Webster, MD, Office of Medical Education and Faculty Development
Feinberg School of Medicine
Northwestern University
Chicago, Illinois

Lori A. Goodhartz, MD
Associate Professor of Radiology
Feinberg School of Medicine
Northwestern University
Chicago, Illinois

Carla B. Harmath, MD
Assistant Professor of Radiology
Feinberg School of Medicine
Northwestern University
Chicago, Illinois

Nancy M. Major, MD
Professor of Radiology and Orthopaedics
Division Musculoskeletal
University of Pennsylvania Health System
Philadelphia, Pennsylvania

Srinivasan Mukundan, Jr., PhD, MD
Section Head of Neuroradiology
Brigham & Women's Hospital;
Associate Professor of Radiology
Harvard Medical School
Boston, Massachusetts

Illustrations by
Frank H. Netter, MD

Contributing Illustrator
Carlos A.G. Machado, MD

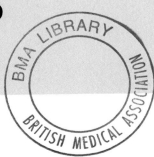

ELSEVIER
SAUNDERS

3251 Riverport Lane
St. Louis, Missouri 63043

NETTER'S INTRODUCTION TO IMAGING   978-1-4377-0759-5

Library of Congress Cataloging-in-Publication Data

Cochard, Larry R.
  Netter's introduction to imaging / Larry R. Cochard ... [et al.] ; illustrations by Frank H. Netter ; contributing illustrator, Carlos A.G. Machado.—1st ed.
    p. ; cm.
  Introduction to imaging
  Includes bibliographical references and index.
  ISBN 978-1-4377-0759-5 (pbk. : alk. paper)   1. Diagnostic imaging.   I. Netter, Frank H. (Frank Henry), 1906-1991.   II. Title.   III. Title: Introduction to imaging.
  [DNLM: 1. Diagnostic Imaging.   WN 180]
  RC78.7.D53C59 2012
  616.07′54—dc23
                                                      2011014087

Editor: Elyse O'Grady
Developmental Editor: Marybeth Thiel
Publishing Services Manager: Deborah L. Vogel
Senior Project Manager: Jodi M. Willard
Design Manager: Steve Stave
Illustrations Manager: Karen Giacomucci
Marketing Manager: Jason Oberacker
Editorial Assistant: Chris Hazle-Cary

Printed in Canada

Last digit is the print number: 9 8 7 6 5 4 3 2 1

To Sue, my wife and best friend, for her support, her love, and her good nature when hearing way too much about teaching, anatomy projects, and the latest news on the book.

Larry R. Cochard, PhD

To all my family and friends who have encouraged me along the way.

Lori A. Goodhartz, MD

To my parents, Carlos and Tania, for teaching me to persevere,
To my husband, Alexandre, for being there for me,
To my son, Lucas, who makes me want to be a better person,
To Dr. Goodhartz, for being a mentor and a friend,
To all students and residents, who inspire me to continue learning!

Carla B. Harmath, MD

To students past and present, who have made me a better teacher,
To Glen Toomayan—thank you for being the most dependable and trusted friend one can have.

Nancy M. Major, MD

To the students who will use this book,
To Shailesh Gaikwad, Pamela Deaver, and Karli Spetzler for their many contributions to this project,
And, finally, to my wife, Dr. Nancy Mukundan, and our sons, Dev and TJ.

Srinivasan Mukundan, Jr., PhD, MD

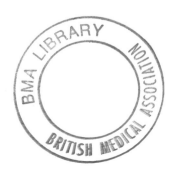

Acknowledgments

The idea for this book originated from Dr. Larry Cochard's participation as a member of an Imaging Task Force chaired by Dr. Amy Kontrick at the Feinberg School of Medicine in 2004. This task force was charged with evaluating the teaching of imaging in all 4 years of medical school, identifying constraints, and suggesting ways it might be improved.

The concept evolved with the development of a password-protected imaging website with Netter anatomy correlations. This website, organized by curricular units, was funded by an Augusta Webster Innovations in Education grant to Dr. Cochard and Dr. Lori Goodhartz.

Many individuals played a valuable role in the production of this book by contributing images or text, labeling images, editing, or general consultation. Our heartfelt thanks go to the following individuals:

Dr. James Baker
David Botos
Dr. James Carr
Dr. Pamela Deaver
Dr. James Donaldson
Dr. Jon Ellison
Dr. Shailesh Gaikwad
Dr. Melina Kibbe
Dr. Randolph Perkins
Angela Del Pino
Dr. Julia Poccia
Karli Spetzler
Dr. Glen Toomayan

A special thanks goes to Senior Developmental Editor Marybeth Thiel for her patience, her good nature, and her skill at guiding a ship that often seemed like a flotilla; and to Jodi Willard, Senior Project Manager, for her attention to detail in page layouts and for her enthusiasm and accommodation, which made the entire corrections process enjoyable.

About the Editors

Larry R. Cochard, PhD, is an Assistant Professor of Medical Education at Northwestern University's Feinberg School of Medicine. He teaches anatomy, embryology, and histology in the M1 curriculum and is a curricular leader. He is a four-time winner of the George H. Joost award for M1 Basic Science Teacher of the Year and has won many other teaching awards. He is also the author of *Netter's Atlas of Human Embryology* (ICON Learning Systems, 2002).

Lori A. Goodhartz, MD, is an Associate Professor of Radiology at Northwestern University's Feinberg School of Medicine and is an attending radiologist at Northwestern Memorial Hospital in Chicago. She has been involved in medical education throughout her career. For 6 years she was the Diagnostic Radiology Residency Program Director. She is currently the Vice Chair for Education in the Department of Radiology.

Carla B. Harmath, MD, is a fellowship-trained body imager and is an Assistant Professor in the Department of Radiology at Northwestern University's Feinberg School of Medicine.

Nancy M. Major, MD, began her career as an MSK radiologist at Duke University Medical Center. After completing her fellowship training at Duke, she remained on the faculty for 13 years. Her research interest is musculoskeletal imaging with a concentration in sports-related injuries, musculoskeletal tumors, and biomechanics associated with injuries. During her tenure at Duke, she educated residents, fellows, and medical students about the nuances of musculoskeletal radiology. She prepared the Duke University radiology residents for their board exams, was Director of Medical Student Radiology Education, and has been voted Teacher of the Year at Duke University School of Medicine multiple times. Her involvement in medical student education and anatomy instruction led to the interest in putting together this volume of the Netter anatomy series.

Dr. Major is a co-editor of the extremely successful *Musculoskeletal MR* and a number of other radiology texts and references, including *Fundamentals of Body CT, Radiology Core Review,* and *A Practical Approach to Radiology.* In addition, she is well-published in peer-reviewed journals.

Dr. Major is Professor and Chief of MSK Radiology with a joint appointment in Orthopaedics at the University of Pennsylvania. She continues to educate residents, fellows, and medical students and lectures nationally and internationally about MSK radiology.

Srinivasan Mukundan, Jr., PhD, MD, is an Associate Professor of Radiology at Harvard Medical School and Section Head of Neuroradiology at the Brigham and Women's Hospital in Boston. Along with Drs. Tracey Milligan (Neurology) and Jane Epstein (Psychiatry), Dr. Mukundan is a Founder and Co-Director of the Integrated Mind-Brain Medicine course at Harvard Medical School. In addition, he has been involved in teaching courses at the undergraduate, graduate, and postgraduate levels at Duke University, where he still is appointed Adjunct Associate Professor of Biomedical Engineering.

About the Artists

Frank H. Netter, MD

Frank H. Netter was born in New York City in 1906. He studied art at the Art Student's League and the National Academy of Design before entering medical school at New York University, where he received his MD degree in 1931. During his student years, Dr. Netter's notebook sketches attracted the attention of medical faculty and other physicians, allowing him to augment his income by illustrating articles and textbooks. He continued illustrating as a side career after establishing a surgical practice in 1933, but he ultimately opted to give up his practice in favor of a full-time commitment to art. After service in the U.S. Army during World War II, Dr. Netter began his long collaboration with the CIBA Pharmaceutical Company (now Novartis Pharmaceuticals). This 45-year partnership resulted in the production of the extraordinary collection of medical art so familiar to physicians and other medical professionals worldwide.

In 2005 Elsevier Inc. purchased the Netter Collection and all publications from Icon Learning Systems. More than 50 publications feature the art of Dr. Netter and are available through Elsevier Inc. (In the United States: www.us.elsevierhealth.com/Netter. Outside the United States: www.elsevierhealth.com.)

Dr. Netter's works are among the finest examples of the use of illustration in the teaching of medical concepts. The 13-book *Netter Collection of Medical Illustrations*, which includes the greater part of the more than 20,000 paintings created by Dr. Netter, became and remains one of the most famous medical works ever published. *The Netter Atlas of Human Anatomy*, first published in 1989, presents the anatomical paintings from the Netter Collection. Now translated into 16 languages, it is the anatomy atlas of choice among medical and health professions students around the world.

The Netter illustrations are appreciated not only for their aesthetic qualities but, more important, for their intellectual content. As Dr. Netter wrote in 1949, "...clarification of a subject is the aim and goal of illustration. No matter how beautifully painted, how delicately and subtly rendered a subject may be, it is of little value as a *medical illustration* if it does not serve to make clear some medical point." Dr. Netter's planning, conception, point of view, and approach are what inform his paintings and make them so intellectually valuable.

Frank H. Netter, MD, physician and artist, died in 1991.

Learn more about the physician-artist whose work has inspired the Netter Reference collection at http://www.netterimages.com/artist/netter.htm.

Carlos Machado, MD

Carlos Machado was chosen by Novartis to be Dr. Netter's successor. He continues to be the main artist who contributes to the Netter collection of medical illustrations.

Self-taught in medical illustration, cardiologist Carlos Machado has contributed meticulous updates to some of Dr. Netter's original plates and has created many paintings of his own in the style of Netter as an extension of the Netter collection. Dr. Machado's photorealistic expertise and his keen insight into the physician/patient relationship informs his vivid and unforgettable visual style. His dedication to researching each topic and subject he paints places him among the premier medical illustrators at work today.

Learn more about Dr. Machado's background and see more of his art at http://www.netterimages.com/artist/machado.htm.

PREFACE

This book is for first- and second-year medical students and other students who are beginning their study of radiology and anatomy. Imaging is usually taught in conjunction with anatomy or a problem-based learning (PBL) component of the curriculum, and it provides a relevant and interesting context for the study of normal structure and function. A lot of images, anatomical sections, and basic descriptions of modalities are included in first-year textbooks, but it is hard to find readings that address the types of questions M1 students ask about imaging. The goal in writing this book was to provide a more comprehensive resource that students can use for introductory imaging lectures, problem-based learning, and any other context in which imaging is addressed in the first 2 years.

Chapter 1 provides an overview of the basic modalities: x-rays and fluoroscopy, computed tomography (CT), magnetic resonance imaging (MRI), nuclear medicine imaging, and ultrasound. Included in this chapter are key physics principles, where and how the modalities are used, and their advantages and disadvantages. An overview of angiography is also provided. An important theme of Chapter 1 is how images are presented and manipulated on the viewing screen and basic principles of their interpretation. This ranges from the interpretation of x-ray densities to topics such as the Hounsfield scale and windows in CT and volume-rendering vs. maximum intensity projection (MIP) computer algorithms for producing images on the screen. Chapter 1 also provides information on the hospital picture archiving and communication system (PACS), radiation safety, and future trends in imaging.

The imaging in the other chapters reinforces the concepts presented in Chapter 1 by showing how the modalities are applied in each body region. The brief text with the images helps explain what can and cannot be seen, emphasizes important landmarks, and offers guiding principles used to interpret the image. Also addressed is information on the timing of image capture with the use of contrast to best view particular vessels or organs, examples of search strategies radiologists use to systematically look for pathology in a study, and some invasive procedures and interventions that are part of radiology.

Although the emphasis of this book is basic radiology, image interpretation is ultimately about anatomy. This book contains the Netter anatomical sections with comparable images plus some additional high-yield anatomy illustrations to help interpret the sections and images. The text with the anatomy plates gives a general overview of the anatomy, with an emphasis on anatomical relationships that are useful in the interpretation of body sections and imaging in general. In addition, learning tools in the thorax and abdomen chapters help students address what structures can be seen at each vertebral level.

Some examples of pathology are included, but they are not about diagnosis. They are intended to illuminate normal radiological anatomy, to show why particular imaging modalities are chosen for a study, and to indicate the types of things radiologists look for in their systematic search strategies. In the thorax chapter, the search strategy is presented in more detail as an example of how a strategy is applied. The pathology presented there and throughout the book will also help to prepare students for cases they will begin to encounter in their first and second years, in their radiology clerkships or electives, and on board exams.

Another feature of the book is a glossary of radiological terms. The glossary serves as a quick "go to" resource and also presents some terms that were not addressed in the book but may be encountered by students. Some pathology and anatomy terms are also included to add a bit of the integration that is a theme of this book.

It may seem strange that the primary author of an imaging book is not a radiologist. I teach anatomy, histology, and embryology to first-year medical students and, like most anatomists, my initial experience with anything radiological was preparing labeled x-rays for display in the anatomy lab. My knowledge of radiology increased a bit over the years as I worked with radiologists on the imaging content of the M1 curriculum, encountered cases with imaging as a PBL facilitator, and co-authored an imaging and radiologic anatomy website. Frustrated with the lack of suitable print resources, I continued to have a vision for a book like this. I am honored, pleased, and fortunate to work with such a talented group of radiologists on this project. Although there are certainly anatomical points I wanted to make in this book, my main task was to keep the information about the imaging within the scope of an M1/M2 curriculum. This was a result of not only editing but also my enjoyment in playing the role of M1 student. I posed my naïve questions about imaging to the co-authors and incorporated or emphasized the pearls, principles, and light bulb moments I found useful in expanding my knowledge of radiology.

The goals throughout this book are to introduce a discipline that is new and potentially difficult to beginning students in a manner that is easy to understand and to give a view of what radiologists do and how they do it.

Larry R. Cochard, PhD
October 2010

CONTENTS

1 INTRODUCTION TO IMAGING MODALITIES   1

2 BACK AND SPINAL CORD   17

3 THORAX   33

4 ABDOMEN   77

5 PELVIS AND PERINEUM   103

6 UPPER LIMBS   121

7 LOWER LIMBS   147

8 HEAD AND NECK   183

Glossary   261

Index   265

1

INTRODUCTION TO IMAGING MODALITIES

1.1   X-RAY OVERVIEW

1.2   INTERPRETATION OF X-RAY DENSITIES

1.3   COMPUTED TOMOGRAPHY OVERVIEW

1.4   THE HOUNSFIELD SCALE: CT WINDOW LEVELS AND WINDOW WIDTHS

1.5   CT USES, ADVANTAGES, AND DISADVANTAGES

1.6   MAGNETIC RESONANCE IMAGING OVERVIEW

1.7   MRI USES, ADVANTAGES, AND DISADVANTAGES

1.8   MRI PULSE SEQUENCES

1.9   NUCLEAR MEDICINE IMAGING

1.10   FLUOROSCOPY

1.11   ULTRASOUND

1.12   ANGIOGRAPHY: COMPUTED TOMOGRAPHY ANGIOGRAM VS. MAGNETIC RESONANCE ANGIOGRAM AND VOLUME RENDERING VS. MAXIMUM INTENSITY PROJECTION

1.13   ANGIOGRAPHY: DIGITAL SUBTRACTION ANGIOGRAPHY

1.14   ARCHIVING AND COMMUNICATION SYSTEM

1.15   FUTURE DEVELOPMENTS IN IMAGING

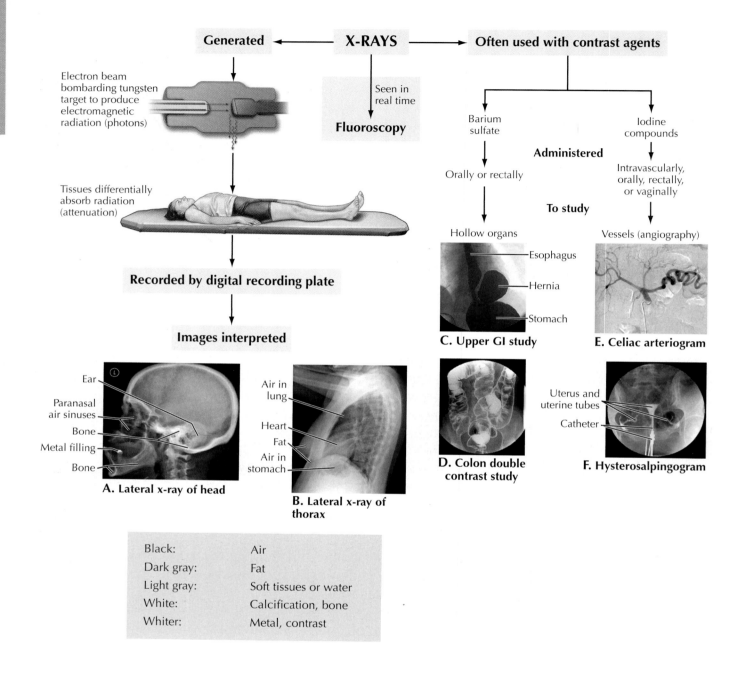

Generated ← **X-RAYS** → **Often used with contrast agents**

Electron beam bombarding tungsten target to produce electromagnetic radiation (photons)

Seen in real time
Fluoroscopy

Tissues differentially absorb radiation (attenuation)

Barium sulfate

Iodine compounds

Administered

Orally or rectally

Intravascularly, orally, rectally, or vaginally

To study

Recorded by digital recording plate

Hollow organs

Vessels (angiography)

Esophagus
Hernia
Stomach

Images interpreted

C. Upper GI study

E. Celiac arteriogram

Ear
Paranasal air sinuses
Bone
Metal filling
Bone

Air in lung
Heart
Fat
Air in stomach

Uterus and uterine tubes
Catheter

A. Lateral x-ray of head

B. Lateral x-ray of thorax

D. Colon double contrast study

F. Hysterosalpingogram

Black:	Air
Dark gray:	Fat
Light gray:	Soft tissues or water
White:	Calcification, bone
Whiter:	Metal, contrast

1.1 X-RAY OVERVIEW

This concept map is an overview of how x-ray images are acquired and interpreted. X-rays (photons) from the tungsten target pass through the body to expose the recording plate (what used to be film). The greater the exposure, the darker the density will be. The greater the attenuation or absorption of the photons by tissues, the whiter the density will appear. Organs with air will appear dark; bone will appear white. Soft tissues and water have intermediate density. A greater thickness of bone or soft tissue results in a whiter density. In **A,** compare the bone densities at the periphery of the neurocranium, the interior of the neurocranium, and the dense cortical bone of the temporal bone at the base of the neurocranium. In **B,** compare the soft tissue densities of the heart and the abdomen. Barium contrast agents are used to study hollow organs (**C** and **D**). Water-soluble iodine compounds are used for vascular studies (**E**) or where contrast might enter a body cavity (**F**).

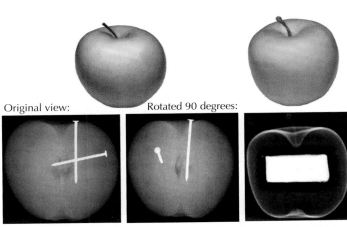

A. **Real apple with nails (left) and plastic apple with center weight (right).**
Compare the densities in the real and plastic apples and the appearance of
the nails in the original and rotated views.

Original view: Rotated 90 degrees:

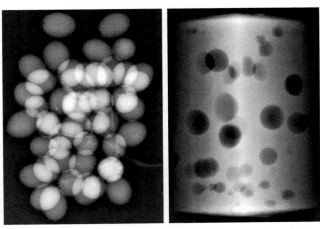

B. **Grapes and a wedge of Swiss cheese with its apex in the midline.**
Note the effect of overlapping grapes and the air spaces in the cheese
on the x-ray densities.

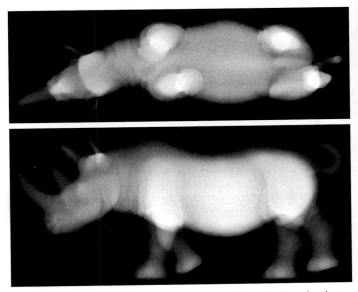

C. **Toy animal.** The obvious shapes in a toy model (bottom) are harder to
interpret in the superior view (top). In both views note that some areas
are brighter than others.

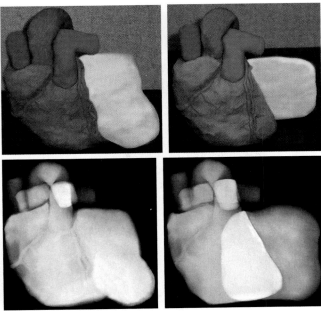

D. **The silhouette sign.** Note how the left margin of the model heart
cannot be discerned in the x-ray where a mass is against the heart (left)
but is visible when the mass is behind the heart (right).

1.2 INTERPRETATION OF X-RAY DENSITIES

The interpretation of x-ray densities is demonstrated with
x-rays of common objects. In **A,** densities ranging from the
metal nails to the air in the plastic apple are seen. Different
views of the apple (or human body) are required to evaluate
the location and shapes of the nails (or anatomical structures
or pathological processes—also see **C**). Like a thin neurocranial bone or a membranelike pleura, the thin shell of the
plastic apple is much denser seen on edge than en face. For
equivalent densities of objects, the x-ray image is denser for
larger or thicker or overlapping objects (**B** and **C**). **D** illustrates
the loss of a boundary of an object or structure if it is against
a structure or fluid of similar density. This is called the *silhouette sign*. The boundary is visible if the object is against air and
the similar density is behind or in front of the object.

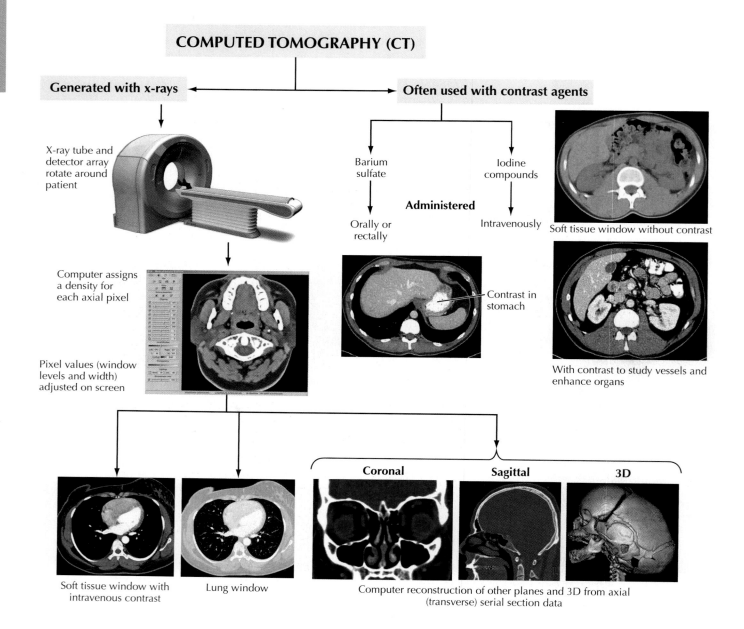

COMPUTED TOMOGRAPHY (CT)

Generated with x-rays

X-ray tube and detector array rotate around patient

Computer assigns a density for each axial pixel

Pixel values (window levels and width) adjusted on screen

Often used with contrast agents

Barium sulfate

Iodine compounds

Administered

Orally or rectally

Intravenously

Soft tissue window without contrast

Contrast in stomach

With contrast to study vessels and enhance organs

Soft tissue window with intravenous contrast

Lung window

Coronal

Sagittal

3D

Computer reconstruction of other planes and 3D from axial (transverse) serial section data

1.3 COMPUTED TOMOGRAPHY OVERVIEW

Current multidetector computed tomography (MDCT) images are generated with x-rays passing through the body in a helical fashion as the patient moves through a gantry containing a rotating x-ray tube. Detectors on the opposite site of the tube collect the x-rays that have passed through the body.

Mathematical algorithms are used to reconstruct axial (transverse plane) images of the body from the data collected by the detectors. Images in the sagittal and coronal planes and three-dimensional renderings can be reconstructed by computer from the serial slices of axial data. The gray-scale image can be manipulated on the monitor.

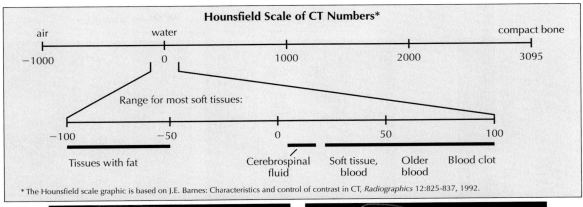

Hounsfield Scale of CT Numbers*

air   water   compact bone

−1000   0   1000   2000   3095

Range for most soft tissues:

−100   −50   0   50   100

Tissues with fat   Cerebrospinal   Soft tissue,   Older   Blood clot
                              fluid   blood   blood

* The Hounsfield scale graphic is based on J.E. Barnes: Characteristics and control of contrast in CT, *Radiographics* 12:825-837, 1992.

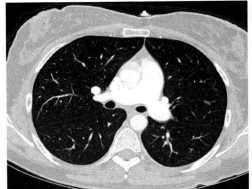

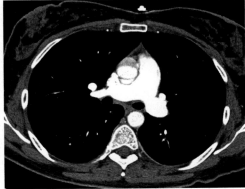

A. Lung window Level −550, width 1600

B. Soft tissue (mediastinal) window
Level 70, width 450, contrast in arterial phase

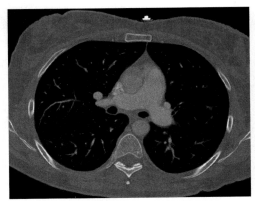

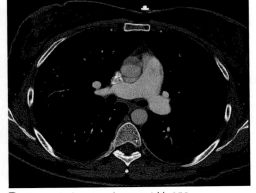

C. Bone window Level 570, width 3077

D. Bone window Level 455, width 958

1.4 THE HOUNSFIELD SCALE: CT WINDOW LEVELS AND WINDOW WIDTHS

Computed tomography (CT) density numbers are attenuation units measured by what is called the *Hounsfield scale*, named after the British engineer who developed the first practical CT scanner in the 1970s. The density of water is set at zero, air (as in the lung or bowel) is −1000, and compact bone is +3095. Most soft tissues in the body have CT numbers between −100 and +100. Computer monitors show 256 levels of gray; thus only a portion of the Hounsfield scale can be displayed, and this "window" can be adjusted on the screen. The number on the Hounsfield scale set to middle gray is referred to as the window level, and the range of the gray scale mapped onto the Hounsfield scale is called the *window width*. All CT numbers below the window width display as black; CT numbers above the window width are white. A wide window width is good for imaging bone; a narrow window is better for soft tissue.

CT IS USEFUL FOR IMAGING:

Bone

Chest and abdomen organs and pathology

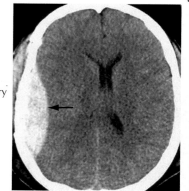

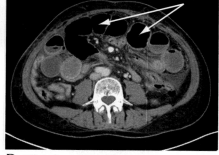

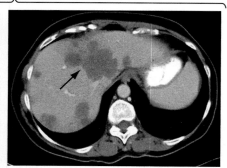

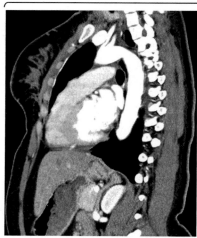

C. Liver metastases

B. Good general organ definition

A. L5 dislocation (spondylolisthesis)

Blood vessels, intracranial bleeding

D. Dilated small intestine

—Left coronary artery

E. Heart and pulmonary vessels

F. Epidural bleeding

Advantages	Disadvantages
• Quick (a few seconds for the whole body)	• Uses ionizing radiation
• Motion not as much of a problem	• Renal function must be evaluated if contrast used
• Gray scale can be manipulated on the viewing screen	• Some patients are allergic to iodine contrast
• Resolution excellent for many areas	
• Widely available and cheaper than magnetic resonance imaging	

1.5 CT USES, ADVANTAGES, AND DISADVANTAGES

Since CT is based on x-rays, CT studies are especially good for evaluating bone and structures containing air, as in the bowel **(D)**. The high speed of acquisition is good for use in the thorax and abdomen since motion artifact is limited. A bone window has excellent discrimination between compact and trabecular bone **(A)** and is useful throughout the body in detecting and evaluating fractures. The majority of CT studies use contrast, and vascular studies (angiography) are commonly done with CT. Vascular contrast also enhances the boundaries between organs and fat or air, and the window levels can be adjusted on the screen. The major disadvantage is the radiation dose. There is increasing concern over the amount of radiation that the U.S. population is being exposed to because of the increased use of CT and nuclear medicine in medical diagnosis. The ALARA principal *(As Low As Reasonably Achievable)* is the basis of radiation safety. This means that, when exposing a patient to radiation for diagnostic purposes, one should always use the lowest radiation dose possible while still ensuring a diagnostic study.

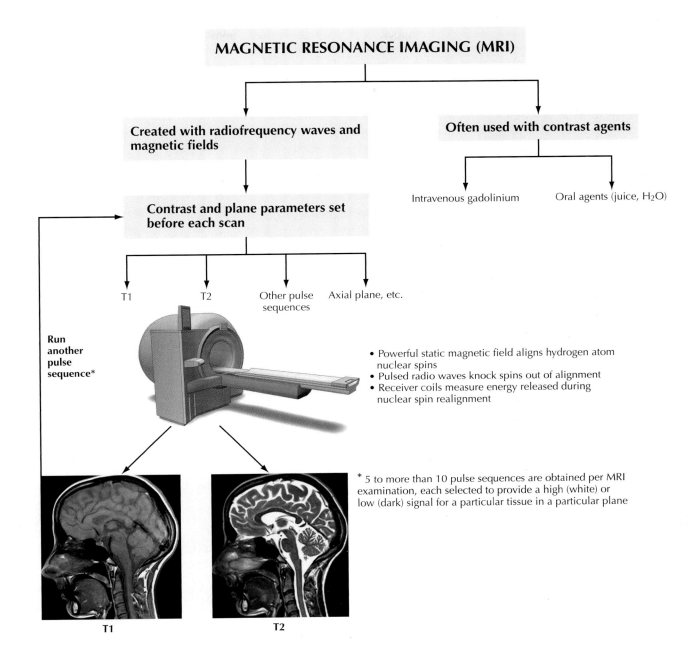

MAGNETIC RESONANCE IMAGING (MRI)

Created with radiofrequency waves and magnetic fields

Often used with contrast agents

Intravenous gadolinium

Oral agents (juice, H_2O)

Contrast and plane parameters set before each scan

T1   T2   Other pulse sequences   Axial plane, etc.

Run another pulse sequence*

- Powerful static magnetic field aligns hydrogen atom nuclear spins
- Pulsed radio waves knock spins out of alignment
- Receiver coils measure energy released during nuclear spin realignment

* 5 to more than 10 pulse sequences are obtained per MRI examination, each selected to provide a high (white) or low (dark) signal for a particular tissue in a particular plane

T1

T2

1.6 MAGNETIC RESONANCE IMAGING OVERVIEW

Magnetic resonance imaging (MRI) does not use ionizing radiation. Images are created using the radiofrequency energy emitted by hydrogen protons when strong magnetic fields generated around a patient are manipulated. Atoms have a property called *nuclear spin* that aligns with the magnetic field. When a radiofrequency pulse is applied, the spin alignments are altered. As they return to equilibrium, the radiofrequency energy emitted by the protons during this "relaxation time" can be measured by the current (MR signal) generated in a receiver coil. Tissues have different relaxation times, depending on their water content and general molecular composition. Additional magnetic field gradients are applied; by varying these and the strength of the radiofrequency pulse, a large library of pulse sequences can be applied to provide the appropriate MR signal contrast to view most any tissue.

MRI Is Useful for Imaging:

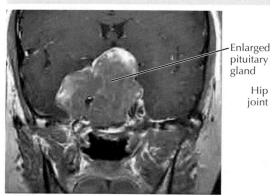

Enlarged pituitary gland

A. Pathologic vs. normal tissue

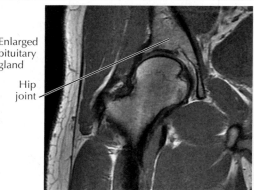

Hip joint

B. Musculoskeletal system

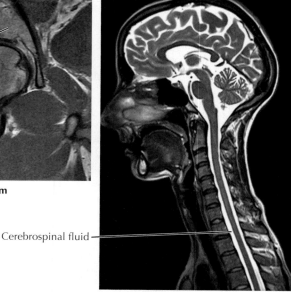

Cerebrospinal fluid

C. Fluid, edema (T2 MRI)

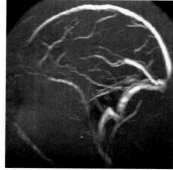

D. Blood vessels and blood flow

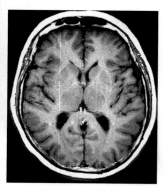

E. Gray vs. white matter in brain

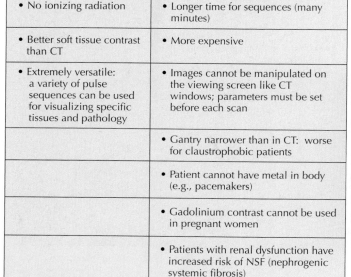

Advantages	Disadvantages
• No ionizing radiation	• Longer time for sequences (many minutes)
• Better soft tissue contrast than CT	• More expensive
• Extremely versatile: a variety of pulse sequences can be used for visualizing specific tissues and pathology	• Images cannot be manipulated on the viewing screen like CT windows; parameters must be set before each scan
	• Gantry narrower than in CT: worse for claustrophobic patients
	• Patient cannot have metal in body (e.g., pacemakers)
	• Gadolinium contrast cannot be used in pregnant women
	• Patients with renal dysfunction have increased risk of NSF (nephrogenic systemic fibrosis)
	• Noisy

1.7 MRI USES, ADVANTAGES, AND DISADVANTAGES

MR images cannot be adjusted on the screen like CT windows. The imaging parameters and planes of section to be viewed must be set at the time of data collection. Two common types of images are based on the T1 and T2 relaxation times of hydrogen protons measured parallel and perpendicular to their axes of spin, respectively. With a T2 pulse sequence fluid is bright white (**C**); with T1 fluid is black. Bone is black (low signal) with both T1 and T2, as are tendons and connective tissue. There is a variety of MR sequences in addition to T1 and T2. For example, there is a fat saturation or "fat-sat" pulse that makes the fat purposely black, and other sequences can reduce the signal of most any tissue. MRI is better than CT for soft tissue contrast, which makes it excellent for studies of the brain, musculoskeletal system, and tumors. The high T2 signal for fluid is good for identifying tissue edema and effusion in joints, tendon sheaths, and other spaces.

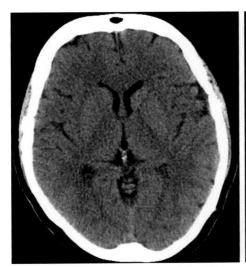

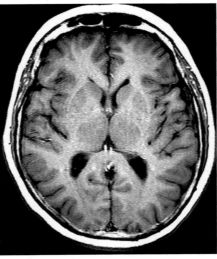

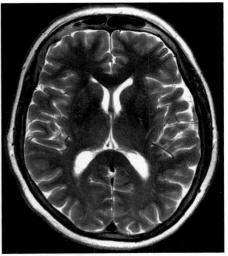

A. CT soft tissue window before contrast. CT images can be distinguished from MRI because bone is bright on CT and has a low signal (black) with MRI.

B. T1-weighted MRI before contrast. What looks like bone in all the MRI sequences is fat or cerebrospinal fluid.

C. T2-weighted MRI where fluid appears bright. This MRI is good for detecting many pathological processes that have fluid accumulation (e.g., edema).

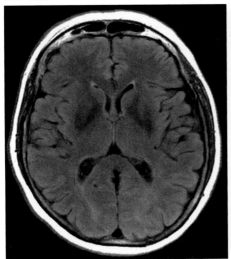

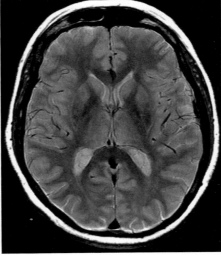

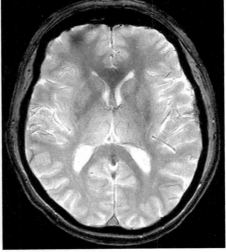

D. FLAIR MRI. FLAIR is an acronym for "fluid attenuation inversion recovery."

E. Proton density MRIs are weighted between T1- and T2-weighted images.

F. GRE MRI. Also called *hemosiderin sequences*, they are exquisitely sensitive to the presence of small amounts of prior hemorrhage that contain the blood breakdown product hemosiderin.

1.8 MRI PULSE SEQUENCES

Imaging of the head and brain is useful for demonstrating a variety of MRI pulse sequences and comparing them with CT (**A**). T1-weighted MR images (**B**) are the mainstay of anatomic imaging. In traditional spin-echo (SE) T1 imaging, fat appears bright, fluid appears dark, and the brain has an intermediate intensity. T2-weighted imaging (**C**) is traditionally known as *pathological imaging*. Typically regions of pathology tend to appear bright on these sequences. On traditional SE T2 imaging, the cerebrospinal fluid (CSF) appears bright, fat appears dark, and the brain appears gray. Traditional fluid attenuation inversion recovery (FLAIR) images (**D**) are T2 weighted but differ from standard T2-weighted imaging in that a special prepulse is used that causes fluid to appear dark. This makes lesions near the periphery of the brain more clear. Proton density images (**E**) are weighted between T1- and T2-weighted images. Before the invention of FLAIR images, they were used to evaluate lesions that may have otherwise been obscured by bright CSF. Gradient recalled images (GRE) (**F**) are another way of creating images that differ from traditional SE imaging. One characteristic that has been exploited is the fact that GRE images turn dark in regions of blood product deposition because of magnetic susceptibility induced by iron-containing hemosiderin, making GRE images good at detecting prior hemorrhage.

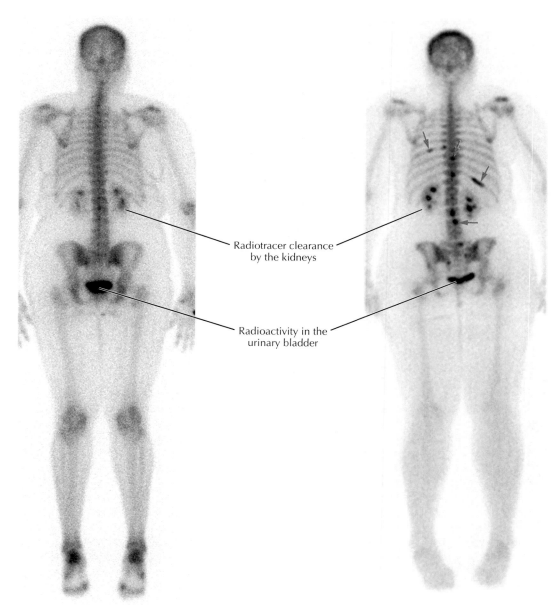

A. Nuclear medicine normal whole-body bone scan, posterior view.

Radiotracer clearance by the kidneys

Radioactivity in the urinary bladder

B. Whole-body bone scan, posterior view, from a patient with breast cancer metastases (*orange arrows*) to some posterior ribs and vertebral bodies.

1.9 NUCLEAR MEDICINE IMAGING

Nuclear medicine imaging measures physiological activity rather than anatomy. Radioactive molecules are attached to other compounds to form radiopharmaceuticals that are administered orally or intravenously. They are designed for binding to and/or uptake by specific cells in specific organs, and their radioactivity is recorded by an external gamma camera. Pathology can be detected by identifying focal areas of increased activity, known as *hot spots,* or decreased activity *(cold spots).* **A** and **B** are whole-body bone scans of patients using the radioactive molecule technetium-99m attached to

methylene-diphosphonate (MDP), a molecule that is taken up by bone cells during formation of hydroxyapatite crystals. Bone scans can be used to detect bone lesions such as infections, microfractures, or in this case (**B**) cancer metastases. There are many nuclear medicine imaging techniques; some can be superimposed on CT or MR images to combine functional and anatomical information. See Chapter 3 (3.21) for an example of single photon emission computed tomography (SPECT), a nuclear medicine imaging technique that can produce slices in different planes by recording the radioactivity from a number of angles.

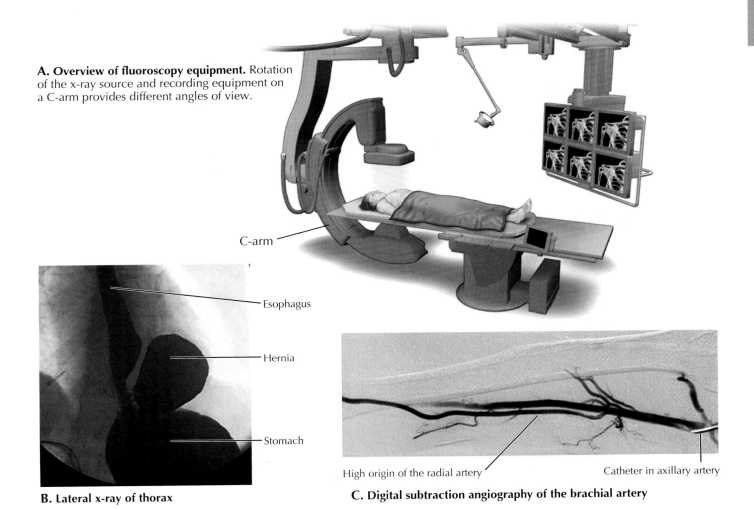

A. Overview of fluoroscopy equipment. Rotation of the x-ray source and recording equipment on a C-arm provides different angles of view.

C-arm

Esophagus

Hernia

Stomach

B. Lateral x-ray of thorax

High origin of the radial artery

Catheter in axillary artery

C. Digital subtraction angiography of the brachial artery

1.10 FLUOROSCOPY

Fluoroscopy uses a continuous stream of x-rays to view the movement of structures in real time. The x-ray source is below the patient, and an image intensifier and data capture equipment are above the patient. With a C-arm the whole apparatus can be rotated to give 3D information (**A**). Fluoroscopy is used for barium contrast studies of the gastrointestinal tract (**B**), a variety of angiographic studies (**C**), catheter and tube placement, fracture repair and apparatus placement in orthopedic surgery, and many other procedures. X-ray images are taken at two to three frames per second for peripheral vascular studies and 15 to 30 frames per second for coronary artery studies.

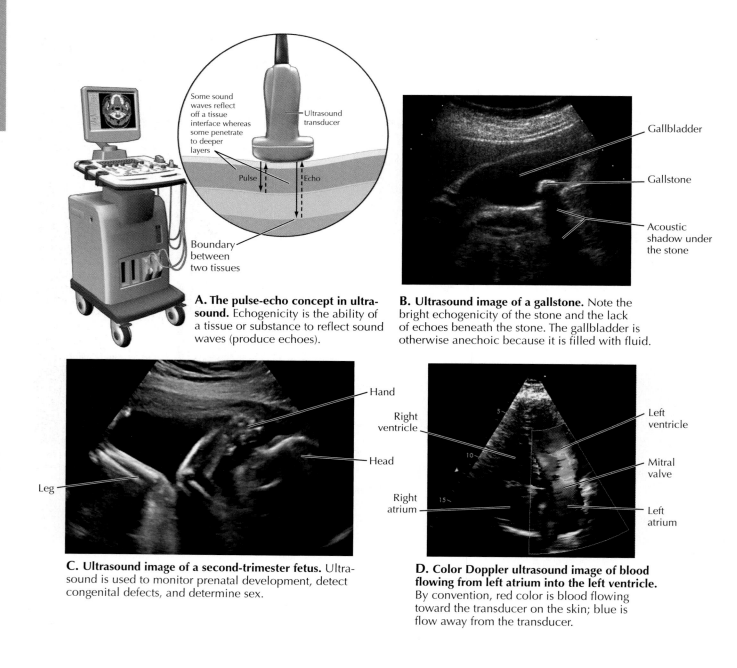

A. The pulse-echo concept in ultra-sound. Echogenicity is the ability of a tissue or substance to reflect sound waves (produce echoes).

B. Ultrasound image of a gallstone. Note the bright echogenicity of the stone and the lack of echoes beneath the stone. The gallbladder is otherwise anechoic because it is filled with fluid.

C. Ultrasound image of a second-trimester fetus. Ultrasound is used to monitor prenatal development, detect congenital defects, and determine sex.

D. Color Doppler ultrasound image of blood flowing from left atrium into the left ventricle. By convention, red color is blood flowing toward the transducer on the skin; blue is flow away from the transducer.

1.11 ULTRASOUND

Ultrasound is a noninvasive imaging technique based on "pulse-echo" sound wave energy. A transducer moving over the skin emits pulses of sound waves into the body and then functions as a receiver that records the energy from the "echo" or reflection of sound waves from tissue interfaces within the body. A computer interprets the sound waves as real-time images. High-frequency transducers (7 to 15 MHz) are used to visualize structures near the surface such as neck vessels and the thyroid gland, breasts, and testes. Lower-frequency sound waves (1 to 3.5 MHz) have greater penetrating power but less resolution and are used for imaging deeper structures in the abdomen and pelvis (**B** and **C**). Tissues deep to bone and air are difficult to visualize because bone absorbs most of the sound energy and air reflects most of it. Doppler ultrasound can visualize and measure blood flow (**D**). Ultrasound is portable, relatively inexpensive, uses no ionizing radiation, and is good at capturing motion.

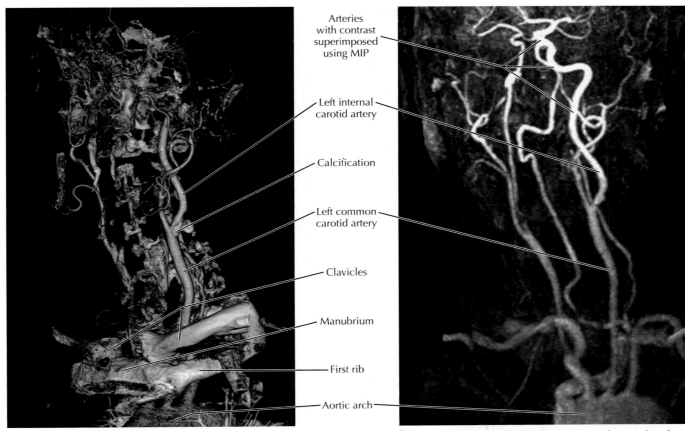

Arteries
with contrast
superimposed
using MIP

Left internal
carotid artery

Calcification

Left common
carotid artery

Clavicles

Manubrium

First rib

Aortic arch

A. CT angiogram of neck arteries with a left anterior oblique (LAO) view of 30 degrees. Volume-rendering algorithms give depth perspective.

B. MR angiogram of the same patient (A) and same view, but using MIP algorithms. Depth perspective can be achieved only by rotating the view.

1.12 ANGIOGRAPHY: COMPUTED TOMOGRAPHY ANGIOGRAM VS. MAGNETIC RESONANCE ANGIOGRAM AND VOLUME RENDERING VS. MAXIMUM INTENSITY PROJECTION

The study of blood vessels and other structures with CT or MRI involves computer reconstruction of 3D images. The images are viewed on the screen using either volume-rendering algorithms that reproduce depth perspective (**A**) or maximum intensity projection (MIP) algorithms that superimpose vessels on each other (**B**). Depth can only be discerned by rotating the view. The technique is called *MIP* because the voxels selected for projection on the monitor have high intensity from the intravascular contrast. With volume-rendering techniques, color, opacity, shading, and other parameters can be manipulated, and other tissues can be viewed for context.

Blood vessels ("angio" means vessel) can be studied with a variety of imaging modalities as demonstrated here by studies of the carotid arteries, which often have stenosis ("narrowing") or occlusion from plaque buildup or calcification. A noninvasive ultrasound study is typically used for screening. If intervention or follow-up is required, computed tomography angiography (CTA) (**A**) or magnetic resonance angiography (MRA) (**B**) may be performed, depending on what equipment and software can produce the best images at a particular hospital. Volume-rendering (**A**) and MIP (**B**) techniques provide similar information, but MIP is easier and quicker and provides clear detail on smaller, peripheral branches and collateral circulation. Volume rendering provides good information on spatial relationships and pathology in the walls of arteries. For any pathology detected by CTA or MRA with volume rendering or MIP, the original data from the serial axial sections should be viewed for the most detailed information.

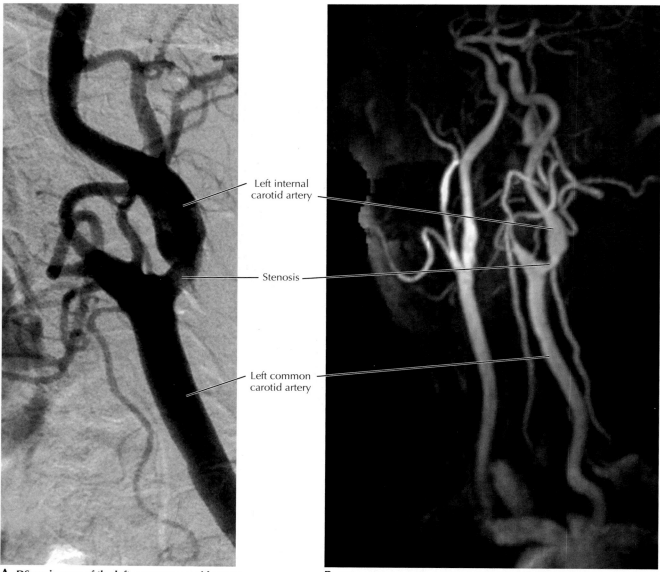

A. DS angiogram of the left common carotid artery and its branches. This is a left anterior oblique view (LAO) of 45 degrees. The view is adjusted by changing the angle of the image intensifier and/or patient, not with the computer.

B. MR angiogram of the same patient (A), also at a 45-degree left anterior oblique (LAO) view.

1.13 ANGIOGRAPHY: DIGITAL SUBTRACTION ANGIOGRAPHY

Angiography of the peripheral vasculature usually refers to digital subtraction angiography (DSA), which has largely replaced the traditional technique of taking an x-ray after injecting the circulation of interest with contrast. DSA is a form of fluoroscopy, a rapid series of x-rays viewed in real time. An image taken before contrast injection is used to digitally "subtract" bones and other tissues from the view after contrast is administered (**A**). This allows for better imaging of the vessels. DSA can be used for diagnostic purposes only, for diagnostic and therapeutic purposes such as balloon angioplasty and stent placement, or to guide catheter placement. A downside of DSA is that it is an invasive procedure in which an artery must be entered percutaneously to gain access to the vasculature. In contrast, CTA and MRA are relatively noninvasive procedures that only require introduction of an intravenous (IV) catheter in an arm vein for contrast injection.

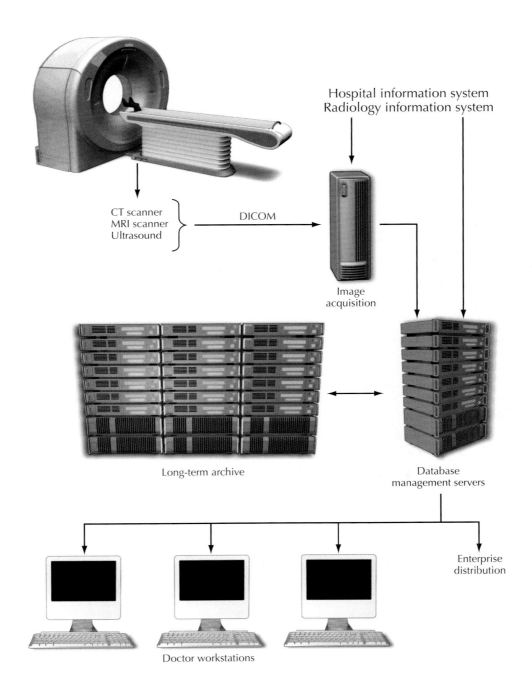

Hospital information system
Radiology information system

CT scanner
MRI scanner
Ultrasound

DICOM

Image
acquisition

Long-term archive

Database
management servers

Enterprise
distribution

Doctor workstations

1.14 ARCHIVING AND COMMUNICATION SYSTEM

As its name implies, a picture archiving and communication system (PACS) incorporates hardware, software, and protocol standards in a digital environment to address all aspects of the use of medical images, from capture, viewing, tagging, and storing to sharing, incorporating reports, and monitoring/managing the workloads of radiologists. It includes workstations connected to a server via a secure local area network (LAN) within a department, hospital, or other unit. The format and protocol standard is DICOM (digital imaging and communications in medicine). This permits pictures from a variety of imaging machines to be viewed directly on workstation screens. The DICOM format groups information into data sets so an image can have an embedded patient ID number, a linked diagnostic report, or other information that facilitates image and workflow management. The format also allows for integration with hospital information systems (HISs) or other systems.

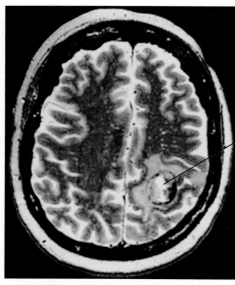

Tumor

A. BOLD imaging. BOLD activation of cerebral cortex related to finger function (orange) is superimposed on a T2 MRI showing a tumor.

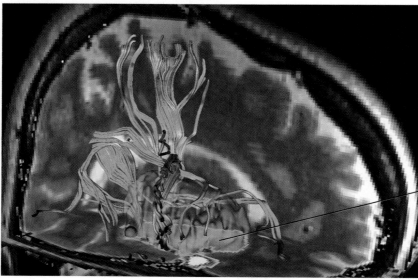

Tumor

B. Multimodal image guidance during surgery. On a T2 backdrop, a tumor (pale green) displaces colored fiber tracts. A BOLD activation of areas responsible for speech is represented by a color scale.

1.15 FUTURE DEVELOPMENTS IN IMAGING

Although future trends in imaging include increasing MRI resolution by increasing the power of the magnets and improving the receiver coils, the most striking developments address the imaging of function in addition to anatomy. Blood oxygen level–dependent contrast, also known as *BOLD imaging*, is a way of evaluating brain activations. When a region of brain is functioning actively, there is a slight increase in blood flow to that region of brain over the baseline that results in a minor increase in signal from that region of brain. By measuring brain signals during periods of rest and periods of performing a task (such as tapping one's fingers), regions of brain activation that are presumably responsible for that task are identified. In this example a region of brain activation (a BOLD activation) is presented as an orange region that is superimposed on a T2-weighted image and overlies the primary motor cortex region responsible for finger movement. A brain tumor

is identified as a complex bright lesion adjacent to the region of brain activation, suggesting that the surgeon may be able to resect the tumor and not destroy finger function.

Another trend in imaging is the use of multimodal guidance during surgery. In this example from the Brigham and Women's Hospital, anatomical information, functional information, and fiber tracking data are combined in a single display. 3D anatomical T2-weighted images serve as the backdrop. Fiber tracts appear as colored "spaghetti" strands that appear to be displaced by the brain tumor, which is displayed in pale green. In addition, a BOLD activation that is responsible for speech is demonstrated as a color scale. In the operating room the surgeon co-registers the patient's brain with the imaging data set. These virtual data points are presented in the dissecting microscope and help guide the surgeon during the operation.

2

BACK AND SPINAL CORD

2.1 VERTEBRAL COLUMN

2.2 THORACIC VERTEBRAE

2.3 LUMBAR VERTEBRAE

2.4 LUMBAR VERTEBRAE IMAGES

2.5 SPINAL MEMBRANES AND NERVE ORIGINS

2.6 SPINAL NERVE ORIGINS: CROSS SECTIONS

2.7 LUMBOSACRAL REGION LIGAMENTS

2.8 NERVE ROOTS

2.9 NORMAL T1 MRI STUDIES OF THE LUMBAR VERTEBRAL COLUMN

2.10 T2 AND FAT SATURATION MRI SEQUENCES

2.11 LUMBAR DISK HERNIATION

2.12 MRI OF A HERNIATED DISK

2.13 CT OF OSTEOPOROSIS IN THE THORACIC SPINE

2.14 MRI OF METASTATIC DISEASE IN THE THORACIC SPINE

2.15 MRI OF SPONDYLOLISTHESIS

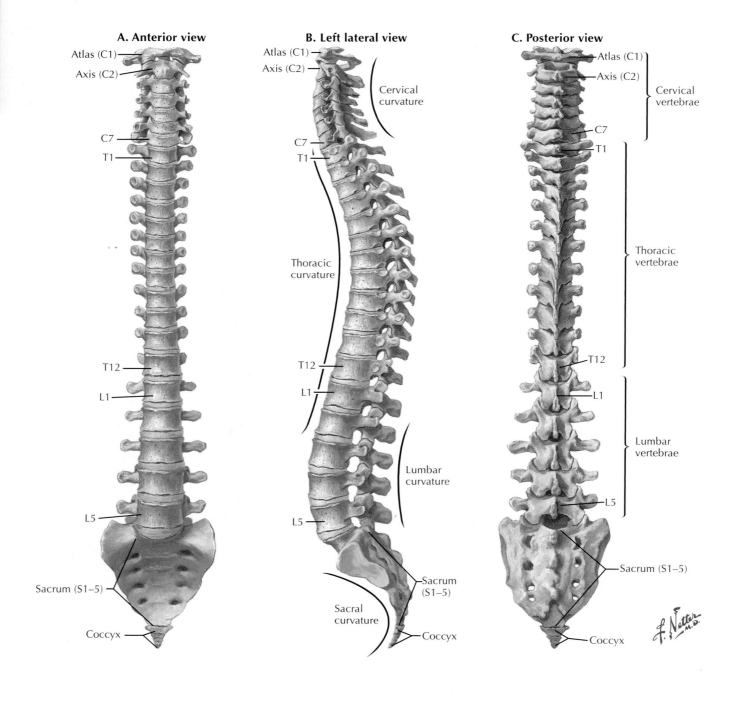

A. Anterior view

Atlas (C1)
Axis (C2)
C7
T1
T12
L1
L5
Sacrum (S1–5)
Coccyx

B. Left lateral view

Atlas (C1)
Axis (C2)
Cervical curvature
C7
T1
Thoracic curvature
T12
L1
Lumbar curvature
L5
Sacral curvature
Sacrum (S1–5)
Coccyx

C. Posterior view

Atlas (C1)
Axis (C2)
Cervical vertebrae
C7
T1
Thoracic vertebrae
T12
L1
Lumbar vertebrae
L5
Sacrum (S1–5)
Coccyx

2.1 VERTEBRAL COLUMN

There are seven cervical vertebrae, twelve thoracic vertebrae defined by their articulation with the twelve pairs of ribs, five lumbar vertebrae, five fused sacral vertebrae that comprise the sacrum, and three to four fused vertebrae that form the coccyx. The cervical and lumbar vertebrae form a curve that is convex anteriorly (lordosis), whereas the thoracic vertebrae have a curve that is convex posteriorly (kyphosis). The two lordoses are secondary curves that develop postnatally.

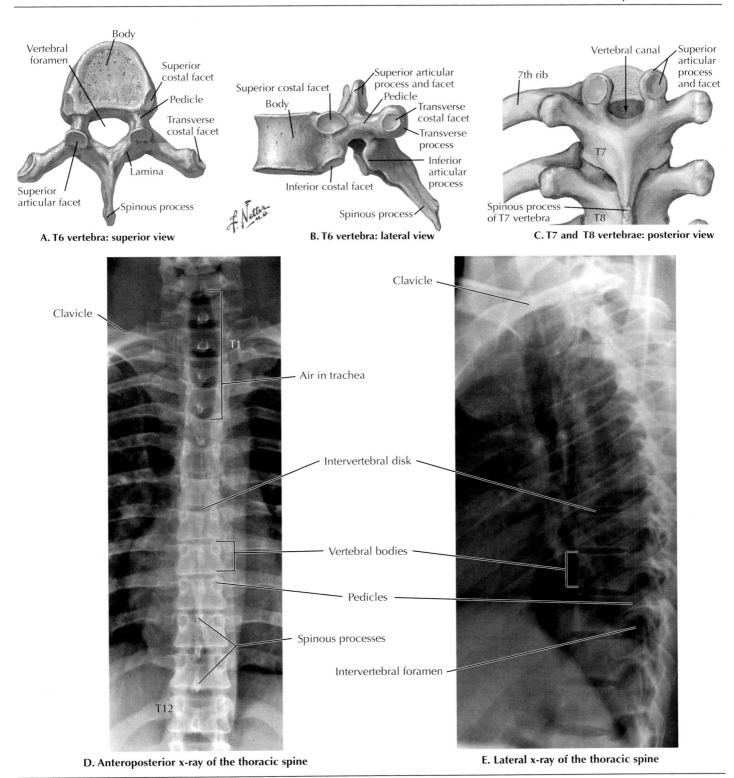

A. T6 vertebra: superior view

Body
Vertebral foramen
Superior costal facet
Pedicle
Transverse costal facet
Lamina
Superior articular facet
Spinous process

B. T6 vertebra: lateral view

Superior articular process and facet
Pedicle
Transverse costal facet
Transverse process
Inferior articular process
Superior costal facet
Body
Inferior costal facet
Spinous process

C. T7 and T8 vertebrae: posterior view

7th rib
Vertebral canal
Superior articular process and facet
T7
Spinous process of T7 vertebra
T8

D. Anteroposterior x-ray of the thoracic spine

Clavicle
T1
Air in trachea
Intervertebral disk
Vertebral bodies
Pedicles
Spinous processes
T12

E. Lateral x-ray of the thoracic spine

Clavicle
Intervertebral disk
Vertebral bodies
Pedicles
Intervertebral foramen

2.2 THORACIC VERTEBRAE

A typical vertebra consists of a body and vertebral arch enclosing a vertebral foramen that contains the spinal cord. The arch consists of pedicles and laminae, and extending from the arch are bony projections called transverse and spinous processes. Thoracic vertebrae are characterized by their facets for the articulation with ribs. The heads of ribs articulate with superior and inferior costal facets on adjacent bodies (two demifacets), and the tubercles of ribs articulate with the facets on the thick transverse processes. The thoracic spinous processes are long and slope inferiorly. The laminae are broad and flat, and the articular facets between vertebrae are oriented in a coronal plane. Lower-density, darker features in the x-rays are the intervertebral disks and the intervertebral foraminae between adjacent pedicles seen in lateral view. Pedicles appear as circular profiles in an anteroposterior view.

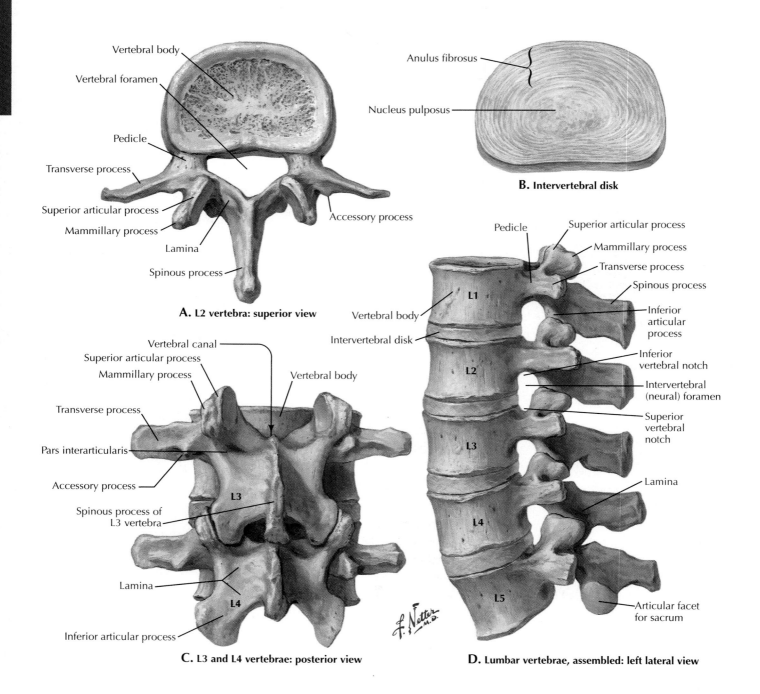

Vertebral body

Vertebral foramen

Pedicle

Transverse process

Superior articular process

Mammillary process

Lamina

Spinous process

A. L2 vertebra: superior view

Anulus fibrosus

Nucleus pulposus

B. Intervertebral disk

Vertebral canal

Superior articular process

Mammillary process

Transverse process

Pars interarticularis

Accessory process

Spinous process of L3 vertebra

Vertebral body

L3

Lamina

L4

Inferior articular process

C. L3 and L4 vertebrae: posterior view

Pedicle

Superior articular process

Mammillary process

Transverse process

Spinous process

Vertebral body

Intervertebral disk

L1

L2

L3

L4

L5

Inferior articular process

Inferior vertebral notch

Intervertebral (neural) foramen

Superior vertebral notch

Lamina

Articular facet for sacrum

D. Lumbar vertebrae, assembled: left lateral view

2.3 LUMBAR VERTEBRAE

Lumbar vertebrae have no rib articulations and are the largest vertebrae because they bear the most weight. Without costal articular facets, their transverse processes are small. Their spinous processes are horizontal in orientation and rectangular in shape. Intervertebral disks are comprised of two parts: a fibrous outer anulus fibrosus and a gelatinous inner nucleus pulposus.

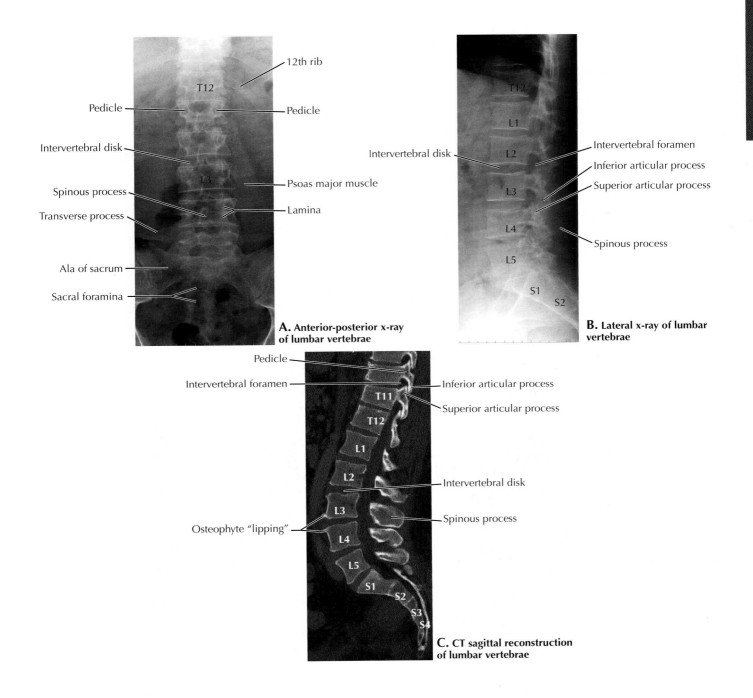

A. Anterior-posterior x-ray of lumbar vertebrae

- 12th rib
- T12
- Pedicle
- Pedicle
- Intervertebral disk
- Psoas major muscle
- Spinous process
- L3
- Transverse process
- Lamina
- Ala of sacrum
- Sacral foramina

B. Lateral x-ray of lumbar vertebrae

- T12
- L1
- L2
- L3
- L4
- L5
- S1
- S2
- Intervertebral disk
- Intervertebral foramen
- Inferior articular process
- Superior articular process
- Spinous process

C. CT sagittal reconstruction of lumbar vertebrae

- Pedicle
- Intervertebral foramen
- Inferior articular process
- Superior articular process
- T11
- T12
- L1
- L2
- L3
- L4
- L5
- S1
- S2
- S3
- S4
- Osteophyte "lipping"
- Intervertebral disk
- Spinous process

2.4 LUMBAR VERTEBRAE IMAGES

Vertebral bodies, spines, pedicles, and intervertebral foramina are evident in the x-rays. Compare the x-rays with the computed tomography (CT) sagittal reconstruction. The latter is a bone window that shows good contrast between the compact cortical bone on the surface of each vertebra and the spongy bone on the interior. Soft tissues such as muscle, intervertebral disks, the spinal cord, and cerebrospinal fluid (CSF) are not seen clearly. X-rays also have soft tissue shadowing superimposed over the bony vertebral column, which is not present in a CT digital reconstruction. Note that the plane of section in the CT is near the midline in the lumbar region but through pedicles and intervertebral foramina higher up, suggesting that there may be some scoliosis present. Abnormal bony growths (osteophytes) are seen anteriorly on the L3 and L4 lumbar vertebral bodies.

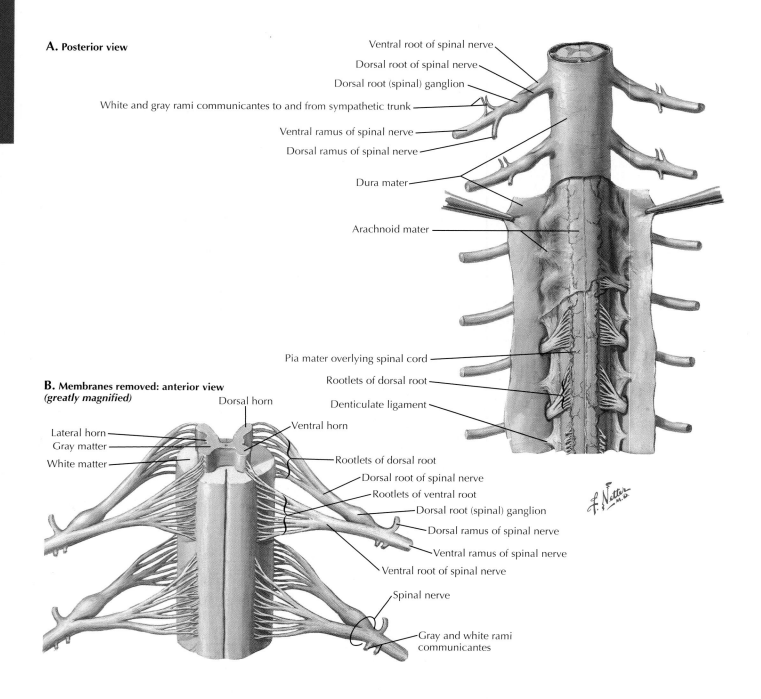

A. Posterior view

Ventral root of spinal nerve

Dorsal root of spinal nerve

Dorsal root (spinal) ganglion

White and gray rami communicantes to and from sympathetic trunk

Ventral ramus of spinal nerve

Dorsal ramus of spinal nerve

Dura mater

Arachnoid mater

Pia mater overlying spinal cord

Rootlets of dorsal root

Denticulate ligament

B. Membranes removed: anterior view
(greatly magnified)

Dorsal horn

Lateral horn

Gray matter

White matter

Ventral horn

Rootlets of dorsal root

Dorsal root of spinal nerve

Rootlets of ventral root

Dorsal root (spinal) ganglion

Dorsal ramus of spinal nerve

Ventral ramus of spinal nerve

Ventral root of spinal nerve

Spinal nerve

Gray and white rami communicantes

2.5 SPINAL MEMBRANES AND NERVE ORIGINS

The spinal cord is surrounded by three membranes: dura mater, arachnoid mater, and pia mater. Dura consists of dense connective tissue. The arachnoid layer is pressed against the dura by cerebrospinal fluid (CSF) that is deep to it, protecting the spinal cord. Pia, the innermost layer, adheres tightly to the brain and spinal cord. Ventral rootlets emerging from the spinal cord merge to form ventral roots, and dorsal roots splay out into dorsal rootlets before their entry into the dorsal spinal cord. Spinal nerves are formed by the joining of dorsal sensory roots with ventral motor roots within the intervertebral foramina. The short spinal nerve quickly branches into dorsal and ventral primary rami, which give rise to the nerves that innervate body wall structures.

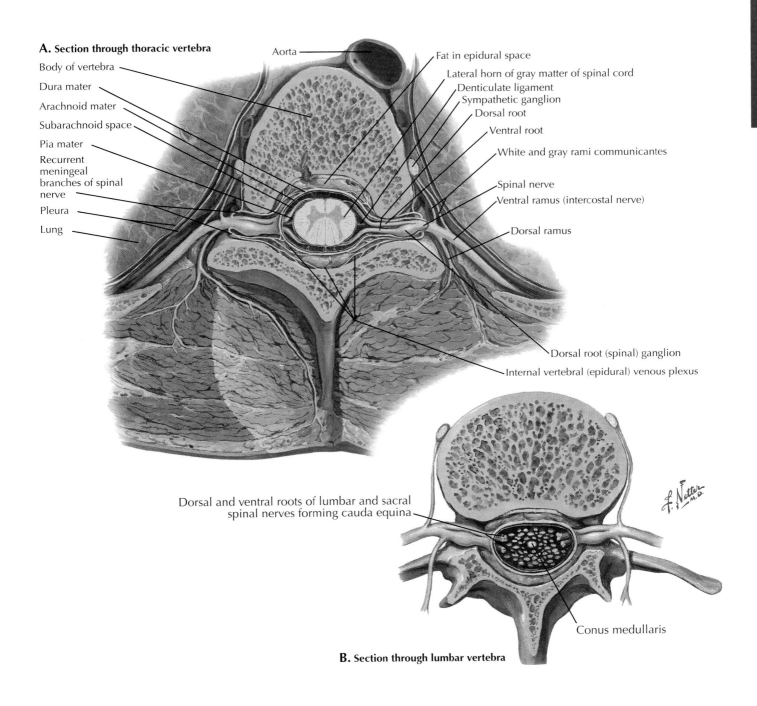

A. Section through thoracic vertebra

Body of vertebra

Dura mater

Arachnoid mater

Subarachnoid space

Pia mater

Recurrent meningeal branches of spinal nerve

Pleura

Lung

Aorta

Fat in epidural space

Lateral horn of gray matter of spinal cord

Denticulate ligament

Sympathetic ganglion

Dorsal root

Ventral root

White and gray rami communicantes

Spinal nerve

Ventral ramus (intercostal nerve)

Dorsal ramus

Dorsal root (spinal) ganglion

Internal vertebral (epidural) venous plexus

Dorsal and ventral roots of lumbar and sacral spinal nerves forming cauda equina

Conus medullaris

B. Section through lumbar vertebra

2.6 SPINAL NERVE ORIGINS: CROSS SECTIONS

The spinal cord and meninges are within the vertebral canal (vertebral foramen of one vertebra). Note the epidural space with fat and a venous plexus, the subarachnoid space with CSF, and the dorsal and ventral roots in the intervertebral foramina. In adults the spinal cord typically ends near the first or second lumbar vertebra. Its termination is known as the *conus medullaris,* which is surrounded by the dorsal and ventral roots passing caudally to their respective exit points. These roots are collectively known as the *cauda equina* because of their resemblance to a horse's tail.

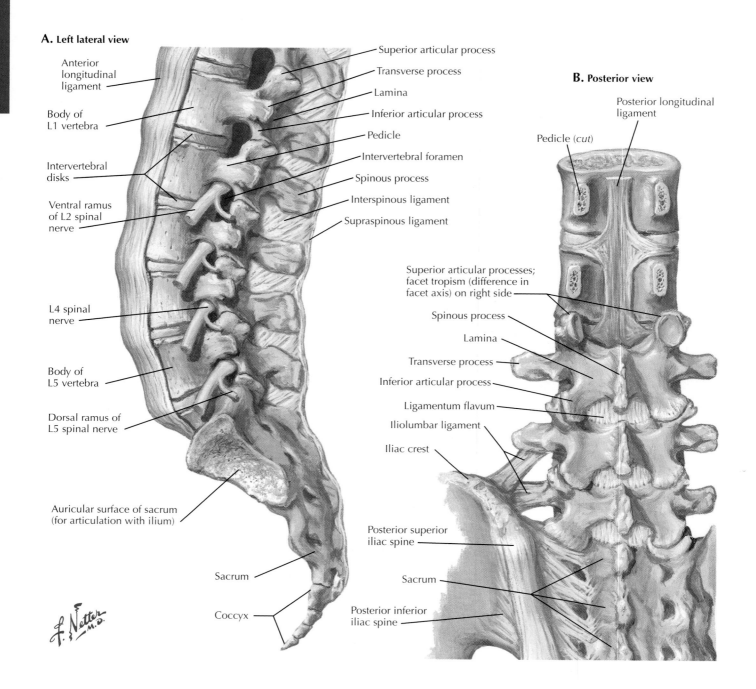

A. Left lateral view

Anterior longitudinal ligament

Body of L1 vertebra

Intervertebral disks

Ventral ramus of L2 spinal nerve

L4 spinal nerve

Body of L5 vertebra

Dorsal ramus of L5 spinal nerve

Auricular surface of sacrum (for articulation with ilium)

Sacrum

Coccyx

Superior articular process

Transverse process

Lamina

Inferior articular process

Pedicle

Intervertebral foramen

Spinous process

Interspinous ligament

Supraspinous ligament

B. Posterior view

Posterior longitudinal ligament

Pedicle (*cut*)

Superior articular processes; facet tropism (difference in facet axis) on right side

Spinous process

Lamina

Transverse process

Inferior articular process

Ligamentum flavum

Iliolumbar ligament

Iliac crest

Posterior superior iliac spine

Sacrum

Posterior inferior iliac spine

f. Netter
M.D.

2.7 LUMBOSACRAL REGION LIGAMENTS

Vertebral bodies are connected by anterior and posterior longitudinal ligaments. The latter are on the anterior surface of the vertebral canal. A ligamentum flavum interconnects lamina and has a considerable amount of elastic connective tissue. Interspinous and supraspinous ligaments interconnect vertebral spines. Note in the posterior view that the profile of a cut pedicle is similar to its appearance in an anteroposterior x-ray.

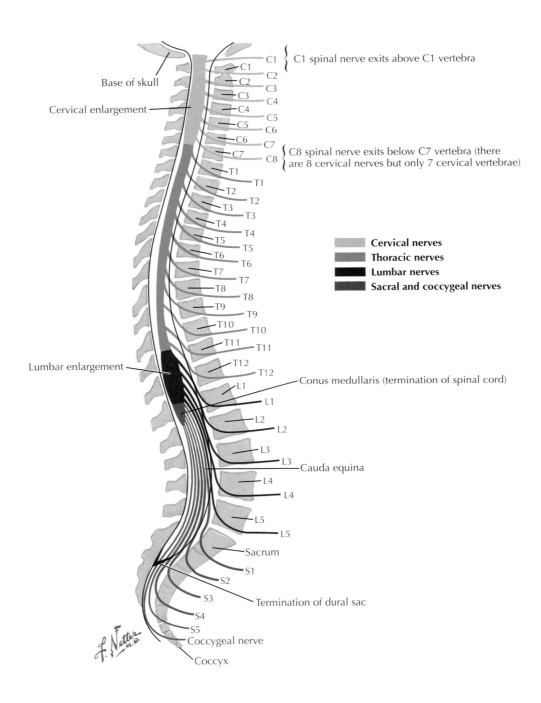

Base of skull

Cervical enlargement

C1
C1
C2
C2
C3
C3
C4
C4
C5
C5
C6
C6
C7
C7
C8
T1
T1
T2
T2
T3
T3
T4
T4
T5
T5
T6
T6
T7
T7
T8
T8
T9
T9
T10
T10
T11
T11
T12
T12
L1
L1
L2
L2
L3
L3
L4
L4
L5
L5
S1
S2
S3
S4
S5

C1 spinal nerve exits above C1 vertebra

C8 spinal nerve exits below C7 vertebra (there are 8 cervical nerves but only 7 cervical vertebrae)

Cervical nerves
Thoracic nerves
Lumbar nerves
Sacral and coccygeal nerves

Lumbar enlargement

Conus medullaris (termination of spinal cord)

Cauda equina

Sacrum

Termination of dural sac

Coccygeal nerve

Coccyx

f. Netter m.d.

2.8 NERVE ROOTS

Imaging studies of the vertebral column and spinal cord are often done to evaluate pain or functional deficits caused by the compression of spinal nerve roots and/or the spinal cord. The spinal cord is larger in diameter in the cervical and lumbosacral regions because of the greater number of neurons required to innervate the upper and lower extremities, respectively. Because the spinal cord ends near L1-L2, upper spinal nerves exit the vertebral column near the level of their origin, whereas lumbar and sacral spinal nerves must travel inferiorly in the vertebral canal to their appropriate exit levels. The subarachnoid space within the dural sac terminates at S2-S3. Lower sacral nerves are in an epidural location.

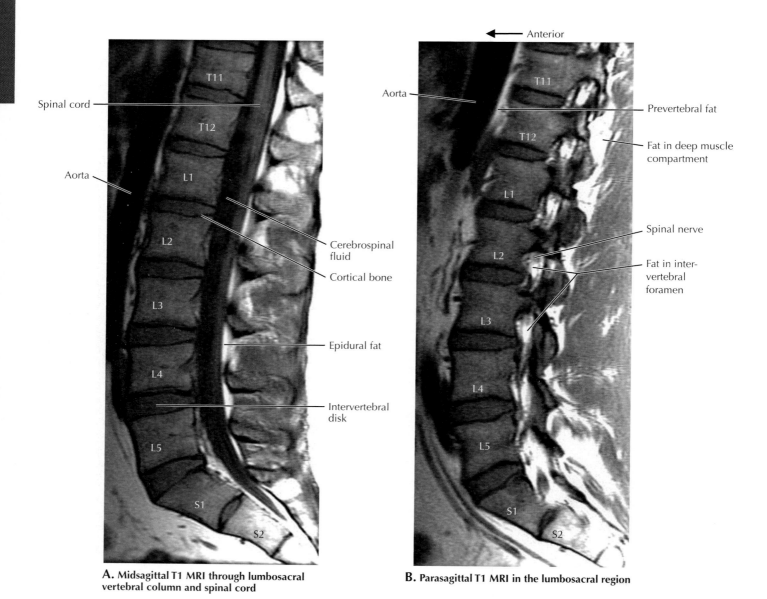

A. Midsagittal T1 MRI through lumbosacral vertebral column and spinal cord

B. Parasagittal T1 MRI in the lumbosacral region

2.9 NORMAL T1 MRI STUDIES OF THE LUMBAR VERTEBRAL COLUMN

Magnetic resonance imaging (MRI) is the optimal imaging tool for spinal cord evaluation, providing more information than myelography/CT myelogram. In **A** (midsagittal T1 MRI), the vertebral bodies have an intermediate signal intensity. The cortical bone of the bodies is dark, and fat is bright in the epidural space. The aorta is dark as a result of the loss of signal in flowing blood (flow void). Spinous processes have a similar signal intensity to the vertebral bodies, although some adjacent tissue is captured in the plane. The CSF is dark. In **B** (parasagittal T1 MRI), note the similar signal intensities for bone compared with **A**. The nerve roots in the intervertebral foramina are gray (isointense); they are surrounded by fat that appears bright on this T1-weighted sequence.

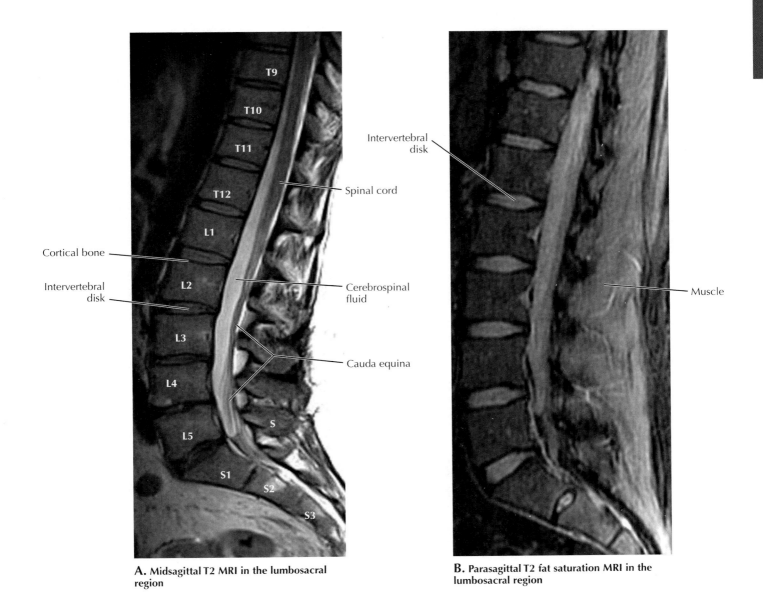

A. Midsagittal T2 MRI in the lumbosacral region

B. Parasagittal T2 fat saturation MRI in the lumbosacral region

2.10 T2 AND FAT SATURATION MRI SEQUENCES

In a spin-echo T2-weighted MRI (**A**), bone marrow typically appears darker, and fluids brighter, when compared with a T1-weighted image. Note the contrast between the signal intensity of the spinal cord and surrounding CSF. A fat saturation sequence (**B**) is obtained to suppress the fat signal, which helps to differentiate pathology that appears isointense to fat on other sequences. This sequence is useful in the evaluation of metastatic disease within the vertebral bodies.

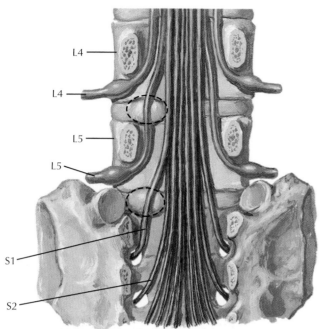

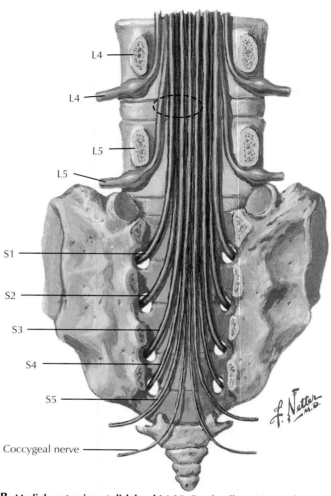

A. Lumbar disk protrusion. Does not usually affect nerve exiting above disk. Lateral protrusion at disk level L4-L5 affects L5 spinal nerve, not L4 spinal nerve. Protrusion at disk level L5-S1 affects S1 spinal nerve, not L5 spinal nerve.

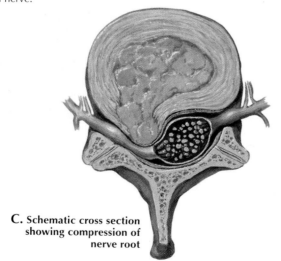

C. Schematic cross section showing compression of nerve root

B. Medial protrusion at disk level L4-L5. Rarely affects L4 spinal nerve but may affect L5 spinal nerve and sometimes S1-S4 spinal nerves.

2.11 LUMBAR DISK HERNIATION

Because of the lumbar lordotic curvature, compression of an intervertebral disk usually results in a posterior herniation of the nucleus pulposus through the anulus fibrosus. The herniation is usually just lateral to the relatively narrow posterior longitudinal ligament, although it may be more medial as well (**B**). Because the nerve roots pass inferiorly to the intervertebral foramina, the disk herniation usually does not affect the nerve that exits at the same level (exiting root) but does affect the root one level caudal to the protrusion (transiting root).

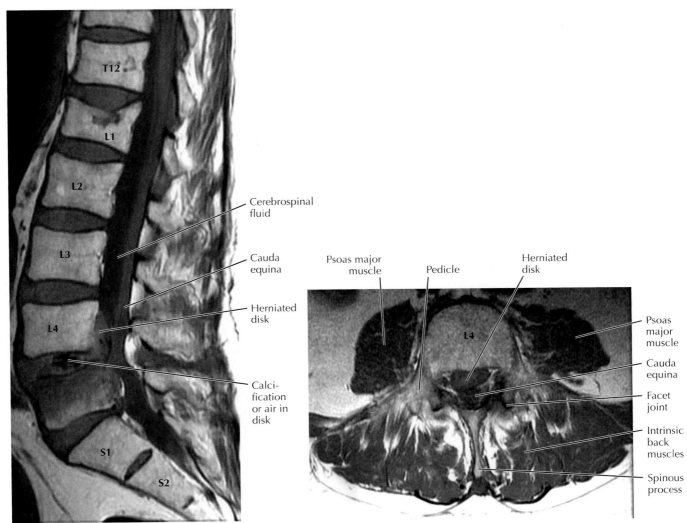

A. Sagittal T1 MRI of the lumbosacral region showing an L4-L5 herniated disk. Inflammatory response in the L5 vertebral body and a collapse of the L1 vertebral body.

B. Axial (transverse) T1 MRI. Same patient showing the herniated disk fragment posterior to the L4 vertebral body.

2.12 MRI OF A HERNIATED DISK

There is a herniation of the intervertebral disk at L4-L5 with cranial migration of disk tissue in the vertebral canal anterior to the cauda equina. Dark signal within the disk suggests the presence of calcifications or air within the disk. The vertebral bodies are brighter than normal and have foci of increased intensity (i.e., whiter) because of the replacement of normal bone marrow signal with fat. Bony changes are seen in the L5 vertebra that may suggest acute inflammatory response in the degenerative spine. Also note collapse of the L1 vertebral body, which could be secondary to osteoporosis. The intrinsic back muscles have an intermediate (isointense) signal, whereas the fat in the superficial fascia and muscle planes appears bright on T1-weighted images.

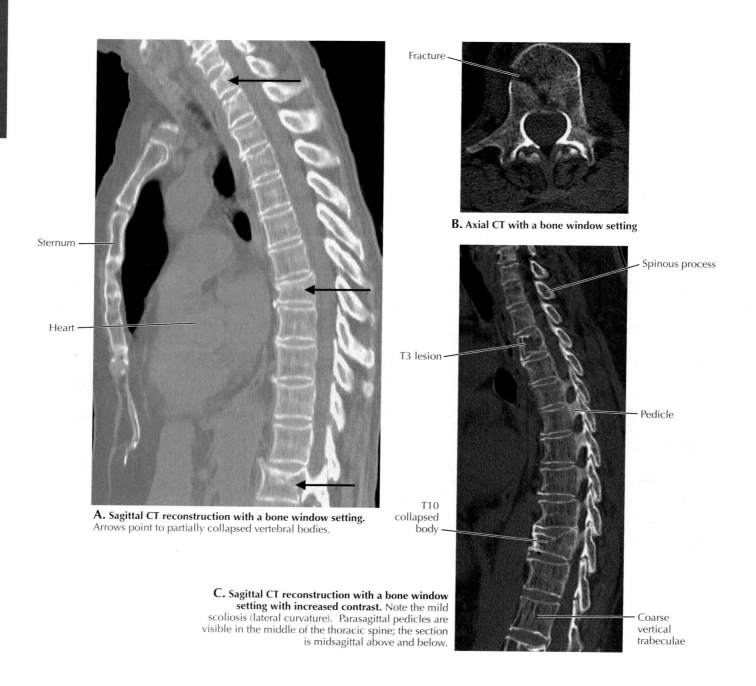

Fracture

B. **Axial CT with a bone window setting**

Sternum

Heart

Spinous process

T3 lesion

Pedicle

T10 collapsed body

A. Sagittal CT reconstruction with a bone window setting.
Arrows point to partially collapsed vertebral bodies.

Coarse vertical trabeculae

C. Sagittal CT reconstruction with a bone window setting with increased contrast. Note the mild scoliosis (lateral curvature). Parasagittal pedicles are visible in the middle of the thoracic spine; the section is midsagittal above and below.

2.13 CT OF OSTEOPOROSIS IN THE THORACIC SPINE

A and B demonstrate CT of the thoracic spine to evaluate the cause for diffuse bone pain and localized tenderness in a patient. The CT scan was done with thin slice acquisition, and sagittal (**A**) and axial (**B**) reformatted images were obtained. There is evidence of generalized osteoporosis in the entire thoracic spine with fractures at multiple levels *(arrows)*. The involved vertebral bodies are partially collapsed, causing them to be shorter than adjacent vertebral bodies. **C** shows a patient with osteoporosis and a hemangioma in the T3 vertebral body, a benign tumor of blood vessel epithelium. There is partial collapse of the T10 vertebral body, and the increased contrast shows prominent, coarse vertical trabeculae in the bodies as a result of relatively greater loss of horizontal trabeculae resulting from the osteopenia.

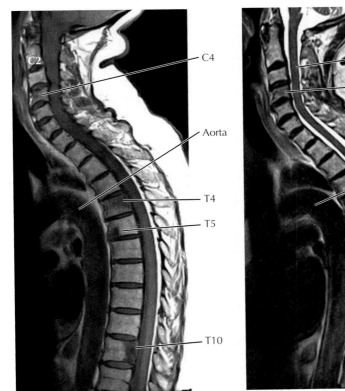

A. Sagittal T1 MRI

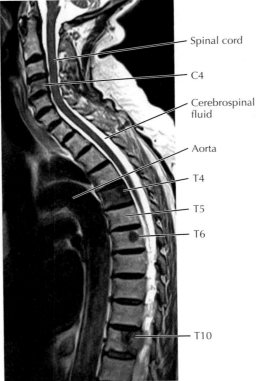

B. Sagittal T2 MRI

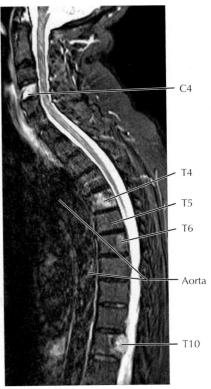

C. Sagittal T2 STIR (fat saturation) MRI

2.14 MRI OF METASTATIC DISEASE IN THE THORACIC SPINE

These images represent parasagittal T1 (**A**), T2 (**B**), and T2 STIR (short tau inversion recovery) (**C**) MRI sequences that were obtained for the evaluation of suspected metastatic disease in the spine. Metastases are demonstrated at C4, T4, T5, T6, and T10 levels. In comparison to bone marrow, the cancerous soft tissue lesions are hypointense (dark) on T1 images (**A**) and appear isointense to hyperintense on T2 images (**B**). These lesions appear more conspicuous on fat suppression (STIR) sequences (**C**).

Compro-
mised
vertebral
canal

Sacroiliac
joint

A. CT sagittal plane reconstruction of the lumbosacral vertebral column with spondylo-listhesis of L5 over S1

B. Axial view of L5/S1 in A

Indicates the plane of section

Ear = superior
articular process

Eye = pedicle

Snout =
transverse
process

Front leg =
inferior
articular
process

Neck = pars
interarticularis

Body = lamina

Tail and hind
leg = spinous
process

C. X-ray of an oblique view of a normal lumbar spine showing a "Scotty dog" profile of the vertebra features. A fracture of the pars interarticularis would appear as a collar on the neck.

2.15 MRI OF SPONDYLOLISTHESIS

Spondylolisthesis ("vertebra-slippage") is defined as the displacement of a vertebral body with respect to the vertebral body below, in this case, the sacrum. Spondylolisthesis may be ventral (anterolisthesis) or dorsal (retrolisthesis). This spine has anterior displacement of L5 over S1 (grades 2 to 3: 50% to 75% displacement). In the axial view the L5 vertebra is seen anterior to S1 (**B**). The vertebral canal is compromised by the body of S1 with possible compression of the cauda equina. There also may be traction of the L5 nerve roots caused by forward displacement of the L5 vertebra. In females the anterior location of L5 reduces the size of the birth canal and may create problems during parturition. Spondylolisthesis may be caused by fracture of the pars interarticularis (**C**) or degenerative changes in the vertebral column.

3

THORAX

3.1 THORACIC TOPOGRAPHY: ANTERIOR AND POSTERIOR VIEWS

3.2 POSTEROANTERIOR AND CHEST X-RAY (MALE AND FEMALE)

3.3 MIDAXILLARY CORONAL SECTION

3.4 ANTERIOR AXILLARY CORONAL SECTION

3.5 ANTERIOR AXILLARY CT AND MRI

3.6 MEDIASTINUM: LEFT LATERAL VIEW AND LEFT MEDIAL LUNG

3.7 MEDIASTINUM: RIGHT LATERAL VIEW AND RIGHT MEDIAL LUNG

3.8 LATERAL CHEST X-RAY

3.9 SAGITTAL CT AND MRI

3.10 LUNG ANATOMY

3.11 POSTEROANTERIOR AND LATERAL X-RAYS: SUPERIMPOSED OUTLINES OF LUNG LOBES

3.12 CT AIRWAY STUDIES

3.13 ANTERIOR AND POSTERIOR VIEWS OF THE HEART

3.14 POSTEROANTERIOR AND LATERAL X-RAYS: VIEWS OF SUPERIMPOSED HEART CHAMBERS

3.15 T8 MEDIASTINUM CROSS SECTION WITH T8 CT AND MRI

3.16 ATRIA, VENTRICLES, AND INTERVENTRICULAR SEPTUM

3.17 RIGHT CORONARY ARTERY STUDY

3.18 LEFT CORONARY ARTERY STUDY

3.19 HEART IMAGING STUDIES

3.20 ECHOCARDIOGRAPHY

3.21 SINGLE PHOTON EMISSION COMPUTED TOMOGRAPHY

3.22 COMPARISON OF CARDIAC IMAGING MODALITIES

3.23   VERTEBRAL LEVELS IN THE THORAX

3.24   T3 CROSS SECTION WITH T3 CT

3.25   T3-T4 CROSS SECTION WITH T3-T4 CT

3.26   T4-T5 CROSS SECTION WITH T4-T5 CT

3.27   T7 CROSS SECTION WITH T7 CT

3.28   SYSTEMATIC CHEST X-RAY EVALUATION

3.29   SEARCH STRATEGY: IDENTIFYING VIEWS

3.30   SEARCH STRATEGY: TECHNICAL QUALITY OF IMAGES

3.31   SEARCH STRATEGY: TUBES, LINES, AND SUPPORT DEVICES

3.32   SEARCH STRATEGY: THORACIC WALL SOFT TISSUES (E.G., AIR, CALCIFICATION, FOREIGN BODIES)

3.33   SEARCH STRATEGY: BONES

3.34   SEARCH STRATEGY: PLEURAL SPACES AND DIAPHRAGM

3.35   SEARCH STRATEGY: PLEURAL SPACES AND DIAPHRAGM (CONT'D)

3.36   SEARCH STRATEGY: UPPER ABDOMEN

3.37   SEARCH STRATEGY: MEDIASTINUM AND HILA

3.38   SEARCH STRATEGY: HEART AND VASCULATURE

3.39   SEARCH STRATEGY: LUNGS—SILHOUETTE SIGN

3.40   SEARCH STRATEGY: LUNGS, ATELECTASIS

3.41   SEARCH STRATEGY: LUNGS, ALVEOLAR VS. INTERSTITIAL OPACITY

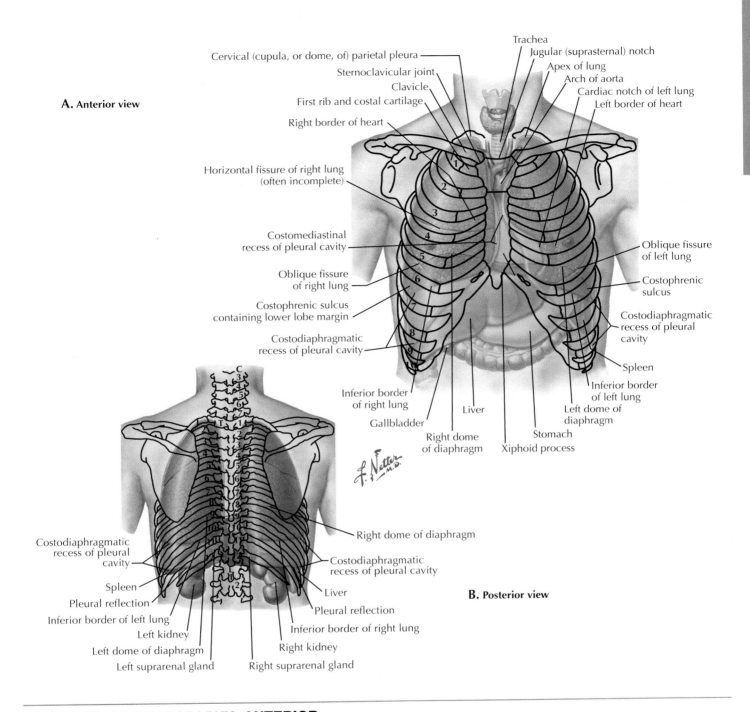

A. Anterior view

Cervical (cupula, or dome, of) parietal pleura
Sternoclavicular joint
Clavicle
First rib and costal cartilage
Right border of heart

Trachea
Jugular (suprasternal) notch
Apex of lung
Arch of aorta
Cardiac notch of left lung
Left border of heart

Horizontal fissure of right lung
(often incomplete)

Costomediastinal
recess of pleural cavity

Oblique fissure
of left lung

Oblique fissure
of right lung

Costophrenic
sulcus

Costophrenic sulcus
containing lower lobe margin

Costodiaphragmatic
recess of pleural
cavity

Costodiaphragmatic
recess of pleural cavity

Spleen

Inferior border
of right lung

Inferior border
of left lung

Gallbladder

Liver

Left dome of
diaphragm

Right dome
of diaphragm

Stomach

Xiphoid process

Right dome of diaphragm

Costodiaphragmatic
recess of pleural
cavity

Costodiaphragmatic
recess of pleural cavity

Spleen

Pleural reflection

Liver

Inferior border of left lung

Pleural reflection

Left kidney

Inferior border of right lung

Left dome of diaphragm

Right kidney

Left suprarenal gland

Right suprarenal gland

B. Posterior view

3.1 THORACIC TOPOGRAPHY: ANTERIOR AND POSTERIOR VIEWS

The thorax is the part of the trunk between the neck and the abdominal cavity. It extends from the first rib to the diaphragm and is bounded by the sternum, twelve thoracic vertebrae, the twelve pairs of ribs, and the muscles that attach to these bones. The thorax contains the lungs surrounded by pleural spaces. It also contains the mediastinum, the block of tissue between the lungs consisting of the heart, esophagus, trachea, vessels, lymph nodes, connective tissue, and nerves. The heart is the approximate length of the body of the sternum. The great vessels and bifurcation of the trachea are behind the manubrium. The dome-shaped diaphragm extends over the liver on the right and spleen and stomach on the left. The apices of the lungs are above the first rib and clavicle. The parietal pleura that lines the pleural cavities extends more inferiorly than the lungs themselves in the recess between the diaphragm and the rib cage. The bases of the lungs during quiet respiration are near the seventh rib, whereas the costodiaphragmatic recess of the parietal pleura extends down to the ninth rib laterally. The right and left hemidiaphragms, pleural cavities, and lungs extend to a lower level in the posterior thorax than they do anteriorly.

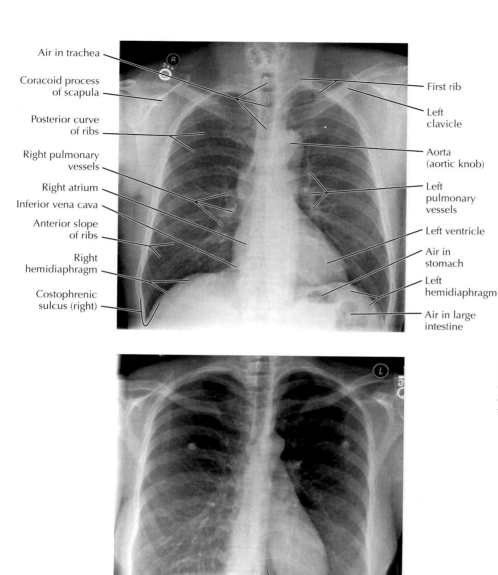

Air in trachea

Coracoid process
of scapula

Posterior curve
of ribs

Right pulmonary
vessels

Right atrium

Inferior vena cava

Anterior slope
of ribs

Right
hemidiaphragm

Costophrenic
sulcus (right)

First rib

Left
clavicle

Aorta
(aortic knob)

Left
pulmonary
vessels

Left ventricle

Air in
stomach

Left
hemidiaphragm

Air in large
intestine

A. Male posteroanterior x-ray

B. Female posteroanterior x-ray
Note the increased density
wherever the mammary glands
overlap with structures posterior
to them.

Contours of the
mammary glands

3.2 POSTEROANTERIOR AND CHEST X-RAY (MALE AND FEMALE)

For a standard posteroanterior (PA) chest x-ray the patient "hugs" the x-ray recording plate. This protracts the shoulder girdles and moves the scapulae off the lungs. Having the x-ray beam pass from posterior to anterior through the patient, with the anterior chest adjacent to the recording plate, minimizes the magnification of the heart by the divergent beam. The lung fields appear dark because of their high air content. The larger pulmonary vessels (arteries and veins) are the white tubular densities near the lung roots. Note the air *(darker area)* in the midline trachea and in the stomach and splenic flexure of the colon under the left hemidiaphragm. Also note the clavicles, scapulae, and arch of each hemidiaphragm. The heart borders are seen clearly against the air-filled lungs. The right margin of the heart on the PA view is the right atrium. The left margin is the left ventricle. The right ventricle and left atrium do not contribute to the heart borders on a PA x-ray. They are better seen in a lateral view.

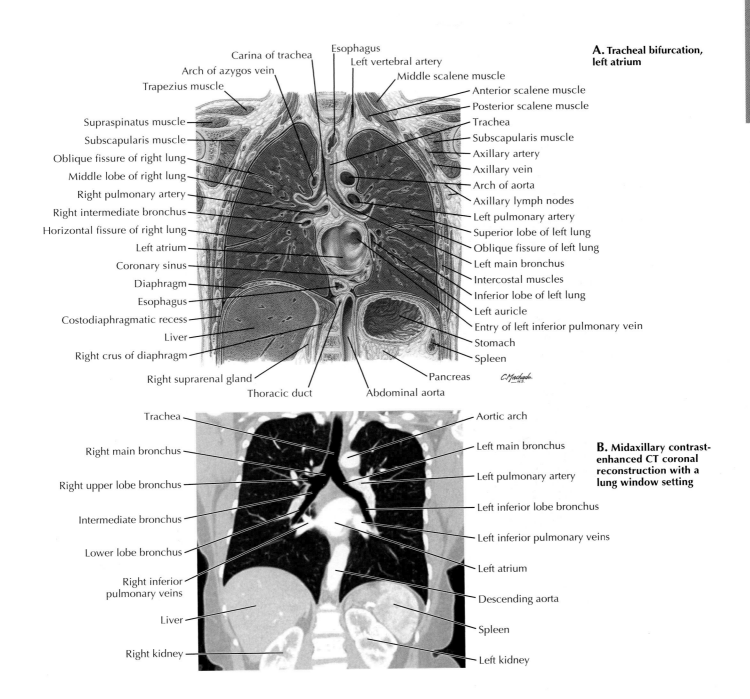

A. Tracheal bifurcation, left atrium

Carina of trachea
Esophagus
Arch of azygos vein
Left vertebral artery
Trapezius muscle
Middle scalene muscle
Anterior scalene muscle
Posterior scalene muscle
Supraspinatus muscle
Trachea
Subscapularis muscle
Subscapularis muscle
Oblique fissure of right lung
Axillary artery
Middle lobe of right lung
Axillary vein
Right pulmonary artery
Arch of aorta
Right intermediate bronchus
Axillary lymph nodes
Horizontal fissure of right lung
Left pulmonary artery
Left atrium
Superior lobe of left lung
Coronary sinus
Oblique fissure of left lung
Diaphragm
Left main bronchus
Esophagus
Intercostal muscles
Costodiaphragmatic recess
Inferior lobe of left lung
Liver
Left auricle
Right crus of diaphragm
Entry of left inferior pulmonary vein
Stomach
Spleen
Right suprarenal gland
Pancreas
Thoracic duct
Abdominal aorta

C.Machado.

B. Midaxillary contrast-enhanced CT coronal reconstruction with a lung window setting

Trachea
Aortic arch
Right main bronchus
Left main bronchus
Right upper lobe bronchus
Left pulmonary artery
Intermediate bronchus
Left inferior lobe bronchus
Lower lobe bronchus
Left inferior pulmonary veins
Right inferior pulmonary veins
Left atrium
Liver
Descending aorta
Spleen
Right kidney
Left kidney

3.3 MIDAXILLARY CORONAL SECTION

Most of the heart is anterior to the midaxillary coronal plane. This section contains the arches of the aorta and azygos vein and the division of the trachea into the primary bronchi. Cervical and lumbar vertebrae are visible. The normal thoracic kyphosis (curvature) is out of the plane of section. The esophagus follows the contour of the vertebral column behind the heart. It is visible above the trachea and below the left atrium. The pulmonary arteries are above the level of the left atrium and the pulmonary veins that drain into it.

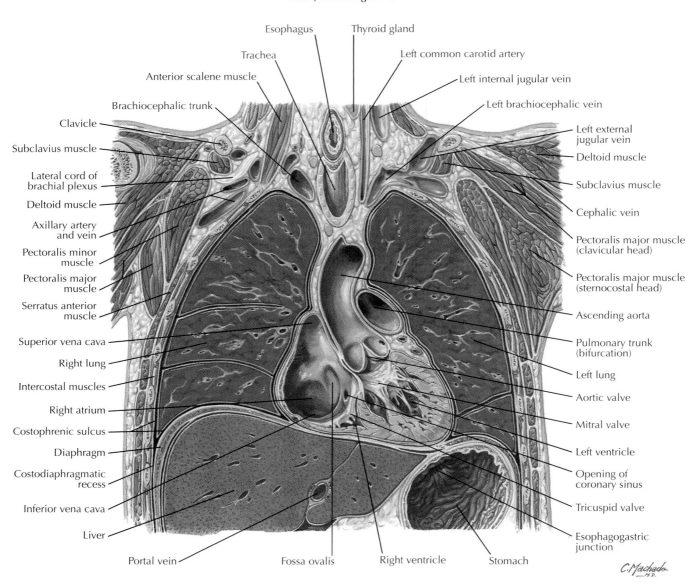

Heart, ascending aorta

Esophagus

Thyroid gland

Trachea

Left common carotid artery

Anterior scalene muscle

Left internal jugular vein

Brachiocephalic trunk

Left brachiocephalic vein

Clavicle

Left external jugular vein

Subclavius muscle

Deltoid muscle

Lateral cord of brachial plexus

Subclavius muscle

Deltoid muscle

Cephalic vein

Axillary artery and vein

Pectoralis major muscle (clavicular head)

Pectoralis minor muscle

Pectoralis major muscle (sternocostal head)

Pectoralis major muscle

Serratus anterior muscle

Ascending aorta

Superior vena cava

Pulmonary trunk (bifurcation)

Right lung

Left lung

Intercostal muscles

Aortic valve

Right atrium

Mitral valve

Costophrenic sulcus

Left ventricle

Diaphragm

Opening of coronary sinus

Costodiaphragmatic recess

Tricuspid valve

Inferior vena cava

Esophagogastric junction

Liver

Portal vein

Fossa ovalis

Right ventricle

Stomach

C. Machado
_M.D.

3.4 ANTERIOR AXILLARY CORONAL SECTION

This more anterior coronal section passes through the middle of the left ventricle and right atrium of the heart. The aortic semilunar valve, ascending aorta, and superior and inferior vena cavae are also seen. The pulmonary trunk is visible under the arch of the aorta. The stomach is visible in the patient's left upper abdomen. The apices of the lungs are close to the brachiocephalic vessels.

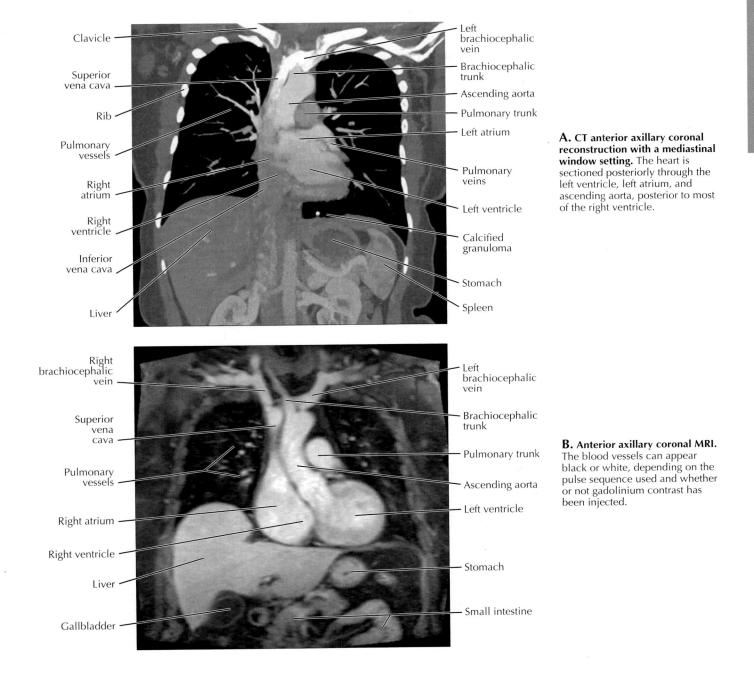

Clavicle

Superior
vena cava

Rib

Pulmonary
vessels

Right
atrium

Right
ventricle

Inferior
vena cava

Liver

Left
brachiocephalic
vein

Brachiocephalic
trunk

Ascending aorta

Pulmonary trunk

Left atrium

Pulmonary
veins

Left ventricle

Calcified
granuloma

Stomach

Spleen

A. CT anterior axillary coronal reconstruction with a mediastinal window setting. The heart is sectioned posteriorly through the left ventricle, left atrium, and ascending aorta, posterior to most of the right ventricle.

Right
brachiocephalic
vein

Superior
vena
cava

Pulmonary
vessels

Right atrium

Right ventricle

Liver

Gallbladder

Left
brachiocephalic
vein

Brachiocephalic
trunk

Pulmonary trunk

Ascending aorta

Left ventricle

Stomach

Small intestine

B. Anterior axillary coronal MRI. The blood vessels can appear black or white, depending on the pulse sequence used and whether or not gadolinium contrast has been injected.

3.5 ANTERIOR AXILLARY CT AND MRI

Both computed tomography (CT) and magnetic resonance imaging (MRI) are used for chest studies, although CT is more common. MRI is used for some heart studies and in cases in which patients may have allergies or other problems with receiving iodinated contrast used in CT. On the CT examination **(A),** the contrast was introduced into a left arm vein, and it is just entering the heart and lungs. The superior vena cava is bright white, and the white profiles in the lungs are blood vessels with some contrast. The very

bright nodule at the left lung base medially is a calcified granuloma.

The window width and level of images can be adjusted on the computer screen to visualize either the soft tissue structures or the lung parenchyma. On this mediastinal window setting, the soft tissue structures of the mediastinum are visualized. The details of the lung parenchyma are poorly seen, and the lungs appear predominantly black. The window width and level can also be adjusted to make the white contrast in the blood vessels look brighter or less intense.

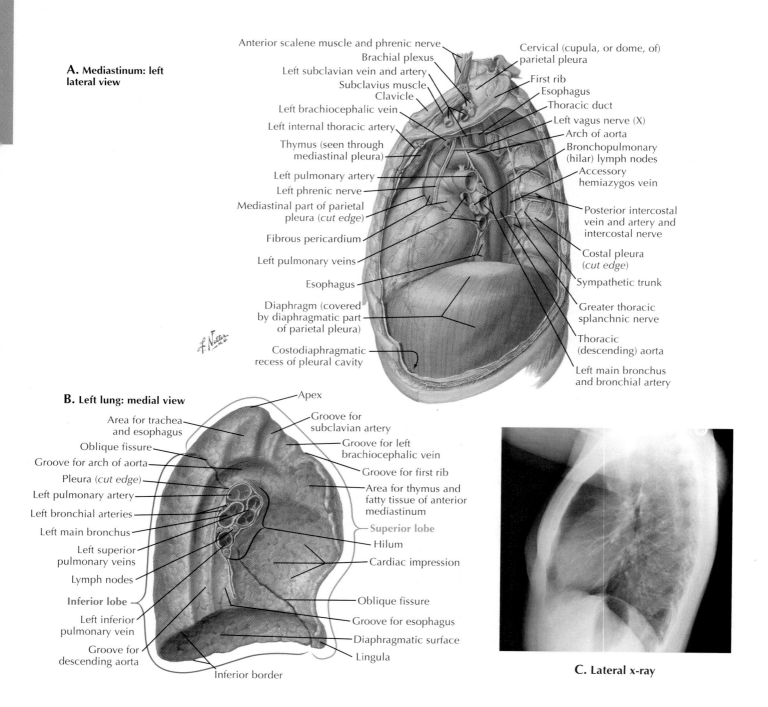

A. Mediastinum: left lateral view

Anterior scalene muscle and phrenic nerve
Brachial plexus
Left subclavian vein and artery
Subclavius muscle
Clavicle
Left brachiocephalic vein
Left internal thoracic artery
Thymus (seen through mediastinal pleura)
Left pulmonary artery
Left phrenic nerve
Mediastinal part of parietal pleura (*cut edge*)
Fibrous pericardium
Left pulmonary veins
Esophagus
Diaphragm (covered by diaphragmatic part of parietal pleura)
Costodiaphragmatic recess of pleural cavity

Cervical (cupula, or dome, of) parietal pleura
First rib
Esophagus
Thoracic duct
Left vagus nerve (X)
Arch of aorta
Bronchopulmonary (hilar) lymph nodes
Accessory hemiazygos vein
Posterior intercostal vein and artery and intercostal nerve
Costal pleura (*cut edge*)
Sympathetic trunk
Greater thoracic splanchnic nerve
Thoracic (descending) aorta
Left main bronchus and bronchial artery

B. Left lung: medial view

Area for trachea and esophagus
Oblique fissure
Groove for arch of aorta
Pleura (*cut edge*)
Left pulmonary artery
Left bronchial arteries
Left main bronchus
Left superior pulmonary veins
Lymph nodes
Inferior lobe
Left inferior pulmonary vein
Groove for descending aorta
Inferior border

Apex
Groove for subclavian artery
Groove for left brachiocephalic vein
Groove for first rib
Area for thymus and fatty tissue of anterior mediastinum
Superior lobe
Hilum
Cardiac impression
Oblique fissure
Groove for esophagus
Diaphragmatic surface
Lingula

C. Lateral x-ray

3.6 MEDIASTINUM: LEFT LATERAL VIEW AND LEFT MEDIAL LUNG

The heart on the left is bounded by the lingula segment of the left upper lobe. There is no middle lobe in the left lung. Most of the left lower lobe is either below or behind the heart. A portion extends superior and posterior to the heart. The arch of the aorta courses over the root of the lung to the left of the trachea. The descending thoracic aorta is posterior to the esophagus. The right main stem bronchus is above the right pulmonary artery (eparterial), whereas the left main stem bronchus is below the left pulmonary artery (hyparterial). The lungs do not extend all the way into the costodiaphragmatic recess, the inferior boundary of the pleural cavity. This recess is a potential space that is not visible on an x-ray.

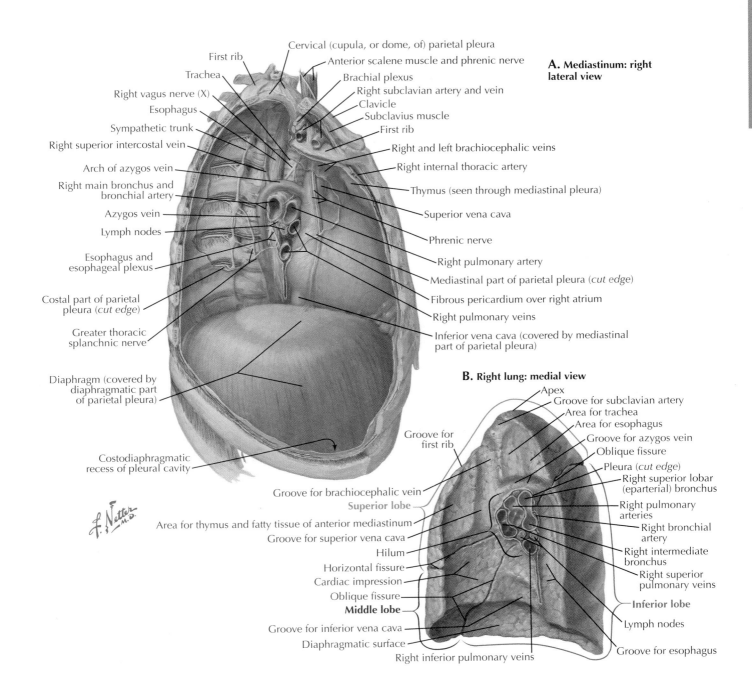

Cervical (cupula, or dome, of) parietal pleura
First rib
Anterior scalene muscle and phrenic nerve
Trachea
Brachial plexus
Right vagus nerve (X)
Right subclavian artery and vein
Esophagus
Clavicle
Sympathetic trunk
Subclavius muscle
Right superior intercostal vein
First rib
Right and left brachiocephalic veins
Arch of azygos vein
Right internal thoracic artery
Right main bronchus and bronchial artery
Thymus (seen through mediastinal pleura)
Azygos vein
Superior vena cava
Lymph nodes
Phrenic nerve
Esophagus and esophageal plexus
Right pulmonary artery
Mediastinal part of parietal pleura (*cut edge*)
Costal part of parietal pleura (*cut edge*)
Fibrous pericardium over right atrium
Greater thoracic splanchnic nerve
Right pulmonary veins
Inferior vena cava (covered by mediastinal part of parietal pleura)
Diaphragm (covered by diaphragmatic part of parietal pleura)

A. Mediastinum: right lateral view

B. Right lung: medial view

Apex
Groove for subclavian artery
Area for trachea
Area for esophagus
Groove for azygos vein
Oblique fissure
Pleura (*cut edge*)
Right superior lobar (eparterial) bronchus
Right pulmonary arteries
Right bronchial artery
Right intermediate bronchus
Right superior pulmonary veins
Costodiaphragmatic recess of pleural cavity
Groove for first rib
Groove for brachiocephalic vein
Superior lobe
Area for thymus and fatty tissue of anterior mediastinum
Groove for superior vena cava
Hilum
Horizontal fissure
Cardiac impression
Oblique fissure
Middle lobe
Groove for inferior vena cava
Diaphragmatic surface
Right inferior pulmonary veins
Inferior lobe
Lymph nodes
Groove for esophagus

3.7 MEDIASTINUM: RIGHT LATERAL VIEW AND RIGHT MEDIAL LUNG

The heart is anteriorly located in the thorax. It is bounded laterally on the right by the middle lobe of the right lung. The right lower lobe extends upward and posterior to the right middle lobe and the heart. The esophagus is posterior to the heart against the left atrium. The right main stem bronchus is above the right main pulmonary artery, unlike the left side where the left main stem bronchus is below the left main pulmonary artery. The arch of the azygos vein passes over the right primary bronchus and pulmonary artery in the root of the right lung.

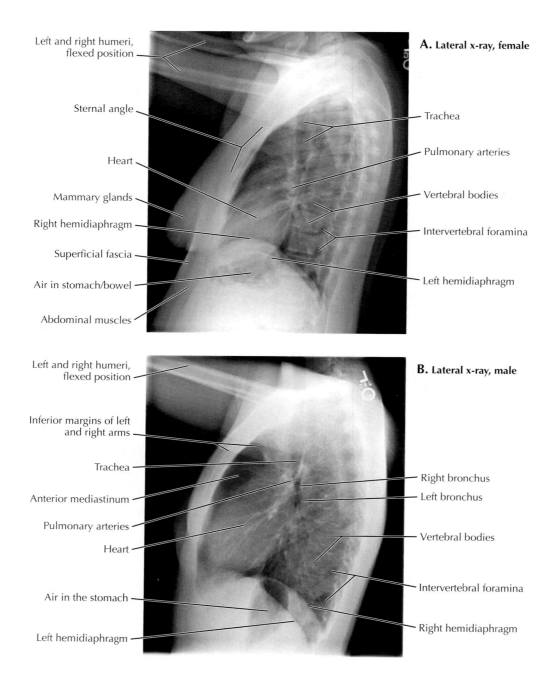

Left and right humeri, flexed position

Sternal angle

Heart

Mammary glands

Right hemidiaphragm

Superficial fascia

Air in stomach/bowel

Abdominal muscles

A. Lateral x-ray, female

Trachea

Pulmonary arteries

Vertebral bodies

Intervertebral foramina

Left hemidiaphragm

Left and right humeri, flexed position

Inferior margins of left and right arms

Trachea

Anterior mediastinum

Pulmonary arteries

Heart

Air in the stomach

Left hemidiaphragm

B. Lateral x-ray, male

Right bronchus

Left bronchus

Vertebral bodies

Intervertebral foramina

Right hemidiaphragm

3.8 LATERAL CHEST X-RAY

Routinely a left lateral chest radiograph (x-ray beam passing from right to left) is obtained to keep the heart closest to the image receptor. The patient's arms are elevated to move the humeri and soft tissues of the arms out of the field of view. Lateral radiographs are used in conjunction with the PA view to evaluate the thorax in three dimensions and better localize any pathology that may be present. The roots of both lungs are superimposed on each other in the middle mediastinum. The right upper lobe bronchus is higher than the left upper lobe bronchus. Each is seen on end where the trachea ends.

The distal arch of the aorta is seen posterior to the trachea. The clear space behind the sternum superiorly corresponds to the anterior mediastinum. The right ventricle is the most anterior heart chamber and makes up the anterior superior margin of the heart on the lateral view. The left atrium comprises the superior posterior border of the heart, and the left ventricle is the inferior posterior border of the heart. The contour of the left hemidiaphragm is not seen anteriorly because it is silhouetted by (against) the heart. The right hemidiaphragm contour can normally be followed along its entire course.

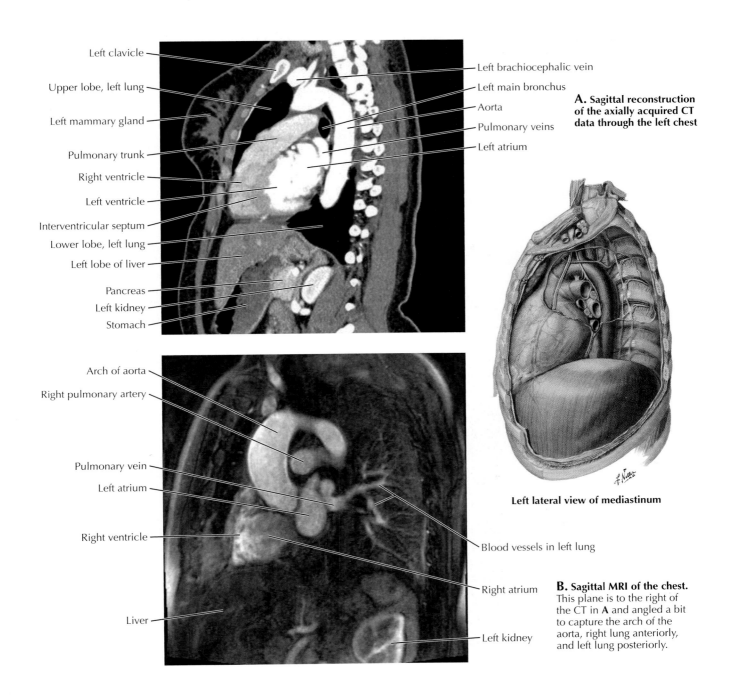

Left clavicle

Upper lobe, left lung

Left mammary gland

Pulmonary trunk

Right ventricle

Left ventricle

Interventricular septum

Lower lobe, left lung

Left lobe of liver

Pancreas

Left kidney

Stomach

Left brachiocephalic vein

Left main bronchus

Aorta

Pulmonary veins

Left atrium

A. Sagittal reconstruction of the axially acquired CT data through the left chest

Arch of aorta

Right pulmonary artery

Pulmonary vein

Left atrium

Right ventricle

Liver

Blood vessels in left lung

Right atrium

Left kidney

Left lateral view of mediastinum

B. Sagittal MRI of the chest. This plane is to the right of the CT in **A** and angled a bit to capture the arch of the aorta, right lung anteriorly, and left lung posteriorly.

3.9 SAGITTAL CT AND MRI

In the CT reconstruction in **A,** the descending aorta, clavicle, and breast indicate that the section is to the left of the midline. Iodinated intravenous contrast is seen in the left ventricle, aortic arch, and descending thoracic aorta and two of the branch arteries of the aortic arch. The lungs appear black on this image viewed with a mediastinal window. The anterior clear space is the upper lobe of the left lung projecting over the anterior mediastinum. The heart and aorta are in the middle mediastinum, and the thoracic vertebral column (spine) is in the posterior mediastinum. In the upper abdomen portions of the left lobe of the liver, stomach, pancreas and left kidney are seen. **B** is a corresponding MRI sagittal section of the chest. Blood vessels can appear white on MRI without the injection of gadolinium contrast, depending on the pulse sequence used. On this image the ascending aorta and aortic arch are seen clearly. The heart is located anteriorly. Some blood vessels are seen in the left lung, and the left kidney is seen in the upper abdomen.

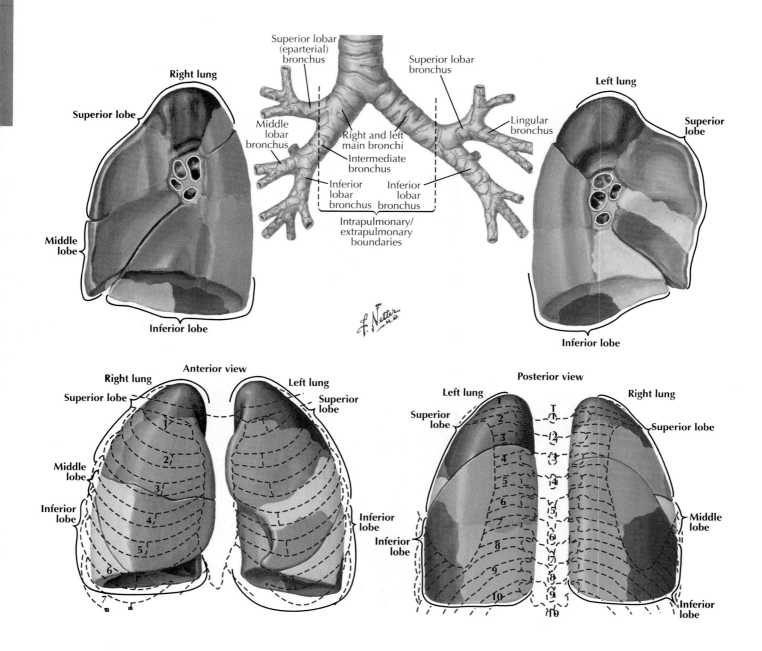

3.10 LUNG ANATOMY

A primary (main stem) bronchus supplies each lung. Secondary (lobar) bronchi supply lobes, and tertiary (segmental) bronchi supply bronchopulmonary segments, the subdivisions of each lobe that are colored in the figures. The right primary bronchus is shorter than the left and has a more vertical orientation in line with the trachea. The right lung has three lobes, with a horizontal (minor) fissure separating the superior and middle lobes and an oblique (major) fissure separating the upper and middle lobes from the inferior lobe. The left lung has only two lobes separated by an oblique fissure. The lingual segment (lingula) of the left upper lobe is equivalent to the middle lobe of the right lung. Note that the inferior lobes of both lungs extend posteriorly to the superior lobes behind the middle lobe of the right lung and lingula of the left lung. At the root of the lungs the pulmonary arteries are above the pulmonary veins.

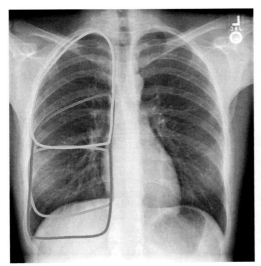

A. Lobes of the right lung in anterior view

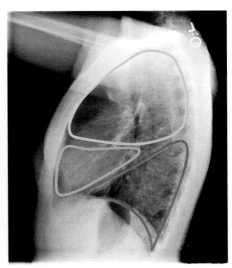

B. Lobes of the right lung in lateral view.
Note the middle lobe adjacent to the heart and
the lower lobe behind it.

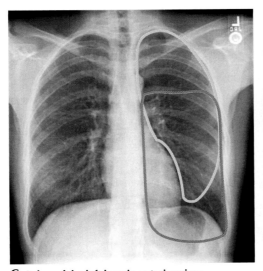

C. Lobes of the left lung in anterior view

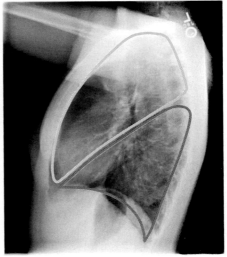

D. Lobes of the left lung in lateral view.
The lingula of the upper lobe is against the heart.

— = Upper lobe   — = Middle lobe   — = Lower lobe

3.11 POSTEROANTERIOR AND LATERAL X-RAYS: SUPERIMPOSED OUTLINES OF LUNG LOBES

The outlines of the lung lobes are distinct in a lateral view but overlap in a PA view. The middle lobe of the right lung and the lingula of the left upper lobe are adjacent to the heart on either side anteriorly. The lower lobes extend to a level higher than the middle lobe and lingula but are posterior to these structures and the heart. Portions of the lower lobe overlap portions of the upper lobes and right middle lobe or lingula segment on the PA view. Both PA and lateral views are necessary to localize an abnormal finding in three dimensions. The fissures are only visible on plain radiographs if they are parallel to the x-ray beam. The horizontal fissure may be seen on both the lateral and PA views. The oblique fissure is usually seen on the lateral view.

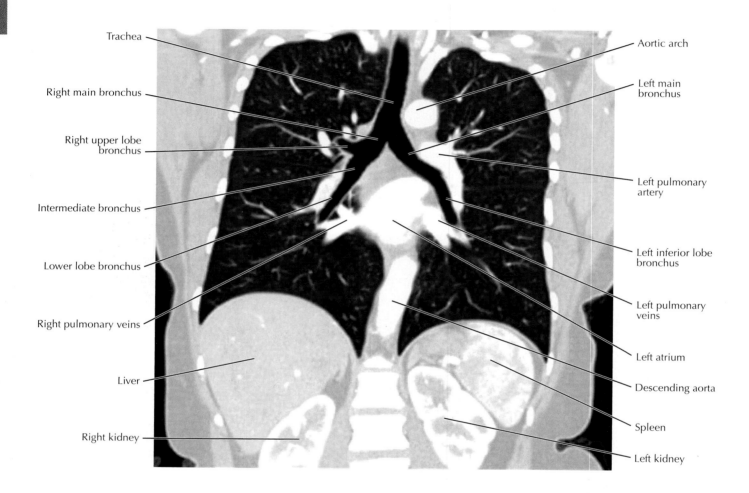

Trachea

Right main bronchus

Right upper lobe bronchus

Intermediate bronchus

Lower lobe bronchus

Right pulmonary veins

Liver

Right kidney

Aortic arch

Left main bronchus

Left pulmonary artery

Left inferior lobe bronchus

Left pulmonary veins

Left atrium

Descending aorta

Spleen

Left kidney

3.12 CT AIRWAY STUDIES

The current standard for the study of the airway is CT. Intravenous contrast is not necessary. Thin collimation serial axial images are obtained using a high-contrast computer algorithm and can be reconstructed in the coronal or sagittal planes. Three-dimensional reconstructions can also be generated on a computer workstation. The slice thickness obtained is thinner than for routine CT chest studies, and slices may be overlapped during reconstruction for higher resolution. CT is better than MRI for evaluating the lung parenchyma. The window width and level are adjusted to highlight air-filled lung tissue, with a resulting decrease in soft tissue contrast outside the lungs. Note the primary and secondary bronchi seen on the coronal reconstruction.

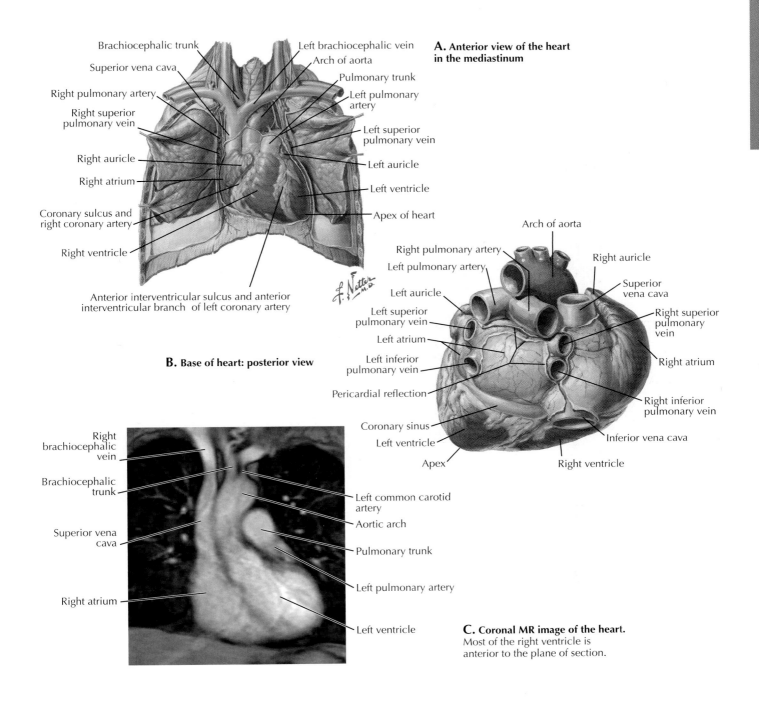

Brachiocephalic trunk

Superior vena cava

Right pulmonary artery

Right superior
pulmonary vein

Right auricle

Right atrium

Coronary sulcus and
right coronary artery

Right ventricle

Left brachiocephalic vein
Arch of aorta
Pulmonary trunk
Left pulmonary artery
Left superior
pulmonary vein
Left auricle
Left ventricle
Apex of heart

**A. Anterior view of the heart
in the mediastinum**

Anterior interventricular sulcus and anterior
interventricular branch of left coronary artery

B. Base of heart: posterior view

Right pulmonary artery
Left pulmonary artery
Left auricle
Left superior
pulmonary vein
Left atrium
Left inferior
pulmonary vein
Pericardial reflection
Coronary sinus
Left ventricle
Apex

Arch of aorta

Right auricle
Superior
vena cava
Right superior
pulmonary
vein
Right atrium
Right inferior
pulmonary vein
Inferior vena cava
Right ventricle

Right
brachiocephalic
vein

Brachiocephalic
trunk

Superior vena
cava

Right atrium

Left common carotid
artery
Aortic arch
Pulmonary trunk
Left pulmonary artery
Left ventricle

C. Coronal MR image of the heart.
Most of the right ventricle is
anterior to the plane of section.

3.13 ANTERIOR AND POSTERIOR VIEWS OF THE HEART

The heart is roughly the length of the body of the sternum. All of the great vessels arise from the aortic arch behind the manubrium of the sternum. The axis of the heart projects 45 degrees anteriorly and 45 degrees to the left. The right margin of the heart is the right atrium. The left margin is the left ventricle. The right ventricle is the most anterior chamber of the heart. The left atrium is the upper posterior margin of the heart, lying against the anterior wall of the esophagus. On the coronal MR image the superior vena cava is clearly seen entering the right atrium. The superior vena cava forms the right border of the mediastinum at the level of the aortic arch. The ascending aorta is seen clearly just to the left of the superior vena cava. The brachiocephalic trunk and left common carotid artery are seen as the first two vessels off the aortic arch. A small portion of the left pulmonary artery is visualized.

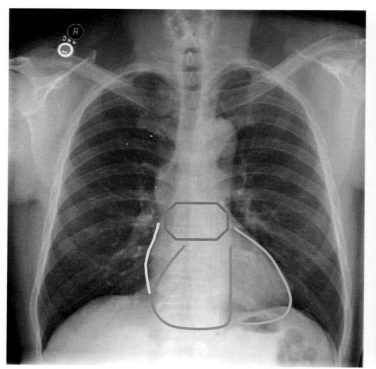

A. Outlines of heart chambers in a PA x-ray

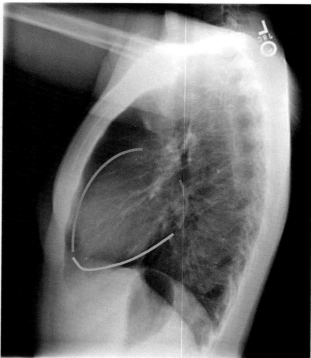

B. Outlines of heart chambers in a lateral x-ray

| Right atrium | Right ventricle | Left atrium | Left ventricle |

3.14 POSTEROANTERIOR AND LATERAL X-RAYS: VIEWS OF SUPERIMPOSED HEART CHAMBERS

The heart occupies the middle mediastinum in the anterior portion of the thoracic cavity. On a PA x-ray of the chest, the left margin of the heart (left ventricle) and right margin (right atrium) are clearly seen because they are bordered by the air-filled lungs that have a different x-ray density. The inferior margin of the heart on the left is not visible because it is against the soft tissue of the left hemidiaphragm that has the same density. The right ventricle forms the anterior margin on the lateral view, and the left atrium is the posterior superior margin bordering the esophagus and posterior mediastinum. The left ventricle is the inferior margin. The boundaries of the right ventricle and left atrium can only be estimated in a PA view.

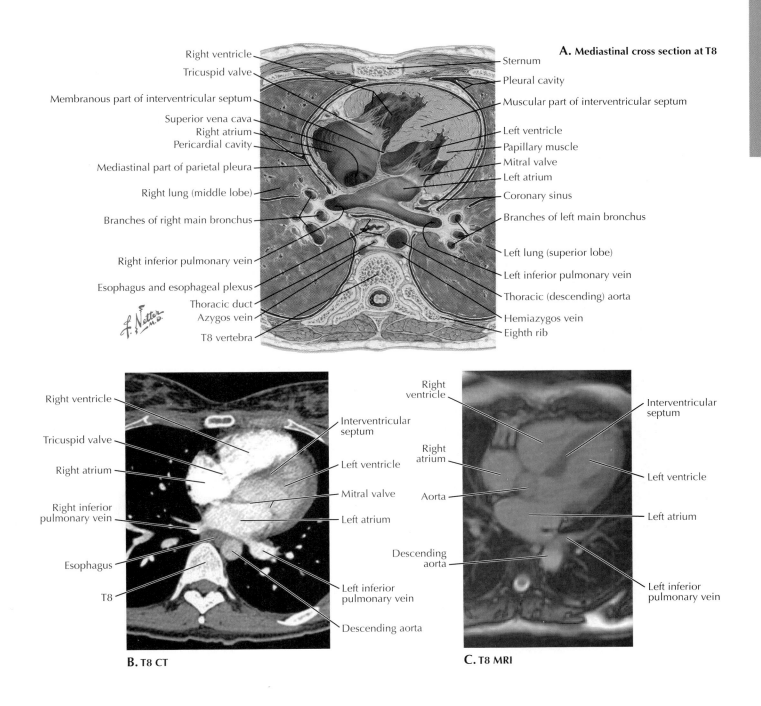

A. Mediastinal cross section at T8

Right ventricle — — Sternum
Tricuspid valve — — Pleural cavity
Membranous part of interventricular septum — — Muscular part of interventricular septum
Superior vena cava — — Left ventricle
Right atrium — — Papillary muscle
Pericardial cavity — — Mitral valve
Mediastinal part of parietal pleura — — Left atrium
Right lung (middle lobe) — — Coronary sinus
Branches of right main bronchus — — Branches of left main bronchus
Right inferior pulmonary vein — — Left lung (superior lobe)
Esophagus and esophageal plexus — — Left inferior pulmonary vein
Thoracic duct — — Thoracic (descending) aorta
Azygos vein — — Hemiazygos vein
T8 vertebra — — Eighth rib

Right ventricle —
Tricuspid valve —
Right atrium —
Right inferior pulmonary vein —
Esophagus —
T8 —
— Interventricular septum
— Left ventricle
— Mitral valve
— Left atrium
— Left inferior pulmonary vein
— Descending aorta

B. T8 CT

Right ventricle —
Right atrium —
Aorta —
Descending aorta —
— Interventricular septum
— Left ventricle
— Left atrium
— Left inferior pulmonary vein

C. T8 MRI

3.15 T8 MEDIASTINUM CROSS SECTION WITH T8 CT AND MRI

At the T8 level all four heart chambers are visible because of the AP orientation of the axis of the heart. The lower lobes of the lungs are posterior to the heart. The thoracic duct is behind the esophagus. The sections in all three figures capture inferior pulmonary veins entering the left atrium. Both CT and MRI are used to study the anatomy and function of the heart, including chamber size, wall thickness, valve structure, and blood flow through the coronary arteries. On the CT image (**B**) there is more contrast in the right side of the heart compared to the left. This is related to the time the image slice is acquired relative to the time after the contrast injection. In the MRI (**C**) the four chambers of the heart and a small portion of the aorta centrally are visualized. No contrast has been injected for this MRI sequence. Blood can appear white or black on MRI, depending on parameters set before the sequence is acquired.

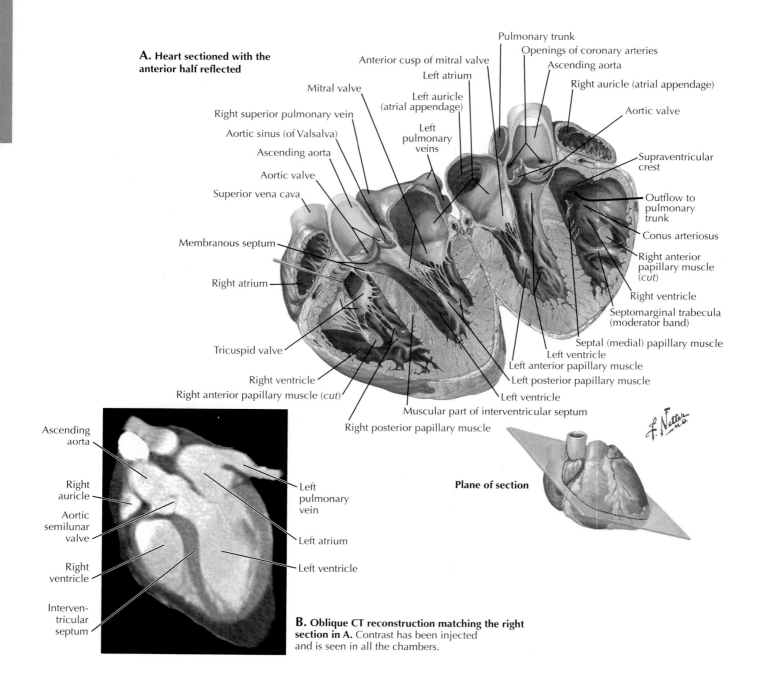

A. Heart sectioned with the anterior half reflected

Pulmonary trunk

Anterior cusp of mitral valve

Openings of coronary arteries

Ascending aorta

Left atrium

Right auricle (atrial appendage)

Mitral valve

Left auricle (atrial appendage)

Aortic valve

Right superior pulmonary vein

Left pulmonary veins

Aortic sinus (of Valsalva)

Ascending aorta

Supraventricular crest

Aortic valve

Superior vena cava

Outflow to pulmonary trunk

Conus arteriosus

Membranous septum

Right anterior papillary muscle (*cut*)

Right atrium

Right ventricle

Septomarginal trabecula (moderator band)

Septal (medial) papillary muscle

Tricuspid valve

Left ventricle

Left anterior papillary muscle

Right ventricle

Left posterior papillary muscle

Right anterior papillary muscle (*cut*)

Left ventricle

Muscular part of interventricular septum

Right posterior papillary muscle

Plane of section

Ascending aorta

Right auricle

Left pulmonary vein

Aortic semilunar valve

Left atrium

Right ventricle

Left ventricle

Interventricular septum

B. Oblique CT reconstruction matching the right section in A. Contrast has been injected and is seen in all the chambers.

3.16 ATRIA, VENTRICLES, AND INTERVENTRICULAR SEPTUM

The heart is sectioned here along an axis from the base of the heart (at the top) to the apex and opened like a book. The section is through all four chambers and the ascending aorta exiting the left ventricle. Not sectioned but visible in the right half is the pulmonary trunk from the right ventricle; it is anterior to the ascending aorta. In the section on the left, pulmonary veins enter the left atrium, and the superior vena cava enters the right atrium. The inferior vena cava is not visible. The right atrioventricular (tricuspid) valve has three flaps connected to papillary muscles in the right ventricle. The left atrioventricular (mitral or bicuspid) valve has two flaps. The valves of the ascending aorta and pulmonary trunk each have three cusps that function like the valves in veins. The CT image (**B**) shows both ventricles, the interventricular septum, two cusps of the aortic valve, a small portion of the left atrium, and one of the left pulmonary veins.

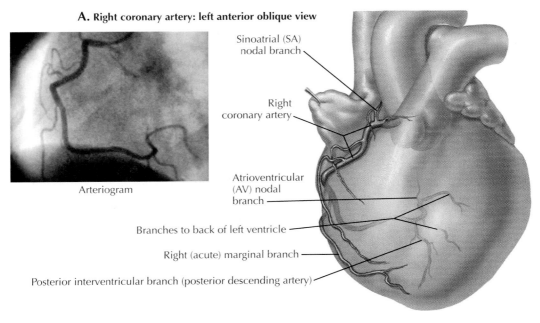

A. Right coronary artery: left anterior oblique view

Arteriogram

Sinoatrial (SA) nodal branch

Right coronary artery

Atrioventricular (AV) nodal branch

Branches to back of left ventricle

Right (acute) marginal branch

Posterior interventricular branch (posterior descending artery)

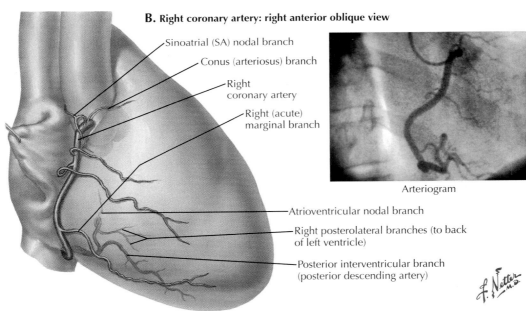

B. Right coronary artery: right anterior oblique view

Sinoatrial (SA) nodal branch

Conus (arteriosus) branch

Right coronary artery

Right (acute) marginal branch

Arteriogram

Atrioventricular nodal branch

Right posterolateral branches (to back of left ventricle)

Posterior interventricular branch (posterior descending artery)

3.17 RIGHT CORONARY ARTERY STUDY

To perform a coronary angiogram, an arterial catheter is usually inserted into one of the femoral arteries and under fluoroscopy advanced into the descending thoracic aorta and around the aortic arch to the level of the aortic sinuses (of Valsalva). Each coronary artery is then injected separately with iodinated contrast, and images of each artery are taken in various projections. The right coronary artery arises from the proximal ascending aorta and travels in the atrioventricular groove between the right atrium and right ventricle to supply the right side and back of the heart. It gives rise to a sinoatrial (SA) branch to the SA node and right atrium, a marginal branch to the right ventricle, and continues as the posterior interventricular artery. Oblique views of the heart show coronary branches to the best advantage, either parallel to the plane of the image or with minimal superimposition of the main branches.

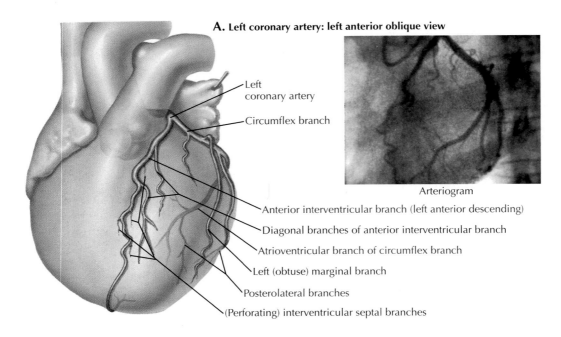

A. Left coronary artery: left anterior oblique view

Left coronary artery

Circumflex branch

Arteriogram

Anterior interventricular branch (left anterior descending)

Diagonal branches of anterior interventricular branch

Atrioventricular branch of circumflex branch

Left (obtuse) marginal branch

Posterolateral branches

(Perforating) interventricular septal branches

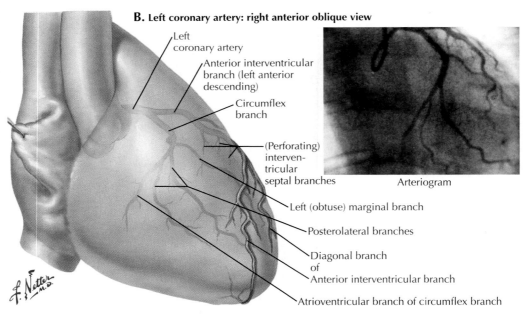

B. Left coronary artery: right anterior oblique view

Left coronary artery

Anterior interventricular branch (left anterior descending)

Circumflex branch

(Perforating) interventricular septal branches

Arteriogram

Left (obtuse) marginal branch

Posterolateral branches

Diagonal branch of Anterior interventricular branch

Atrioventricular branch of circumflex branch

3.18 LEFT CORONARY ARTERY STUDY

The left coronary artery arises from the ascending aorta to supply the anterior and left sides of the heart. It divides into anterior interventricular (left anterior descending) and circumflex branches, with many branches to the left ventricle and interventricular septum.

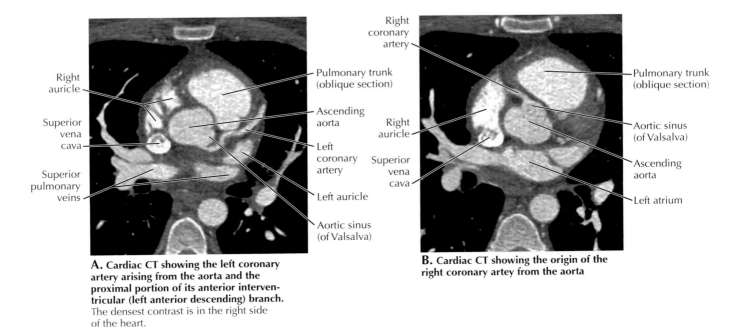

Right
auricle

Superior
vena
cava

Superior
pulmonary
veins

Pulmonary trunk
(oblique section)

Ascending
aorta

Left
coronary
artery

Left auricle

Aortic sinus
(of Valsalva)

A. Cardiac CT showing the left coronary
artery arising from the aorta and the
proximal portion of its anterior interventricular (left anterior descending) branch.
The densest contrast is in the right side
of the heart.

Right
coronary
artery

Right
auricle

Superior
vena
cava

Pulmonary trunk
(oblique section)

Aortic sinus
(of Valsalva)

Ascending
aorta

Left atrium

B. Cardiac CT showing the origin of the
right coronary artey from the aorta

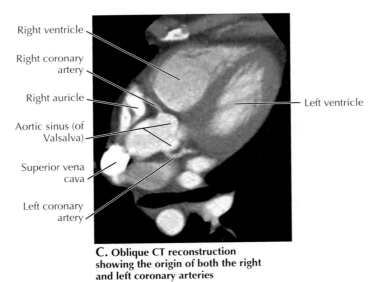

Right ventricle

Right coronary
artery

Right auricle

Aortic sinus (of
Valsalva)

Superior vena
cava

Left coronary
artery

Left ventricle

C. Oblique CT reconstruction
showing the origin of both the right
and left coronary arteries

3.19 HEART IMAGING STUDIES

CT and MRI can both be used to study the heart. CT is also used to study the coronary arteries. Motion imaging of the heart gated (synchronized) to the cardiac cycle can be performed using MRI and CT. Images can be obtained in multiple planes with MRI and reconstructed in multiple planes with CT. Three-dimensional reconstructions can also be generated and evaluated. Cardiac chamber size can be calculated with both CT and MRI.

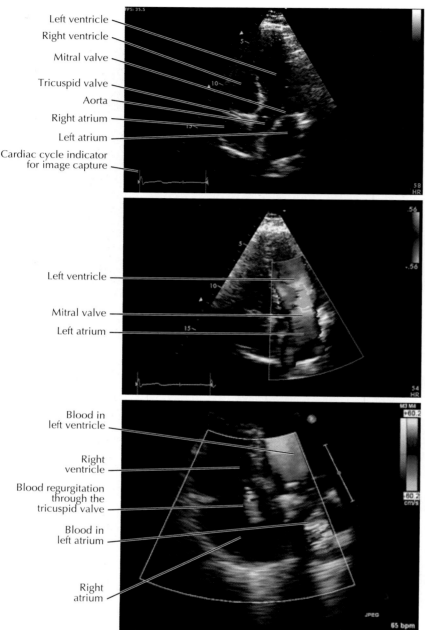

Left ventricle
Right ventricle
Mitral valve
Tricuspid valve
Aorta
Right atrium
Left atrium
Cardiac cycle indicator for image capture

A. Gray-scale echocardiogram showing all four chambers. The apex of the heart is at the top of the image. The transducer is on the patient's skin anteriorly. Different views of the heart are obtained by placing the ultrasound transducer in different positions on the chest wall.

Left ventricle
Mitral valve
Left atrium

B. Color enhancement in a four-chamber view. Shows blood flow from left atrium to left ventricle through the open mitral valve. Blue is flow away from the transducer on the patient's skin, and red is toward the transducer. There is some turbulent/ bidirectional flow in the left ventricle as evidenced by both the red and blue colors being present.

Blood in left ventricle
Right ventricle
Blood regurgitation through the tricuspid valve
Blood in left atrium
Right atrium

C. Color Doppler four-chamber view showing reversed flow (regurgitation) from the right ventricle into the right atrium through a leaky tricuspid valve during systole. Turbulent flow is seen in the left atrium located posteriorly on the right side of the image.

3.20 ECHOCARDIOGRAPHY

Echocardiography provides real-time ultrasound imaging of the heart without radiation. Portable examinations can be performed on very sick patients. Wall motion and ventricular contractility can be assessed, and the left ventricular output can be calculated. Chamber size, wall thickness, and the morphology of the heart valves can be evaluated. Blood flow through the heart can be further evaluated with the injection of a microbubble contrast agent that makes the blood flow more obvious and can help to evaluate intracardiac shunts. The cost relative to cardiac catheterization, cardiac CT, and MRI is much less. With color Doppler imaging the direction and magnitude of the blood flow through the heart can be visualized (**B** and **C**). By convention, red, is flow toward the transducer on the anterior chest wall, and blue is away from the transducer.

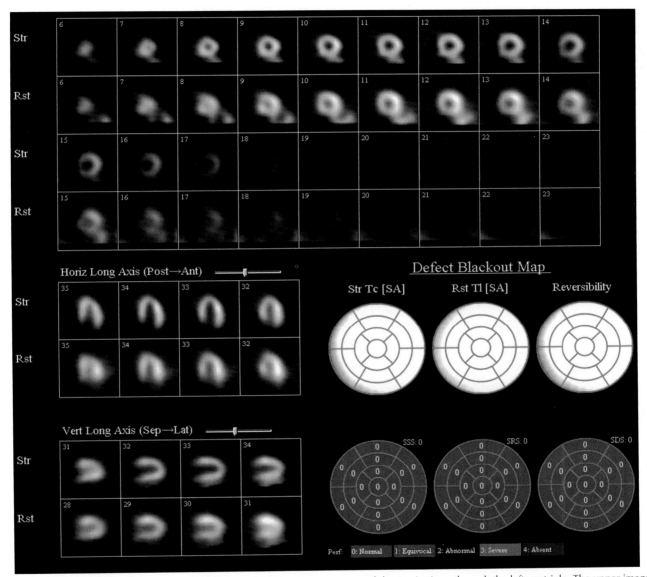

Normal SPECT examination. The upper two rows of images are a sequence of short-axis views through the left ventricle. The upper images are immediately after exercise, and the next row at rest. They are continued in the third and fourth rows. These views show the anterior, inferior, and lateral walls and the septum. The middle set of images are horizontal long-axis views. The lateral wall, apex, and septum are visualized. The bottom set of images are vertical long-axis views and show the anterior and inferior walls and the apex. Defects, if present, can be mapped onto the polar maps of the heart in the lower right corner.

3.21 SINGLE PHOTON EMISSION COMPUTED TOMOGRAPHY

Nuclear medicine studies are also used to study the heart. Myocardial function and perfusion can be studied by tagging red blood cells with a radioactive tracer such as thallium 201, technetium (Tc)-99m, or Tc-99m sestamibi. Single photon emission computed tomography (SPECT) is used to generate images of the heart in different projections and can be performed with the patient at maximal exercise and then at rest. Thallium 201 is a potassium analog and is taken up by the

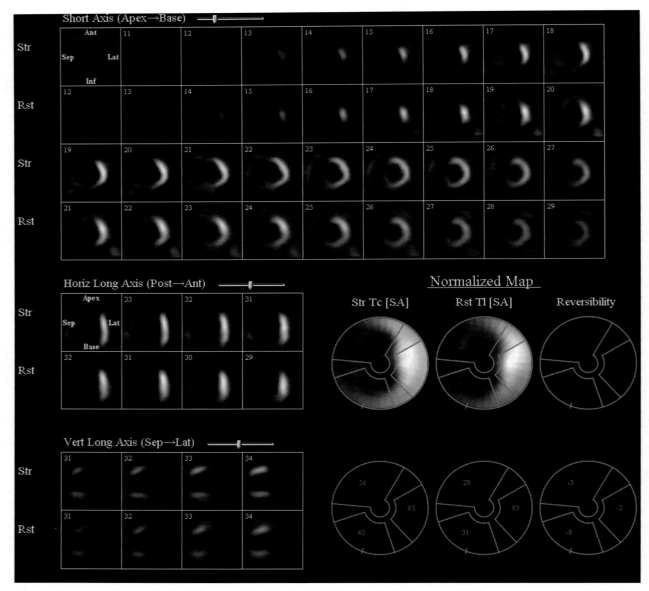

Abnormal SPECT study. Note that the left ventricle is dilated and the entire wall of the left ventricle does not take up the radiopharmaceutical on either the stress or resting images. This indicates areas of infarction. With ischemic myocardium there would be no uptake on the stress images but uptake on the resting images. This is called a *reversible defect*.

3.21 SINGLE PHOTON EMISSION COMPUTED TOMOGRAPHY (CONT'D)

myocytes. Decreased perfusion to a portion of the wall appears as an empty area on the scan images. Different portions of the left ventricular wall are imaged as sections along three planes oriented to the axis of the heart, referred to as the *long axis*.

In short-axis views perpendicular to the long axis, the ventricular wall appears as a doughnut with the chamber in the center. In vertical and horizontal long-axis views, the ventricular wall looks like a horseshoe. Multiple slices (tomograms) are created along each axis to represent all areas of the ventricular wall.

Comparison of Cardiac Imaging Modalities

Structure	Echo	Nuclear	CMR	CT
Anatomy	+ +	– – –	+ + + +	+ + + +
Chamber size	+ + +	+	+ + + +	+ + + +
Muscle thickness	+ + +		+ + + +	+ + + +
Valve structure	+ + + +	– – –	+ +	+ +
Coronary arteries	– – –	– – –	+ +	+ + + +
Pericardium	+ + +	– – –	+ + +	+ + + +
Function				
Stroke volume	+ +	+ +	+ + + +	+ + + +
Ejection fraction	+ +	+ + + +	+ + + +	+ + + +
Regional fraction	+ + +	+	+ + + +	+ + + +
Diastolic function	+ + +	– – –	+ +	– – –
Valve function	+ + + +	– – –	+ +	+
Coronary flow	– – –	+ + +	+	– – –
Muscle perfusion	+	+ + + +	+ + + +	+
Practicality				
Availability	+ + + +	+ + +	+ +	+ +
Portability	+ + +	– – –	– – –	– – –
Radiation	– – –	+ +	– – –	+ + + +
Cost	$	$$	$$$$	$$$$

Echo, Echocardiography; *nuclear*, nuclear cardiology; *CMR*, cardiac magnetic resonance; *CT*, computed tomography.
Printed with permission from Robert O. Bonow, MD.

3.22 COMPARISON OF CARDIAC IMAGING MODALITIES

Echocardiography, the cheapest and most available and portable imaging modality, is the best modality for evaluating valve structure and function because it captures (real-time) motion. It is also nearly as good as MRI and CT for overall heart structure and function. Nuclear studies are best for evaluating blood flow in the heart and within the myocardium. MRI and CT offer the best resolution but are the most expensive.

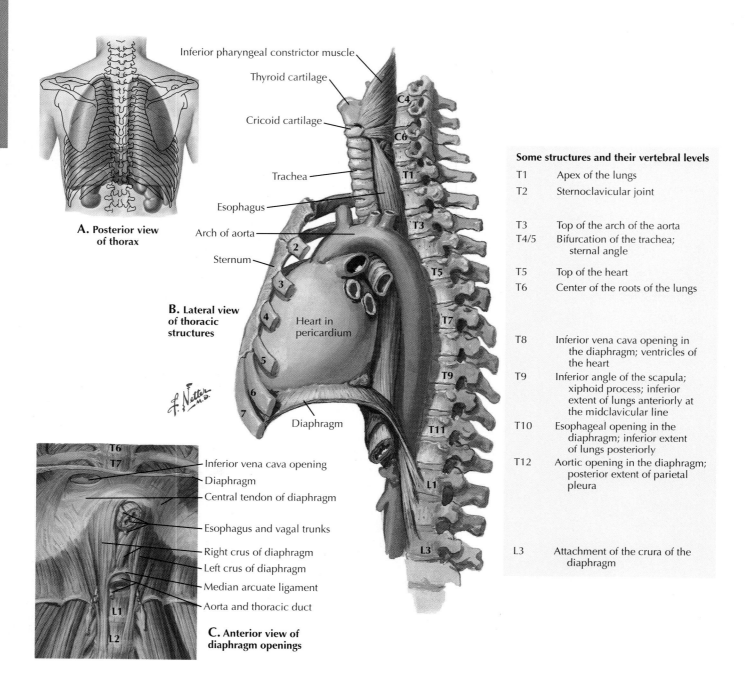

Inferior pharyngeal constrictor muscle

Thyroid cartilage

Cricoid cartilage

Trachea

Esophagus

Arch of aorta

Sternum

B. Lateral view of thoracic structures

Heart in pericardium

Diaphragm

A. Posterior view of thorax

C. Anterior view of diaphragm openings

Inferior vena cava opening
Diaphragm
Central tendon of diaphragm
Esophagus and vagal trunks
Right crus of diaphragm
Left crus of diaphragm
Median arcuate ligament
Aorta and thoracic duct

Some structures and their vertebral levels

T1	Apex of the lungs
T2	Sternoclavicular joint
T3	Top of the arch of the aorta
T4/5	Bifurcation of the trachea; sternal angle
T5	Top of the heart
T6	Center of the roots of the lungs
T8	Inferior vena cava opening in the diaphragm; ventricles of the heart
T9	Inferior angle of the scapula; xiphoid process; inferior extent of lungs anteriorly at the midclavicular line
T10	Esophageal opening in the diaphragm; inferior extent of lungs posteriorly
T12	Aortic opening in the diaphragm; posterior extent of parietal pleura
L3	Attachment of the crura of the diaphragm

3.23 VERTEBRAL LEVELS IN THE THORAX

The vertebral bodies are convenient indicators (e.g., T1, L2) of the level of anatomical cross sections on CT and MRI studies. Indicated in this figure are the vertebral levels of major structures and landmarks in the thorax. Although not used for clinical interpretation of images, they can help the novice to identify structures and relationships. Do not confuse vertebral levels with the levels of ribs, spinal cord segments, dermatomes, and visceral sensory innervation of organs. The spinal cord is shorter than the vertebral column, and both ribs and nerves course inferiorly from the vertebral column. For example, the T7 level of the spinal cord is higher than vertebral body T7, and the latter is higher than the seventh rib, the T7 dermatome, and T7 innervation of the stomach. The levels of the structures indicated in the illustration are average levels. There is considerable human variation with the confounding influences of posture and breathing.

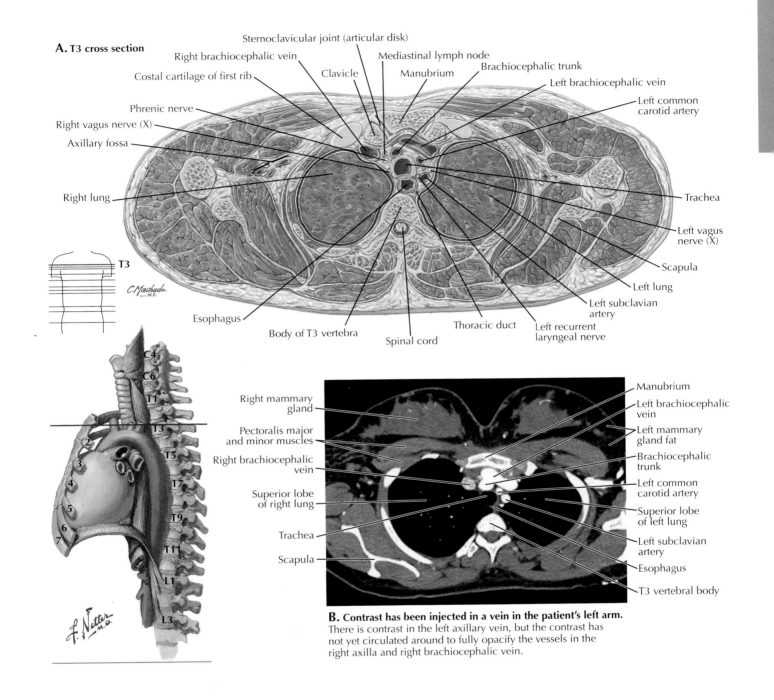

A. T3 cross section

Sternoclavicular joint (articular disk)
Right brachiocephalic vein
Mediastinal lymph node
Clavicle
Manubrium
Brachiocephalic trunk
Left brachiocephalic vein
Costal cartilage of first rib
Left common carotid artery
Phrenic nerve
Right vagus nerve (X)
Axillary fossa
Right lung
Trachea
Left vagus nerve (X)
Scapula
Left lung
Left subclavian artery
Esophagus
Body of T3 vertebra
Spinal cord
Thoracic duct
Left recurrent laryngeal nerve

C4
C6
T1
T3
T5
T7
T9
T11
L1
L3

Right mammary gland
Pectoralis major and minor muscles
Right brachiocephalic vein
Superior lobe of right lung
Trachea
Scapula

Manubrium
Left brachiocephalic vein
Left mammary gland fat
Brachiocephalic trunk
Left common carotid artery
Superior lobe of left lung
Left subclavian artery
Esophagus
T3 vertebral body

B. Contrast has been injected in a vein in the patient's left arm.
There is contrast in the left axillary vein, but the contrast has not yet circulated around to fully opacify the vessels in the right axilla and right brachiocephalic vein.

3.24 T3 CROSS SECTION WITH T3 CT

Cross sectional imaging studies such as CT and MRI are usually obtained with the patient lying supine on a movable table. It is a radiological convention to view axial cross-sectional images as if looking at the supine patient from the feet up. The right side of the patient is on the left side of the image. It is the same as when you are standing face to face with another person. Their right side is opposite your left side. The large vessels in the center of these figures indicate that this is an upper thoracic section above the level of the heart.

Posterior to the left brachiocephalic vein are the great arteries arising from the aortic arch: the brachiocephalic artery, the left common carotid artery, and the left subclavian artery. The brachiocephalic artery is larger because it gives rise to the right common carotid and right subclavian arteries. The patient in **B** has a normal variant: a fourth vessel arising from the arch, the left vertebral artery. Note the black, round, air-filled trachea in the CT. Posterior and to the left of the trachea is the esophagus. Sometimes air can be seen in the esophageal lumen.

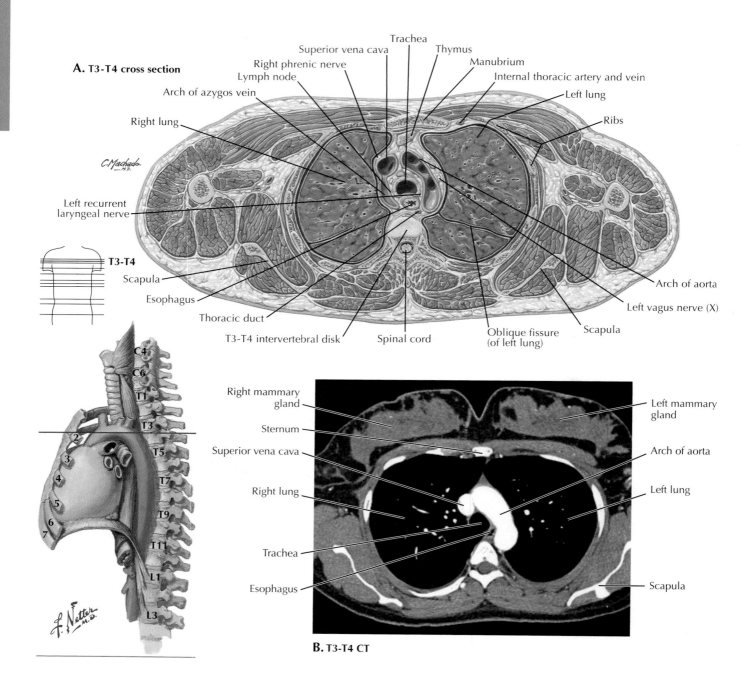

A. T3-T4 cross section

Trachea
Superior vena cava
Right phrenic nerve
Thymus
Lymph node
Manubrium
Arch of azygos vein
Internal thoracic artery and vein
Left lung
Right lung
Ribs
Left recurrent
laryngeal nerve
Arch of aorta
T3-T4
Left vagus nerve (X)
Scapula
Esophagus
Oblique fissure
(of left lung)
Scapula
Thoracic duct
T3-T4 intervertebral disk
Spinal cord

C4
C6
T1
T3
T5
T7
T9
T11
L1
L3

Right mammary
gland
Left mammary
gland
Sternum
Arch of aorta
Superior vena cava
Right lung
Left lung
Trachea
Esophagus
Scapula

B. T3-T4 CT

3.25 T3-T4 CROSS SECTION WITH T3-T4 CT

At T3-T4 this cross-sectional image is still above the level of the heart. The arch of the aorta is on the left, and the arch of the azygos vein entering the superior vena cava is on the right. The primary bronchi and pulmonary arteries in the root of the lungs would be just below the azygos vein and aorta. The oblique fissures of both lungs separate the upper and lower lobes of the lungs. The superior aspects of these fissures are seen in **A** but not on the CT that is viewed at mediastinal soft tissue window settings. The right middle lobe and the lingula of the left upper lobe are more inferiorly located at the level of the heart. On the CT (**B**) the aortic arch is well opacified with intravenous contrast, as is the adjacent superior vena cava. The azygos vein is not seen on this CT image.

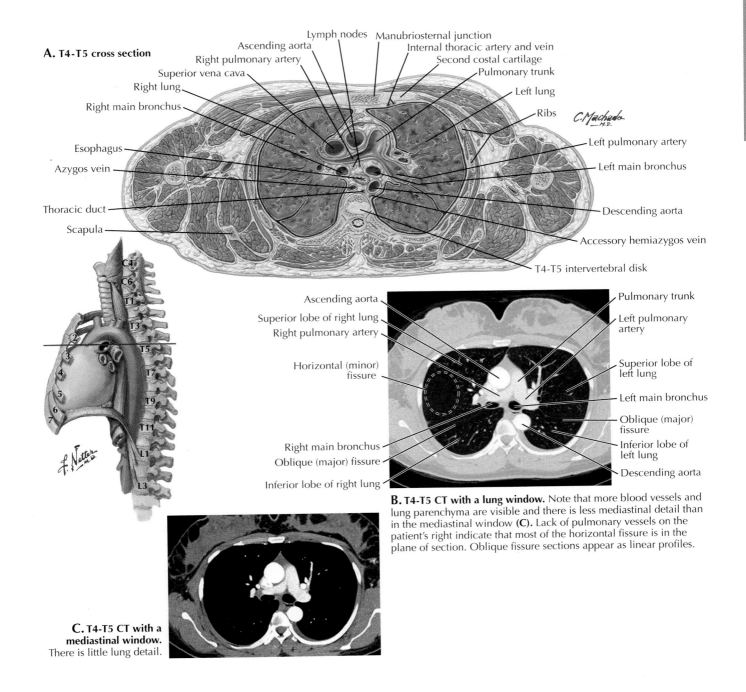

A. T4-T5 cross section

Lymph nodes

Ascending aorta

Right pulmonary artery

Superior vena cava

Right lung

Right main bronchus

Esophagus

Azygos vein

Thoracic duct

Scapula

Manubriosternal junction

Internal thoracic artery and vein

Second costal cartilage

Pulmonary trunk

Left lung

Ribs

Left pulmonary artery

Left main bronchus

Descending aorta

Accessory hemiazygos vein

T4-T5 intervertebral disk

C. Machado M.D.

f. Netter M.D.

Ascending aorta

Superior lobe of right lung

Right pulmonary artery

Horizontal (minor) fissure

Right main bronchus

Oblique (major) fissure

Inferior lobe of right lung

Pulmonary trunk

Left pulmonary artery

Superior lobe of left lung

Left main bronchus

Oblique (major) fissure

Inferior lobe of left lung

Descending aorta

B. T4-T5 CT with a lung window. Note that more blood vessels and lung parenchyma are visible and there is less mediastinal detail than in the mediastinal window (**C**). Lack of pulmonary vessels on the patient's right indicate that most of the horizontal fissure is in the plane of section. Oblique fissure sections appear as linear profiles.

C. T4-T5 CT with a mediastinal window. There is little lung detail.

3.26 T4-T5 CROSS SECTION WITH T4-T5 CT

In this section at T4-T5, the pulmonary trunk divides into the left and right pulmonary arteries. The left and right primary (main stem) bronchi are just posterior to the pulmonary arteries. Anterior to the right pulmonary artery are the larger ascending aorta and smaller superior vena cava. Posterior to the bronchi are the collapsed esophagus, descending aorta, thoracic duct, and azygos vein. The latter two are not seen clearly in this CT. The intravenous contrast is brighter in the ascending and descending aorta compared to the contrast in the pulmonary arteries because it has already circulated through the lungs and heart and the main portion of the bolus is now in the aorta. Different blood vessels can be preferentially enhanced with CT by varying the time at which an image is obtained with respect to the start of the contrast injection. Note the surrounding muscles and ribs and the anterior breast tissue bilaterally.

A. T7 cross section

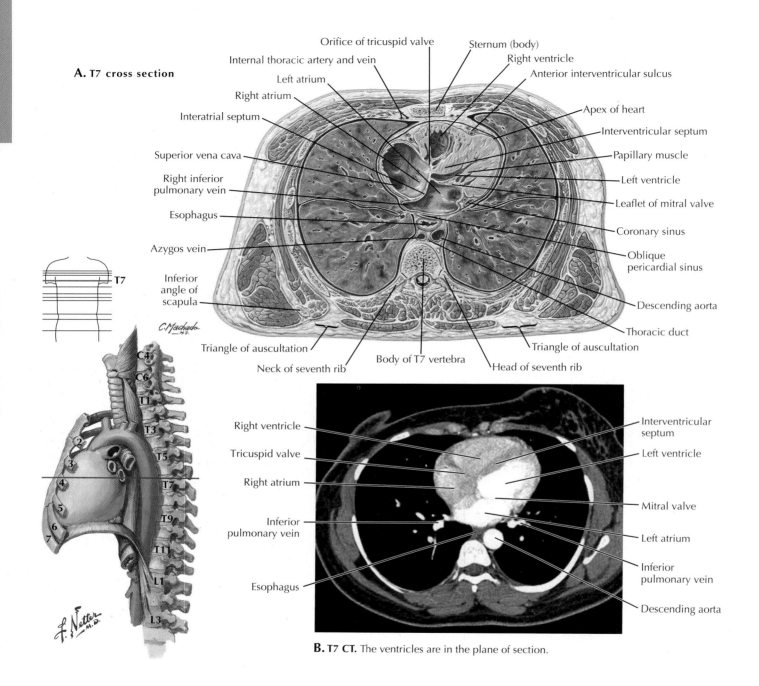

Orifice of tricuspid valve

Internal thoracic artery and vein

Left atrium

Right atrium

Interatrial septum

Superior vena cava

Right inferior pulmonary vein

Esophagus

Azygos vein

T7

Inferior angle of scapula

Triangle of auscultation

Neck of seventh rib

Sternum (body)

Right ventricle

Anterior interventricular sulcus

Apex of heart

Interventricular septum

Papillary muscle

Left ventricle

Leaflet of mitral valve

Coronary sinus

Oblique pericardial sinus

Descending aorta

Thoracic duct

Triangle of auscultation

Body of T7 vertebra

Head of seventh rib

C.Machado _M.D._

C4

C6

T1

T3

T5

T7

T9

T11

L1

L3

F. Netter M.D.

Right ventricle

Tricuspid valve

Right atrium

Inferior pulmonary vein

Esophagus

Interventricular septum

Left ventricle

Mitral valve

Left atrium

Inferior pulmonary vein

Descending aorta

B. T7 CT. The ventricles are in the plane of section.

3.27 T7 CROSS SECTION WITH T7 CT

This T7 section is through both atria at the top of the heart. Part of the atrioventricular valves, the superior portion of the right ventricle anteriorly, and some of the left ventricle are seen. The middle lobe of the right lung and lingula of the left upper lobe are on either side of the heart. The lower (inferior) lobes of the lungs are located posteriorly. On the CT the contrast is predominantly in the left side of the heart (related to

timing of the contrast bolus). The atrioventricular valve plane is identified on both the right and left sides of the heart. The descending thoracic aorta is posterior to the heart on the left and anterior to the poorly opacified azygos vein on the patient's right. The soft tissue of the esophagus is posterior to the left atrium. The superior and inferior vena cava are above and below the plane of section, respectively.

Search Strategy for the Systematic Interpretation of Chest X-rays

1. Identify which views were taken.
2. Evaluate technical quality of images.
3. Look for any tubes, lines, and support devices that may be present and note location.
4. Soft tissues
5. Bones
6. Pleural spaces and diaphragm
7. Upper abdomen
8. Mediastinum and hila of lungs
9. Heart and vasculature
10. Lungs

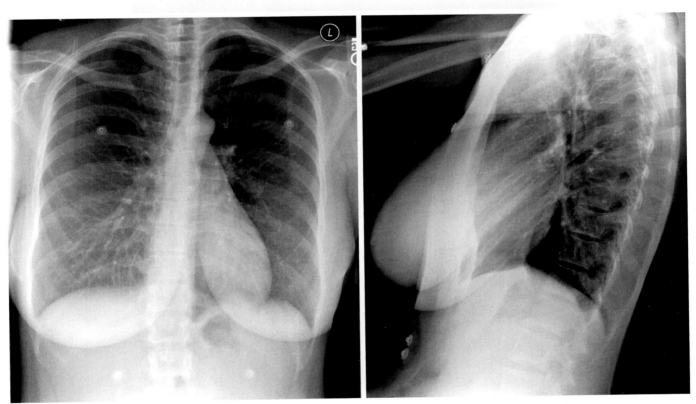

A. Normal PA x-ray

B. Normal lateral x-ray

3.28 SYSTEMATIC CHEST X-RAY EVALUATION

The list above summarizes one method for evaluating chest radiographs. The following pages provide more detail about what to evaluate for each step. It is important to develop a systematic pattern of looking at each of the structures visible on the images. The exact order of looking at the different structures can vary among individuals, but whatever order is chosen should be followed every time you look at chest radiographs. This helps to prevent missing an important finding. In any region look for what is present and what is missing. An understanding of normal anatomical structures and their relationships is essential for correct image interpretation.

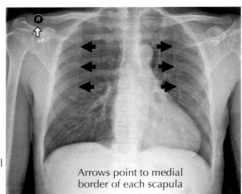

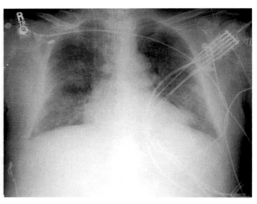

A. Normal AP view. Note the medial border of the scapulae over the upper lungs.

Arrows point to medial border of each scapula

B. More typical AP view in a sicker patient. This patient is intubated and has a right central venous catheter. The lungs appear hazy. This may be caused by the low lung volumes, but it may also be caused by edema and/or infection.

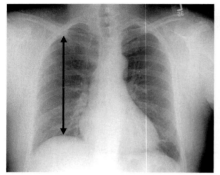

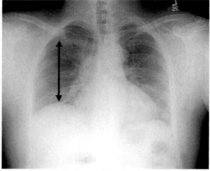

Arrows in both figures (C and D) show the position of the diaphragm in relation to the clavicle.

C. Inspiration view with diaphragm positioned lower. At least nine posterior ribs can be counted, and the heart appears relatively small and the lungs less dense compared with the expiration view. Most chest x-rays are inspiration views in which the anatomy is better evaluated.

D. Expiration view with elevated diaphragm. Only seven ribs are seen; the heart appears relatively large and the lungs denser than in the inspiration view. The relatively large heart may give the (false) impression of pathology.

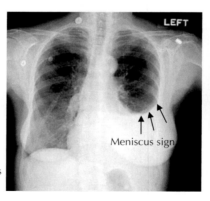

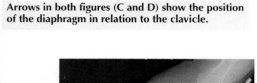

Fluid level

E. Initial PA view of the patient in F. There is opacity obscuring the left lower lobe and left diaphragm. A meniscus sign is seen laterally *(arrows).*

Meniscus sign

F. Left lateral decubitus view of the patient in E. With the patient lying on the left side, the fluid layers out along the lowest point of the lateral surface of the left pleural space.

3.29 SEARCH STRATEGY: IDENTIFYING VIEWS

PA and lateral views (see 3.28) are the preferred projections because there is less magnification of the heart. The patient has to be able to stand for these views. The scapulae project off the lungs on PA views, in which the imaging plate is put against the front of the patient and the x-ray beam transits from the back of the patient (posterior) to the front (anterior). AP radiographs are obtained on sicker patients and can be obtained portably, with the patient sitting upright or supine.

The recording plate is put behind the patient for an AP view, and the scapulae project over the upper lungs (**A**). Decubitus ("lying down") views (**F**) with the patient lying either on his or her right or left side can be obtained to look for layering of pleural fluid. Expiration views can be obtained to look for a small pneumothorax, which appears relatively larger in a smaller thoracic volume during expiration. This is usually done after an interventional procedure such as a central line placement or lung biopsy.

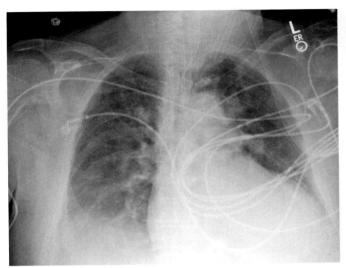

A. The inferior portion of the chest, especially on the right, is cut off in this AP view. This patient probably has bilateral effusions, but this is difficult to discern for sure without the lower thorax on the image. Most of the wires seen are monitoring devices overlying the patient.

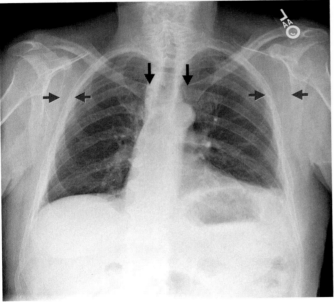

C. Complete situs inversus with dextrocardia, a mirror image reversal of the left-right positioning of organs in the body. This technically satisfactory image shows the heart on the right side of the thorax. The left side of the patient is labeled with a metallic marker and the technologist's personal number. Note the positions of the left ventricle *(black arrow)* and aortic arch *(red arrow)*.

B. The patient is rotated to the left on this PA view. Note the position of each scapula relative to the chest wall *(red arrows)*. The heads of the clavicles are not centered with respect to the trachea and thoracic spine *(black arrows)*. The medial head of the left clavicle is better seen than the right.

3.30 SEARCH STRATEGY: TECHNICAL QUALITY OF IMAGES

Images need to be of satisfactory quality for accurate interpretation. Technical factors to be considered include: (1) Is the entire chest included in the image? (2) Is the image too dark or too light? With digital displays this can be corrected to some extent by the computer. (3) Is the patient rotated? Look to see if the medial heads of the clavicles are centered on either side of the upper thoracic spine. (4) Has the patient taken a good inspiration? Vessels appear crowded, the diaphragm is elevated, and the heart appears larger if there are small lung volumes because of a poor inspiration. (5) Look for patient motion, especially on CT examinations. (6) Look to see that the right or left side of the radiograph is labeled. You cannot depend on which side of the body the heart is located to determine right from left, as indicated in **C.**

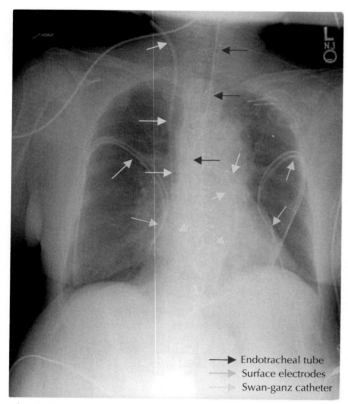

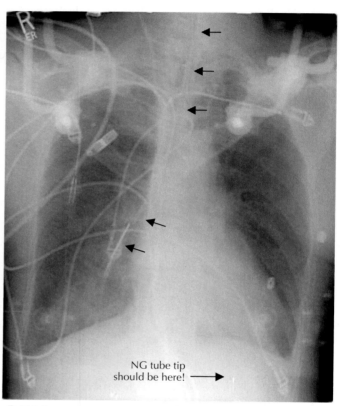

→ Endotracheal tube
→ Surface electrodes
→ Swan-ganz catheter

NG tube tip
should be here! →

A. **AP view of a patient with a right Swan-Ganz catheter used to measure central venous pressures, with its tip in the left pulmonary artery.** There is an endotracheal tube with its tip in the proximal right mainstem bronchus. This needs to be pulled back. Sternal wires in the midline and nonattached pacemaker electrodes are seen overlying the shoulder from prior cardiac surgery.

B. **This image shows a metallic halo device overlying the upper thorax used to stablize the cervical spine after severe injury.** A nasogastric (NG) feeding tube has been placed (*arrows*), and the tip is seen in the right lower lobe bronchus instead of the expected position in the stomach.

3.31 SEARCH STRATEGY: TUBES, LINES, AND SUPPORT DEVICES

Patients may have multiple tubes, drains, and/or intravenous central lines inserted while they are in the hospital. They may also have permanent support devices such as a pacemaker or automatic intracardiac defibrillator (AICD) in place. It is important to check where the tip of the central line is located and if there is a pneumothorax after placement. You also need to check where the tip of an endotracheal tube is located. If the tip is in one of the main stem bronchi, the other lung will not be aerated and will collapse. The tip and side holes of an enteric feeding tube should be in the stomach below the left hemidiaphragm. A patient aspirates food if the tip of a malpositioned tube is in a bronchus or the esophagus (with reflux into the airway). You can also look for any discontinuity in the pacemaker or defibrillator leads from the battery pack to their termination in the heart.

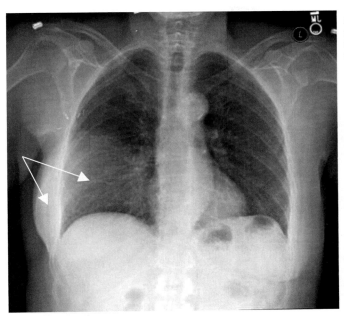

A. This AP view shows increased density (more white) over the right mid to lower lung and surgical clips in the right axilla. This is consistent with a right breast implant (compare with **B**) and lymph node removal in a patient with breast cancer post mastectomy.

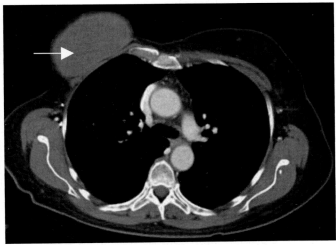

B. Right breast implant seen anterior to the bony thorax on the CT

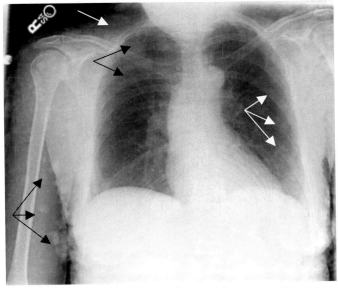

C. PA x-ray of a patient with neurofibromatosis, a neurocutaneous syndrome. Note the multiple soft tissue skin nodules (*arrows*) consistent with neurofibromas.

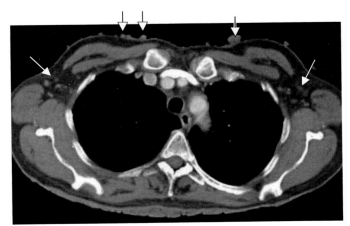

D. Axial CT using a soft tissue window of the patient in C. The location of the nodules (*arrows*) in the superficial body wall is verified.

3.32 SEARCH STRATEGY: THORACIC WALL SOFT TISSUES (E.G., AIR, CALCIFICATION, FOREIGN BODIES)

The thoracic wall includes the skin; subcutaneous fat; breasts; and muscles of the neck, proximal arms, thorax, upper abdomen, and axillae. Evaluation of the overlying soft tissues can give an idea about the overall health of the patient. Is the patient very sick and cachectic with no subcutaneous tissue, or is he or she very obese? Check for the presence of both breasts in adult female patients. Asymmetry to the breast tissue and surgical clips in the axilla (**A**) can suggest a history of breast cancer. Absence of both breasts can be hard to detect. Also look for air in the soft tissues, foreign bodies, asymmetrical swelling, or masses (**C** and **D**).

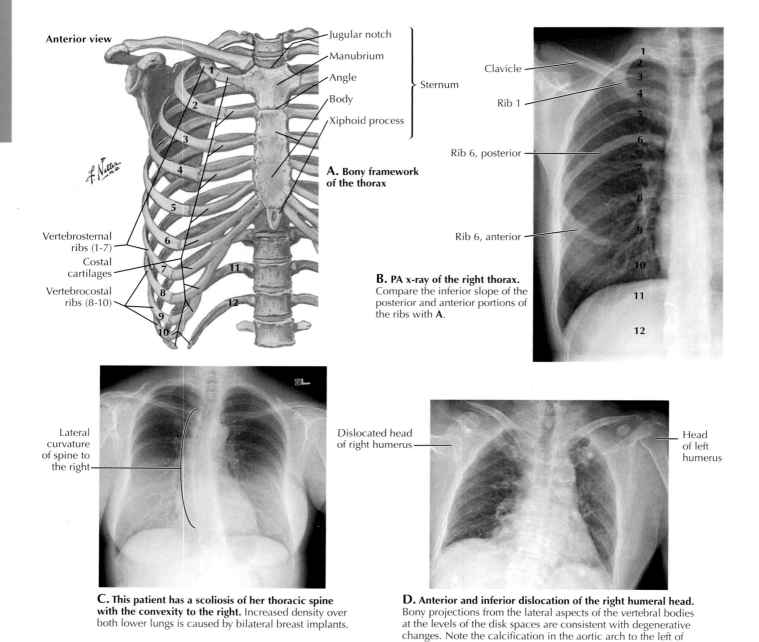

Anterior view

Jugular notch

Manubrium

Angle

Body } Sternum

Xiphoid process

A. Bony framework of the thorax

Vertebrosternal ribs (1-7)

Costal cartilages

Vertebrocostal ribs (8-10)

Clavicle

Rib 1

Rib 6, posterior

Rib 6, anterior

B. PA x-ray of the right thorax.
Compare the inferior slope of the posterior and anterior portions of the ribs with **A**.

Lateral curvature of spine to the right

C. This patient has a scoliosis of her thoracic spine with the convexity to the right. Increased density over both lower lungs is caused by bilateral breast implants.

Dislocated head of right humerus

Head of left humerus

D. Anterior and inferior dislocation of the right humeral head. Bony projections from the lateral aspects of the vertebral bodies at the levels of the disk spaces are consistent with degenerative changes. Note the calcification in the aortic arch to the left of the air-filled trachea.

3.33 SEARCH STRATEGY: BONES

The clavicle and scapulae form the shoulder girdle of the appendicular skeleton of the limbs. The sternum and ribs are parts of the axial skeleton, along with the vertebral column and skull. The sternum consists of the manubrium with its articulation with the clavicle and first rib, the body, and the xiphoid process most inferiorly. There are twelve pairs of ribs defined by their articulation with the twelve thoracic vertebrae. Ribs 1 to 7 are called vertebrosternal ribs because their cartilages attach directly to the sternum anteriorly. Ribs 8 to 10 are vertebrocostal because they attach to the sternum indirectly via the costal cartilage of rib 7. Ribs 11 and 12 are vertebral or "floating" ribs that have no anterior attachment. Note the downward slope of all the ribs. Bony abnormalities can include fractures and shoulder or clavicle dislocations (**C**), rib notching, findings related to metabolic bone diseases, and lytic or sclerotic metastases from different cancers.

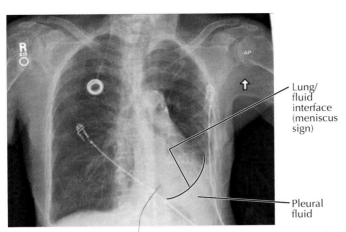

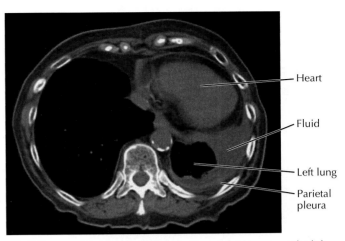

A. AP film showing a right port-a-cath that allows repetitive central venous access for chemotherapy. There is a meniscus sign at the left lung base with increased opacity from the fluid, obscuring visualization of the left diaphragm. There is blunting of the right costophrenic angle from fluid accumulation in the recess.

B. CT image of the same patient in A. Pleural fluid is seen at the left lung base posterior to the heart. The aerated lung appears black on this mediastinal window. There is some pleural thickening around the pleural fluid.

C. This patient has a left port-a-cath with its tip in the superior vena cava. What appears to be an elevated right hemidiaphragm with its peak shifted laterally is actually pleural fluid.

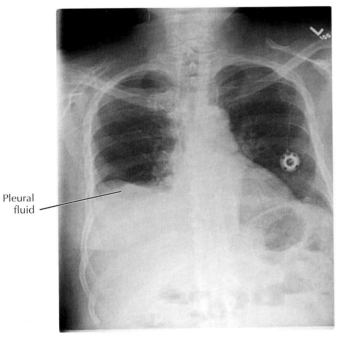

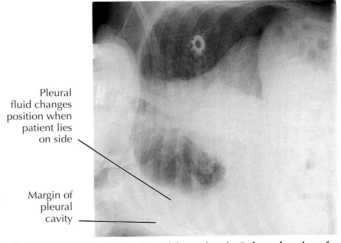

D. Right lateral decubitus view of the patient in C shows layering of a moderate right effusion

3.34 SEARCH STRATEGY: PLEURAL SPACES AND DIAPHRAGM

Visceral pleura covers the surface of the lungs, and parietal pleura abuts the mediastinum (mediastinal pleura) and diaphragm (diaphragmatic pleura) and is the inner layer of the thoracic wall (costal pleura). There is a potential space between visceral and parietal pleura that extends inferiorly to the costodiaphragmatic recess (costophrenic sulcus) of parietal pleura surrounding the periphery of the diaphragm. The position of the diaphragm depends on the degree of inspiration and whether any mass displaces it on either side. Fluid in the pleural space indicates an effusion. This fluid may be simple (hydrothorax), such as occurs with congestive heart failure, or complex and associated with infection (empyema), hemorrhage (hemothorax), or tumor. There is volume loss in the lung on the side of the fluid. Fluid in the pleural space can be seen on routine views with blunting of the sulci (**A**) or, if more fluid is present, a meniscus sign (**A**) with fluid extending superiorly along the lateral chest wall (see p. 64, **E**). Subpulmonic fluid can mimic the diaphragm but with an abnormal shape, either flattened or with its peak shifted laterally (**C**). Pleural fluid that is not loculated (locally contained) can be confirmed with decubitus views (**D**), which shift the fluid with change in the patient's position. Ultrasound can also be used to locate pleural fluid and guide aspiration.

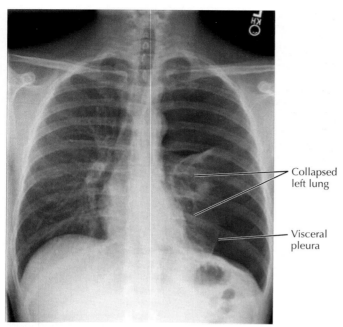

A. A complete left pneumothorax, without mediastinal shift. The trachea is in the midline, centered over the upper vertebral bodies. The collapsed left lung is against the left heart border, and the majority of the left hemithorax is totally black, indicating air.

Collapsed left lung

Visceral pleura

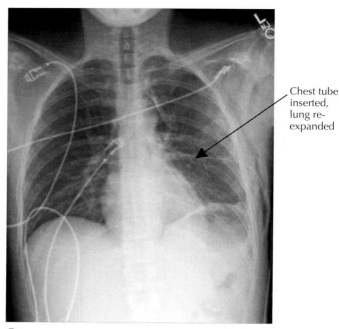

B. Same patient as in A with a chest tube inserted to reinflate the lung

Chest tube inserted, lung re-expanded

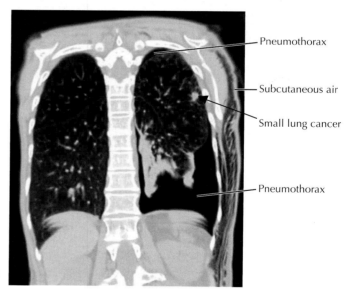

Pneumothorax

Subcutaneous air

Small lung cancer

Pneumothorax

C. Coronal reconstruction CT using lung window settings. This shows a moderate left pneumothorax, most marked in the inferior chest but also involving the left apex. There is extensive left subcutaneous emphysema (air). The pneumothorax was the result of biopsy of the small irregular nodule in the left upper lobe, suspicious for a lung cancer.

3.35 SEARCH STRATEGY: PLEURAL SPACES AND DIAPHRAGM (CONT'D)

Air in the pleural space is called a *pneumothorax*. This can be spontaneous, as can occur when a bleb on the surface of the lung ruptures in patients with asthma or emphysema. It can also be associated with trauma or a penetrating wound through the thoracic wall. Pneumothoraces may be small or large and cause volume loss on the affected side. A sharp white line of the visceral pleura is visible if a pneumothorax is present. There are no lung markings outside the confines of the pleural line. Usually vascular markings extend to the periphery of the lungs, where they underlie the thoracic wall.

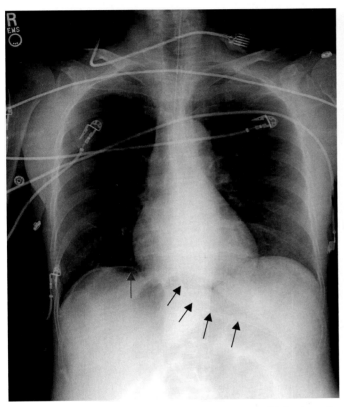

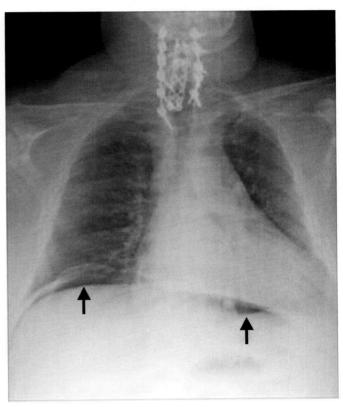

A. This patient has a nasogastric tube *(black arrows)* **with its tip and side hole in the stomach below the left hemidiaphragm.** There is lucency in the right upper abdomen just below the diaphragm. The right hemidiaphragm is outlined by air, indicating free air in the abdomen *(red arrow)*. In this case the patient recently had abdominal surgery, and the air was expected.

B. There is a larger amount of air under both the right and left hemidiaphragms *(arrows)* **in this patient.** A percutaneous tube was recently inserted into the stomach for feeding purposes (PEG tube). Note the internal fixation hardware in the lower cervical spine.

3.36 SEARCH STRATEGY: UPPER ABDOMEN

A portion of the upper abdomen is usually included on chest radiographs. The air bubble from the stomach is usually seen just below the left hemidiaphragm. A portion of the splenic flexure of the colon may be seen in the left upper quadrant as well. The liver is under the right hemidiaphragm. Free air in the abdomen (pneumoperitoneum) rises to just beneath the hemidiaphragms if the patient is upright (**A** and **B**). Look for abnormal bowel in the upper abdomen and soft tissue masses, displacement of the gastric air bubble, and abnormal calcifications. The tip of an enteric feeding tube should extend at least into the left upper quadrant of the abdomen.

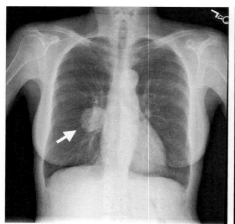

A. PA x-ray of a right infrahilar lung mass (arrow). The pulmonary vasculature can be seen through the mass, suggesting it is not adenopathy (lymph node enlargement among the vessels).

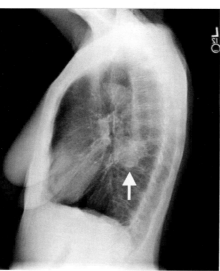

B. Lateral x-ray of the same patient in A. This view confirms that the mass (arrow) projects posteriorly behind the larger vessels. Biopsy showed this to be a lung cancer.

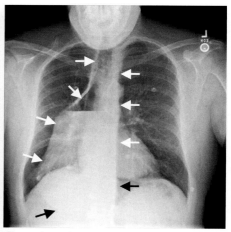

C. PA view of a markedly dilated esophagus (arrows) containing fluid. Note the widened mediastinum in the right lower chest and an air-fluid level within this region. The masslike opacity does not obscure the right heart border or the right diaphragm. This patient has achalasia, in which the lower esophageal sphincter does not relax normally.

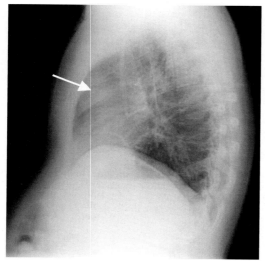

D. Lateral view of soft tissue in the anterior mediastinum. The anterior clear space is not clear (arrow). This suggests an anterior mediastinal mass.

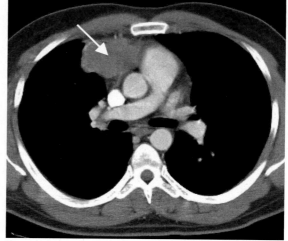

E. Subsequent CT of the same patient in D. There is a soft tissue mass in the anterior mediastinum (arrow), anterior to the superior vena cava and ascending aorta and to the right of the pulmonary outflow tract. This patient had lymphoma (cancer of the lymph nodes).

3.37 SEARCH STRATEGY: MEDIASTINUM AND HILA

The mediastinum contains multiple structures, including the trachea, heart, great vessels, lymph nodes, and esophagus. Enlargement of the mediastinum may be caused by a mass, often adenopathy (enlargement of lymph nodes), or a vascular problem. The pulmonary arteries, pulmonary veins, bronchi, and lymph nodes compose the hilar regions. The hila can appear enlarged as a result of abutting lung masses, lymphadenopathy, or vascular problems. The left hilum is usually higher than the right, although either may be displaced by a mass or volume loss in the adjacent lung.

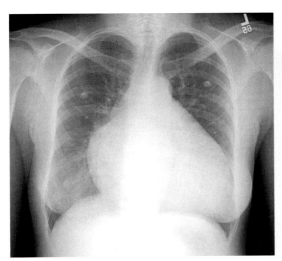

A. PA radiograph of a markedly enlarged heart. The left heart border is straightened. This can be seen with an enlarged left atrium.

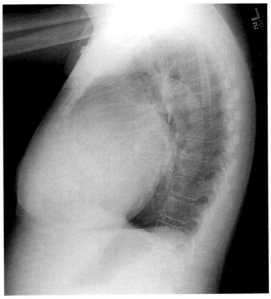

B. Lateral radiograph of the same patient in A. All of the heart chambers are enlarged in this patient with a cardiomyopathy.

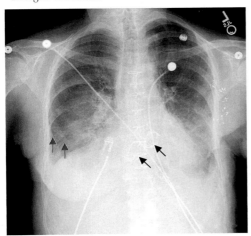

C. This patient had two heart valve replacements *(black arrows).* The heart is enlarged, and there is increased vascularity centrally in the upper lung lobes. Kerley B lines are seen in the periphery of the right lower lobe *(red arrows).* These findings are consistent with interstitial edema.

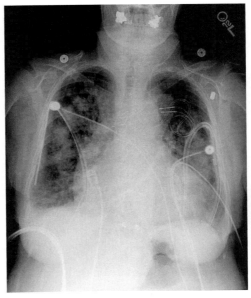

D. This is a different patient, with patchy alveolar opacities in both lungs consistent with more severe alveolar edema. This patient also has right pleural effusion (the right costophrenic angle is blunted) and cardiomegaly.

3.38 SEARCH STRATEGY: HEART AND VASCULATURE

The heart size appearance can vary with the degree of inspiration and the view obtained. Usually the width of the heart is less than 50% of the width of the chest on a PA view. Pericardial effusions are hard to detect on routine chest x-rays unless they are quite large. They are easy to see on CT or echocardiography. Pneumopericardium is unusual unless the patient has had recent heart surgery or trauma. Increased vascular markings are associated with elevated heart pressures and may be seen with congestive heart failure (CHF). In classic CHF the heart is enlarged, and there are bilateral pleural effusions. As the vascular pressure increases in the lungs, fluid begins to leak out of the vessels into the interstitium. Kerley B lines (dilated lymphatic vessels) caused by fluid in the interstitium appear as thin horizontal lines at the lateral periphery of the lower lungs. Decreased pulmonary vascularity is harder to detect. It can be seen diffusely with destructive lung processes such as emphysema and focally with pulmonary emboli (thrombus in pulmonary arteries). Atherosclerotic calcifications involving the aorta and its major branch vessels may also be found.

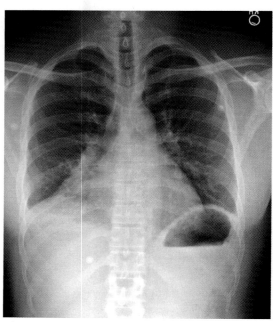

A. PA radiograph showing right middle lobe opacity. The right heart border is not seen because of adjacent opacity in the right middle lobe (the silhouette sign). The left heart margin is sharp.

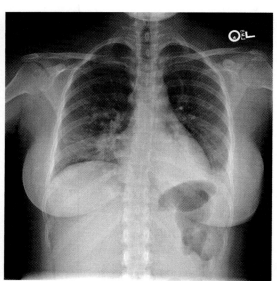

C. PA radiograph demonstrating bilateral areas of alveolar opacity. The one on the right partially obscures the right heart border. The process on the left is in the left lower lobe, posterior to the heart. Note the added opacity in the region of the heart on the left. The left medial diaphragm is poorly seen.

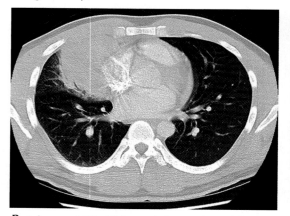

B. Subsequent CT with lung window settings of the same patient in A. The right middle lobe shows alveolar opacity abutting the right heart border. The inferior portion of the right oblique fissure is seen anteriorly. This patient had blastomycosis, a fungal disease.

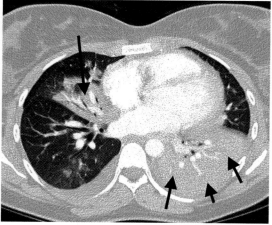

D. Subsequent CT of the chest of the same patient in C. Both the right middle lobe pneumonia and the left lower lobe pneumonia are seen clearly (*arrows*).

3.39 SEARCH STRATEGY: LUNGS— SILHOUETTE SIGN

The silhouette sign refers to the obscuration of a normal border in an x-ray, such as the heart margins or contour of the diaphragm, caused by an abutting area of similar density.

It is used to identify the presence and location of an abnormality. Common examples of pathology that may produce a silhouette sign are the presence of pleural fluid, pneumonia, or atelectasis (focal area of nonaerated lung).

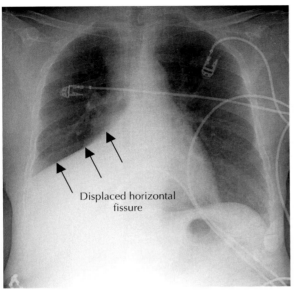

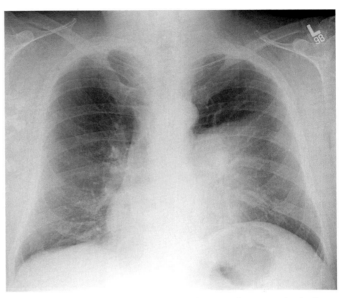

A. Atelectasis of the right middle and lower lobes. There is increased opacity in the right lower lobe and right middle lobe with a sharp line demarcating this area from the aerated right upper lobe. The sharp line is the minor (horizontal) fissure. The right middle lobe and right lower lobe are completely collapsed.

B. PA view of left upper lobe collapse. There is a hazy opacity in the region of the left lung medially. This is called the *veil sign* and indicates left upper lobe collapse. The left upper lobe collapses anteriorly, and the aerated left lower lobe expands posterior to it.

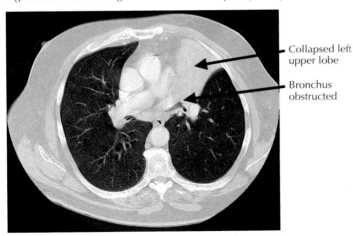

C. CT of the same patient in B. There is abrupt obstruction of the left upper lobe bronchus. This turned out to be caused by lung cancer.

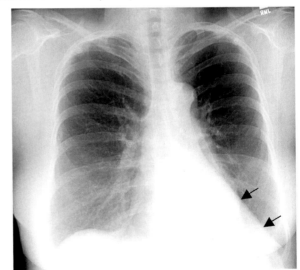

D. PA view of left lower lobe collapse. There is increased opacity behind the heart with a sharp lateral border *(arrows).*

3.40 SEARCH STRATEGY: LUNGS, ATELECTASIS

Atelectasis means collapse. This refers to a portion of the lung that is not aerated. There can be total collapse of a lung or partial collapse of either a lobe or segment. Subsegmental atelectasis refers to small focal areas of nonaerated lung and is most common at the lung bases. Atelectasis may be caused by bronchial obstruction from a foreign body or mass, compression by pleural fluid or pleural air, or contraction from scarring. Signs of atelectasis include increased opacity, displaced fissure, vascular and bronchial crowding, elevated diaphragm, and a displaced hilum. With collapse of a lobe or part of the lung, the rest of the lung expands with a decrease in opacity (density) compared with the opposite normal lung.

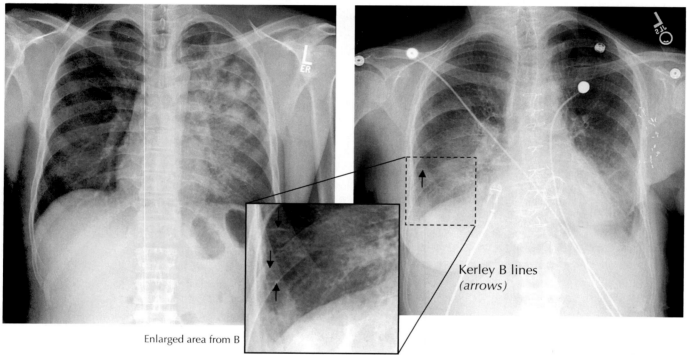

A. PA x-ray of diffuse pneumonia in the left lung. Note the fluffy white opacity in the majority of the left lung compared with the clear right lung. The left ventricular border is partially obscured, indicating involvement of the lingula of the left upper lobe.

B. Interstitial edema is indicated by the horizontal lines at the lung bases. These are Kerley B lines that are dilated lymphatic vessels.

Enlarged area from B

Kerley B lines
(arrows)

3.41 SEARCH STRATEGY: LUNGS, ALVEOLAR VS. INTERSTITIAL OPACITY

Abnormal opacity in the lungs can be caused by blood, pus, water, or cells. This opacity may be within the alveoli and look cloudlike or fluffy. Air bronchograms may be visible, with the air-filled bronchi surrounded by the densely filled air sacs. Abnormal opacity from the same causes can also be within the interstitium, the supporting structure of the lungs composed of connective tissue, nerves, lymphatics, and pulmonary vessels. An interstitial disease process appears linear (reticular) or micronodular. With a reticular pattern there are lines in the lungs that do not follow the normal course of the pulmonary vessels. Many processes have both alveolar and interstitial components. Bacterial pneumonia tends to have an alveolar pattern, whereas viral pneumonias tend to be interstitial. Pulmonary edema starts out as fluid in the interstitium and looks linear; but, as the pulmonary venous pressures rise, fluid enters the alveoli, and the pattern changes to alveolar. Lymphangitic spread from cancer can appear as irregular thickened lines within the lungs, especially at the periphery of the lung bases.

4

ABDOMEN

4.1 BONY FRAMEWORK: CT THREE-DIMENSIONAL RECONSTRUCTION

4.2 USE OF CONTRAST IN ABDOMINAL IMAGING STUDIES

4.3 CT VS. MRI IN ABDOMINAL STUDIES

4.4 SEARCH STRATEGY: SYSTEMATIC INTERPRETATION OF IMAGING STUDIES

4.5 DIAPHRAGM RELATIONSHIPS

4.6 PANCREAS RELATIONSHIPS

4.7 CROSS SECTION AT T10 WITH CT

4.8 CROSS SECTION AT T12 WITH CT

4.9 CROSS SECTION VARIATION AT T12 WITH CT

4.10 CROSS SECTION AT T12-L1 WITH CT

4.11 CROSS SECTION AT L1-L2 WITH CT

4.12 KIDNEY RELATIONSHIPS

4.13 L3-L4 CROSS SECTION WITH CT

4.14 SAGITTAL SECTION THROUGH AORTA WITH CT SAGITTAL RECONSTRUCTION

4.15 STOMACH IN SITU

4.16 UPPER GASTROINTESTINAL CT STUDIES

4.17 HIATAL HERNIA

4.18 LARGE INTESTINE IMAGING STUDIES

4.19 GALLBLADDER, BILE DUCTS, AND PANCREATIC DUCT

4.20 ABDOMINAL FOREGUT ARTERIES

4.21 MIDGUT AND HINDGUT ARTERIES

4.22 ANGIOGRAMS OF THE SUPERIOR AND INFERIOR MESENTERIC VESSELS

4.23 PERITONEAL/RETROPERITONEAL RELATIONSHIPS

4.24 GASTROINTESTINAL PATHOLOGY

3D Reconstruction of the Bones from a CT Scan of the Abdomen and Pelvis

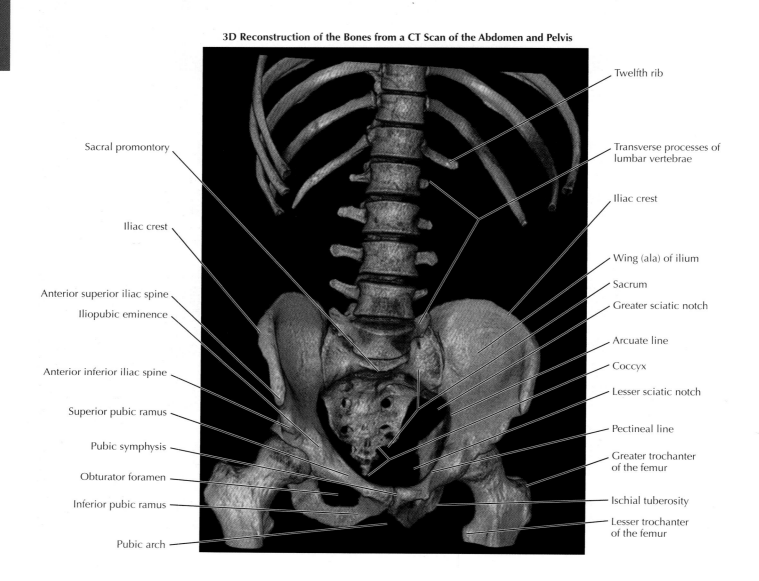

Sacral promontory

Iliac crest

Anterior superior iliac spine

Iliopubic eminence

Anterior inferior iliac spine

Superior pubic ramus

Pubic symphysis

Obturator foramen

Inferior pubic ramus

Pubic arch

Twelfth rib

Transverse processes of lumbar vertebrae

Iliac crest

Wing (ala) of ilium

Sacrum

Greater sciatic notch

Arcuate line

Coccyx

Lesser sciatic notch

Pectineal line

Greater trochanter of the femur

Ischial tuberosity

Lesser trochanter of the femur

4.1 BONY FRAMEWORK: CT THREE-DIMENSIONAL RECONSTRUCTION

This three-dimensional (3D) image is reconstructed with a computer from individual computed tomography (CT) axial images, much like a pile of flat rings form a cylinder. Radiologists may not use images like this routinely for diagnosis, but it is very helpful for surgeons to have a 3D plan of the anatomy to reconstruct fractured bones. Cartilage is not demonstrated on the image because it is not as radiopaque as bone. Without the mineral content of bone, cartilage has a density similar to that of water and soft tissues.

CTs Demonstrating Time Sequence from Organs Without Contrast to Clearance of Contrast By Kidneys

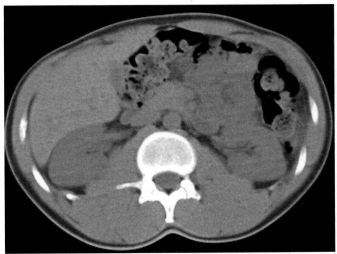

A. Noncontrast CT study. Note the subtle differences between the shades of grey in the solid viscera. Blood vessels in the liver are not well seen.

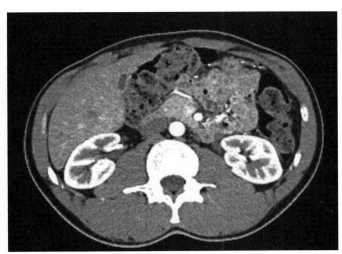

B. Arterial phase image. After 30 seconds of the injection, the contrast is predominantly in the arteries, which are seen as white rounded and linear structures.

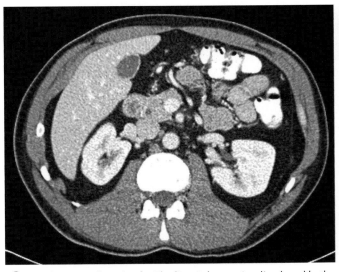

C. Portal-venous phase image. The liver is better visualized, and both the portal veins and the hepatic veins are opacified *(white)*. Contrast has also reached both the renal cortex and the medulla.

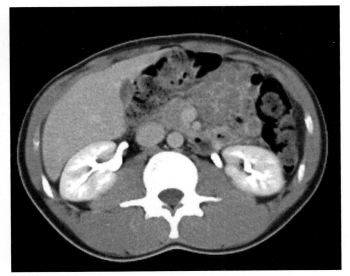

D. Contrast clearance by the kidneys and ureters at approximately 120 seconds. Contrast in the organs is "washing out" and is excreted by the kidneys. The renal calices, renal pelvis, and ureters become white with the concentrated contrast.

4.2 USE OF CONTRAST IN ABDOMINAL IMAGING STUDIES

Computed tomography can be performed with or without oral and/or intravenous (IV) contrast. Oral contrast helps the evaluation of the hollow viscera; agents include water, barium, and iodinated contrast. IV contrast is used to better evaluate the solid viscera, lesions, vasculature, and wall of the hollow viscera. Iodinated contrast is injected into a vein, usually an antecubital vein. It goes to the heart, to the lungs, and then to the aorta, which appears white from the contrast. In **B,** note that contrast has also reached arteries in the renal cortex, which is also white. As time goes by, the contrast is drained by veins in the organs, and everything becomes a little lighter shade of gray (**C**) compared to a noncontrast study. The contrast is filtered by the kidneys and opacifies the renal collecting systems, which become very bright *(white)* from the concentrated contrast (**D**).

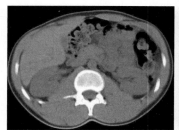 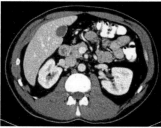 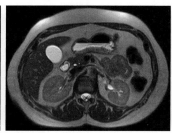 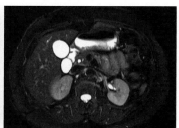

A. CT without contrast

B. CT with oral and intravenous contrast

C. T2 MRI sequence without saturation of the fat signal (fat is light)

D. T2 MRI sequence with fat saturation (fat is dark)

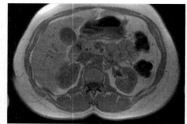 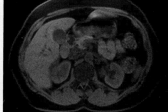 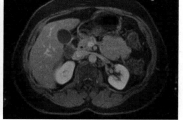

E. T1 MRI sequence without fat saturation

F. T1 MRI sequence with fat saturation

G. T1 MRI sequence with fat saturation and intravenous contrast

CT

Radiation
Fast (less than 5 minutes)
Good overall look at solid organs, fat planes
Best spatial resolution ("thinner" images, can "resolve" small things that are close to each other)
Excellent for calcification (i.e., small renal stones)
Good for overall look of pelvic organs, but with limited detail
Iodine-based intravenous (IV) contrast

MRI

No radiation
Not so fast (usually more than 20 minutes)
Good for characterization of lesions
Best tissue resolution (different tissues have different concentrations of hydrogen (water))
Not good for calcification (i.e., small renal stones)
Excellent for pelvic organs (uterus, ovaries, prostate, seminal vesicles)
Gadolinium-based IV contrast

4.3 CT VS. MRI IN ABDOMINAL STUDIES

These figures give an overview of the differences in appearance in a variety of CT and magnetic resonance imaging (MRI) sequences. A T2-weighted sequence is very fluid sensitive, and the fluid is seen as white. In T1-weighted sequences the fluid is dark. Settings for fat saturation (where fat is dark) help to identify edema (swelling from fluid accumulation) and hemorrhage and distinguish them from fat. Fat saturation also helps to identify lesions that are located within the fat and bone marrow, plus other pathology. Usually several sequences are needed to obtain a diagnosis.

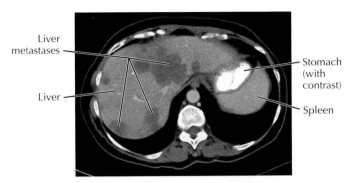

A. Upper abdominal CT with oral and intravenous (IV) contrast. The vascular contrast lightens the liver parenchyma to better visualize liver metastases.

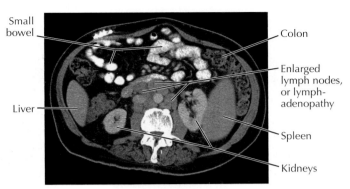

B. CT with oral and IV contrast showing enlarged retroperitoneal lymph nodes

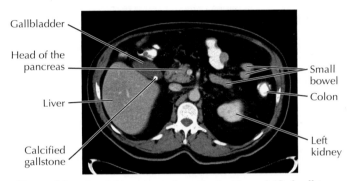

C. CT with oral and IV contrast of a patient with a calcified gallstone. The contrast has no effect on visualizing the stone.

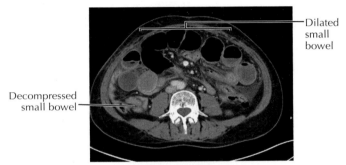

D. CT with IV contrast that demonstrates small bowel obstruction. Compare the dilated small bowel anteriorly with decompressed (normal) bowel.

Search Strategy for Image Interpretation:

Solid organs: liver, spleen, pancreas, adrenal glands, kidneys

Gallbladder/biliary system

Lymph node chains: hepatogastric ligament, periportal region, mesentery

Stomach, duodenum, rest of small bowel, colon

Fat planes, abdominal wall, bones

4.4 SEARCH STRATEGY: SYSTEMATIC INTERPRETATION OF IMAGING STUDIES

As with each body region, every radiologist has his or her own search pattern to interpret a study. The table in this figure contains a useful sequence to follow to look for pathology in a systematic way. Each organ is inspected in great detail before going to the next. Examples of pathology are given in the four figures.

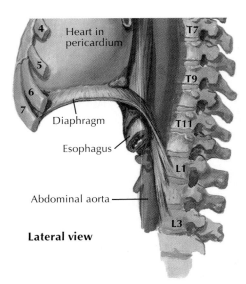

A. Lateral view of diaphragmatic openings at T8, T10, and T12 (the right hemidiaphragm is at a higher level)

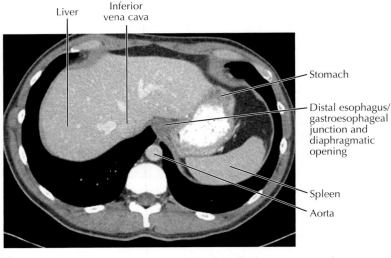

C. CT at a level above the aortic opening of the diaphragm. Note oral contrast *(white)* in the stomach.

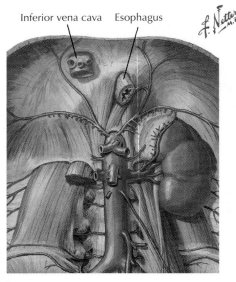

B. Anterior view. Openings from top to bottom are for: inferior vena cava, esophagus, and aorta.

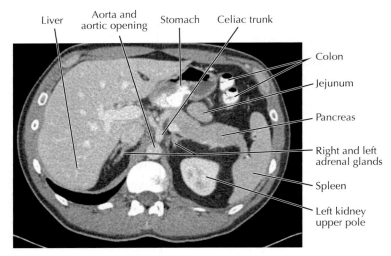

D. CT at the level of the aortic opening in the diaphragm. Some contrast has passed from the small to the large intestine; the small bowel is collapsed and appears as gray structures anterior to the tail of the pancreas.

4.5 DIAPHRAGM RELATIONSHIPS

These figures emphasize the relationships between abdominal organs and the position of the diaphragm. The abdominal cavity extends under the diaphragm to the T8 vertebral level, where the inferior vena cava passes through the central tendon of the right hemidiaphragm. The esophagus passes through its muscle at T10, and the aorta through the crura at T12, where the celiac trunk branches originate. In (**C**), the liver, stomach and spleen are prominent in the image; but the origin of their arteries off the celiac trunk is at a lower level (**D**). The T8, T10, and T12 openings for the three large structures are averages. There is considerable individual variation plus variation caused by posture and position of the diaphragm in the breathing cycle.

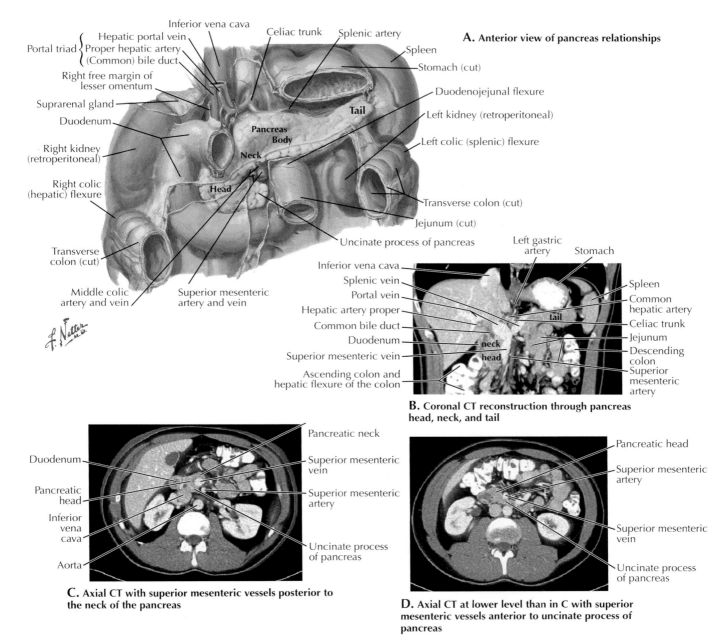

A. **Anterior view of pancreas relationships**

B. **Coronal CT reconstruction through pancreas head, neck, and tail**

C. **Axial CT with superior mesenteric vessels posterior to the neck of the pancreas**

D. **Axial CT at lower level than in C with superior mesenteric vessels anterior to uncinate process of pancreas**

Note: The Netter illustration is a dissection with 3D perspective; and with human variation, not all structures are captured in a CT plane.

4.6 PANCREAS RELATIONSHIPS

The pancreas has anatomical relationships that are clinically important and useful in the identification of structures in the abdominal foregut. The head of the pancreas lies in the curve of the duodenum, and its tail courses upward to the spleen. The celiac trunk originates just above the pancreas, and the splenic artery and vein follow the body and tail of the pancreas to the spleen, giving off numerous pancreatic branches along the way. The superior mesenteric artery originates immediately below the celiac trunk posterior to the neck of the pancreas. It appears medial to the head of the pancreas and passes anterior to the uncinate ("hooklike") process, the most inferior extent of the pancreas. The portal vein is formed behind the pancreas by the union of the splenic and superior mesenteric veins. The common bile duct joins the pancreatic duct in the head of the pancreas to form the ampulla in the second part of the duodenum.

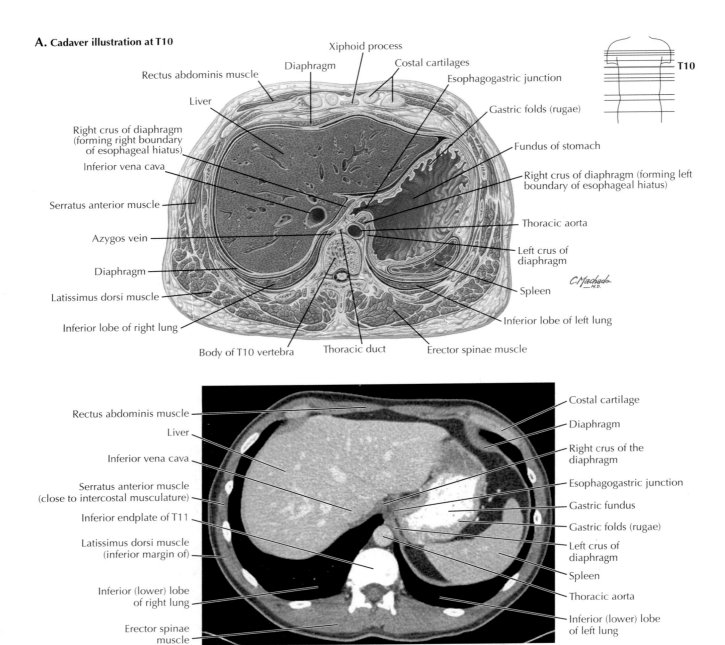

A. Cadaver illustration at T10

Rectus abdominis muscle

Diaphragm

Xiphoid process

Costal cartilages

Esophagogastric junction

Liver

Gastric folds (rugae)

Right crus of diaphragm (forming right boundary of esophageal hiatus)

Fundus of stomach

Inferior vena cava

Right crus of diaphragm (forming left boundary of esophageal hiatus)

Serratus anterior muscle

Thoracic aorta

Azygos vein

Left crus of diaphragm

Diaphragm

Spleen

Latissimus dorsi muscle

Inferior lobe of right lung

Inferior lobe of left lung

Body of T10 vertebra

Thoracic duct

Erector spinae muscle

C. Machado M.D.

T10

Rectus abdominis muscle

Costal cartilage

Liver

Diaphragm

Inferior vena cava

Right crus of the diaphragm

Serratus anterior muscle (close to intercostal musculature)

Esophagogastric junction

Inferior endplate of T11

Gastric fundus

Latissimus dorsi muscle (inferior margin of)

Gastric folds (rugae)

Left crus of diaphragm

Inferior (lower) lobe of right lung

Spleen

Thoracic aorta

Erector spinae muscle

Inferior (lower) lobe of left lung

B. Similar living anatomy from inferior T11 (axial CT with oral and IV contrast)

4.7 CROSS SECTION AT T10 WITH CT

The CT image is at the level of the inferior endplate of T11, but it corresponds closely to the T10 Netter illustration (**A**). The differences in level are likely caused by a breath hold by the patient for the CT study; during a deep breath the diaphragm lowers toward the abdomen. In both figures the esophagus pierces the diaphragm to join the stomach. The liver, the spleen, and the fundus of the stomach dominate the section. The aorta is behind the crura above the level of the celiac trunk. From T8 to T12, the pleural cavities overlap the abdominal cavity at its periphery, and the lungs can be seen around the diaphragm. In the CT the gastric contents are partly white as a result of the oral contrast. The hepatic and portal veins are whiter than the parenchyma of the liver. The hepatic arteries course along the portal veins together with the bile ducts. The arteries are small and are better seen when a purely arterial phase image is obtained. The bile ducts usually are not seen unless dilated.

A. Schematic cross section of abdomen at T12

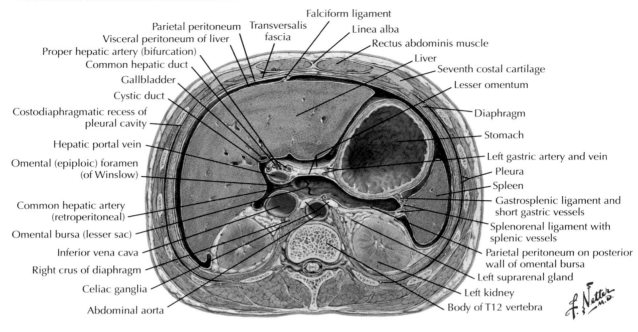

Falciform ligament
Parietal peritoneum
Visceral peritoneum of liver
Transversalis fascia
Linea alba
Proper hepatic artery (bifurcation)
Rectus abdominis muscle
Common hepatic duct
Liver
Gallbladder
Seventh costal cartilage
Cystic duct
Lesser omentum
Costodiaphragmatic recess of pleural cavity
Diaphragm
Hepatic portal vein
Stomach
Omental (epiploic) foramen (of Winslow)
Left gastric artery and vein
Pleura
Common hepatic artery (retroperitoneal)
Spleen
Omental bursa (lesser sac)
Gastrosplenic ligament and short gastric vessels
Inferior vena cava
Splenorenal ligament with splenic vessels
Right crus of diaphragm
Parietal peritoneum on posterior wall of omental bursa
Celiac ganglia
Left suprarenal gland
Abdominal aorta
Left kidney
Body of T12 vertebra

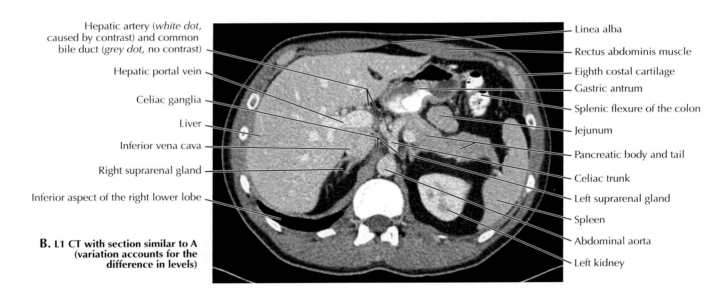

Hepatic artery (*white dot, caused by contrast*) and common bile duct (*grey dot, no contrast*)
Linea alba
Hepatic portal vein
Rectus abdominis muscle
Celiac ganglia
Eighth costal cartilage
Liver
Gastric antrum
Inferior vena cava
Splenic flexure of the colon
Right suprarenal gland
Jejunum
Inferior aspect of the right lower lobe
Pancreatic body and tail
Celiac trunk
Left suprarenal gland
Spleen
Abdominal aorta
Left kidney

B. L1 CT with section similar to A (variation accounts for the difference in levels)

4.8 CROSS SECTION AT T12 WITH CT

A section at T12-L1 is through the middle of the stomach, lesser omentum with the portal triad in its free edge, and lesser peritoneal sac (omental bursa) behind the stomach and lesser omentum. It is close to the origin of the celiac trunk where the aorta pierces the diaphragm. The most inferior parts of the pleural cavities are visible next to the diaphragm. The several "potential" spaces demonstrated in **A** are not visualized on a CT or MRI study. These can become apparent in the case of fluid accumulation (ascites). The fascial planes and peritoneal lining can sometimes be seen as a very thin line but are also not usually visible unless thickened by infection/inflammation or cancer (peritoneal carcinomatosis).

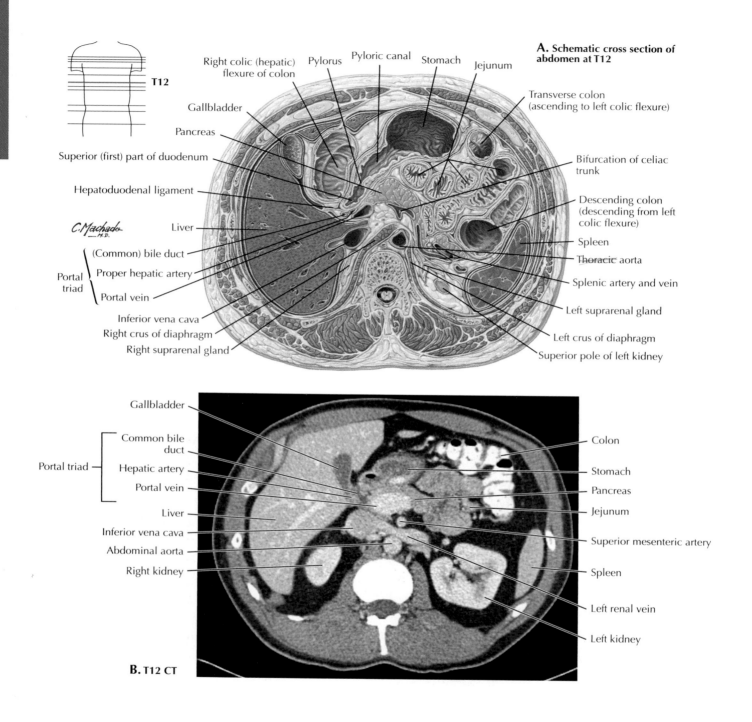

A. Schematic cross section of abdomen at T12

T12

Right colic (hepatic) flexure of colon
Pylorus
Pyloric canal
Stomach
Jejunum

Gallbladder

Pancreas

Superior (first) part of duodenum

Hepatoduodenal ligament

C.Machado ─M.D.

Liver

(Common) bile duct

Portal triad
Proper hepatic artery

Portal vein

Inferior vena cava

Right crus of diaphragm

Right suprarenal gland

Transverse colon (ascending to left colic flexure)

Bifurcation of celiac trunk

Descending colon (descending from left colic flexure)

Spleen

Thoracic aorta

Splenic artery and vein

Left suprarenal gland

Left crus of diaphragm

Superior pole of left kidney

Gallbladder

Portal triad
Common bile duct
Hepatic artery
Portal vein

Liver

Inferior vena cava

Abdominal aorta

Right kidney

Colon

Stomach

Pancreas

Jejunum

Superior mesenteric artery

Spleen

Left renal vein

Left kidney

B. T12 CT

4.9 CROSS SECTION VARIATION AT T12 WITH CT

This level is at the junction of the pyloric part of the stomach with the duodenum. The pancreas and celiac trunk with splenic vessels are in the plane (**A**), and the portal triad is close to the formation of the portal vein behind the pancreas (**B**). There are many ways to distinguish the large intestine (colon) and small intestine. The liquid contents of the small intestine appear homogeneous in a CT, whereas the more solid contents of the large intestine have a more bubbly appearance. Haustra of the colon are lobulations along the outer contour, whereas the mucosal folds of the small intestine have minimal effect on the relatively smooth contour of the outer wall. The colon usually "frames" the small bowel. It is posterior on the right and left for the ascending and descending colon and anterior and superior for the transverse colon. Sections of the colon, predominantly the sigmoid and transverse colon, can be very long in some people.

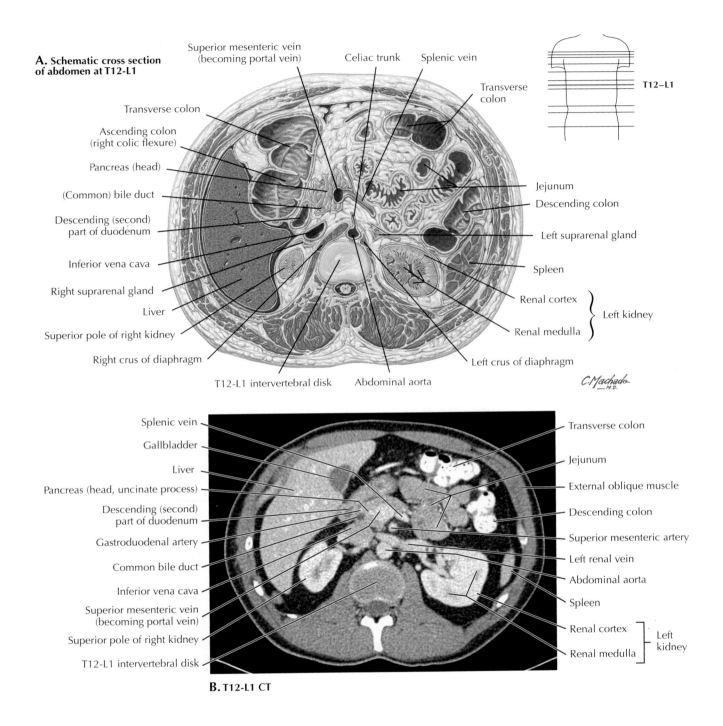

A. Schematic cross section of abdomen at T12-L1

Superior mesenteric vein (becoming portal vein)

Celiac trunk

Splenic vein

Transverse colon

Transverse colon

Ascending colon (right colic flexure)

Pancreas (head)

(Common) bile duct

Descending (second) part of duodenum

Inferior vena cava

Right suprarenal gland

Liver

Superior pole of right kidney

Right crus of diaphragm

T12-L1 intervertebral disk

Abdominal aorta

Left crus of diaphragm

Renal medulla

Renal cortex

Left kidney

Spleen

Left suprarenal gland

Descending colon

Jejunum

T12–L1

C. Machado M.D.

B. T12-L1 CT

Splenic vein

Gallbladder

Liver

Pancreas (head, uncinate process)

Descending (second) part of duodenum

Gastroduodenal artery

Common bile duct

Inferior vena cava

Superior mesenteric vein (becoming portal vein)

Superior pole of right kidney

T12-L1 intervertebral disk

Transverse colon

Jejunum

External oblique muscle

Descending colon

Superior mesenteric artery

Left renal vein

Abdominal aorta

Spleen

Renal cortex

Renal medulla

Left kidney

4.10 CROSS SECTION AT T12-L1 WITH CT

T12 is the aortic opening of the diaphragm and the origin of the celiac trunk. The head of the pancreas is visible, but not the tail. The splenic vein and superior mesenteric vein join to form the portal vein. The left kidney, extending up to the eleventh rib, is higher than the right and therefore appears larger in section. The suprarenal glands have a characteristic wedge shape in section and are separated from the kidneys by fat that is not apparent on dissection in the anatomy laboratory. The duodenum is next to the pancreas, and the colon is at the periphery surrounding the small intestine. In the CT the renal cortex is whiter than the medulla. In about 10 more seconds the contrast would also be present in the medulla, and the kidney would be homogeneous in density.

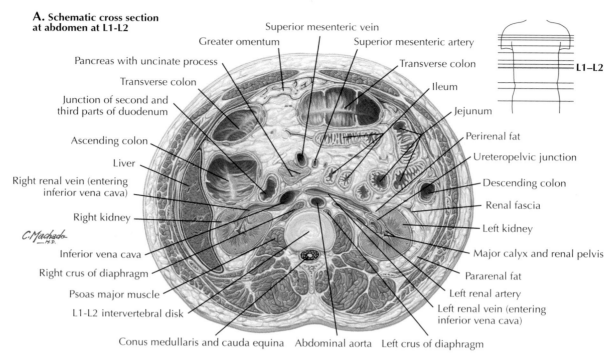

A. Schematic cross section at abdomen at L1-L2

Superior mesenteric vein
Greater omentum
Superior mesenteric artery
Pancreas with uncinate process
Transverse colon
Transverse colon
Ileum
Junction of second and third parts of duodenum
Jejunum
Ascending colon
Perirenal fat
Liver
Ureteropelvic junction
Right renal vein (entering inferior vena cava)
Descending colon
Renal fascia
Right kidney
Left kidney
Inferior vena cava
Major calyx and renal pelvis
Right crus of diaphragm
Pararenal fat
Psoas major muscle
Left renal artery
L1-L2 intervertebral disk
Left renal vein (entering inferior vena cava)
Conus medullaris and cauda equina   Abdominal aorta   Left crus of diaphragm

C. Machado M.D.

L1–L2

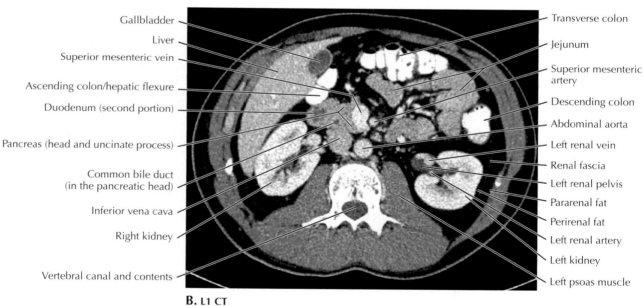

Gallbladder
Transverse colon
Liver
Jejunum
Superior mesenteric vein
Superior mesenteric artery
Ascending colon/hepatic flexure
Descending colon
Duodenum (second portion)
Abdominal aorta
Pancreas (head and uncinate process)
Left renal vein
Common bile duct (in the pancreatic head)
Renal fascia
Left renal pelvis
Inferior vena cava
Pararenal fat
Right kidney
Perirenal fat
Left renal artery
Left kidney
Vertebral canal and contents
Left psoas muscle

B. L1 CT

4.11 CROSS SECTION AT L1-L2 WITH CT

L2 is the most inferior extent of the liver and the uncinate process of the pancreas. The superior mesenteric vessels are anterior to it after passing behind the neck of the pancreas. Next to the pancreas is the duodenum. The renal vessels are visible. The most anterior bowel is the transverse colon, although it can be at a much lower level. At any abdominal section below the stomach, the most anterior structure is the greater omentum that originates from the greater curvature of the stomach and drapes over the intestines. In the CT it is seen as the dark fat anteriorly. Normal fascial planes in fat cannot usually be distinguished, although a thin line of the left renal fascia is visible. The spinal cord and nerve roots cannot be identified discretely on a routine CT unless contrast is introduced into the cerebrospinal fluid. Otherwise the best way to evaluate them is with MRI.

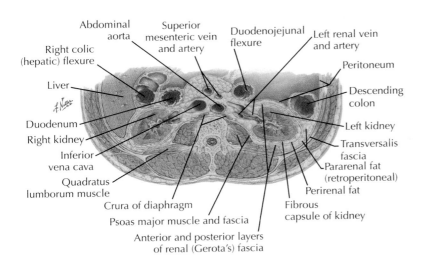

A. Cross section at the level of the kidneys. Transverse section through second lumbar vertebra demonstrates horizontal disposition of fascia.

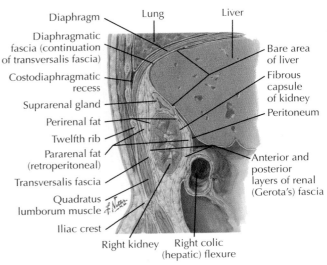

B. Sagittal section through the right kidney. Sagittal section through right kidney and lumbar region demonstrates vertical disposition of renal fascia.

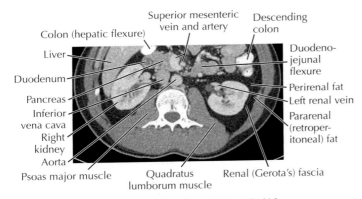

C. Axial CT reconstruction through the right kidney

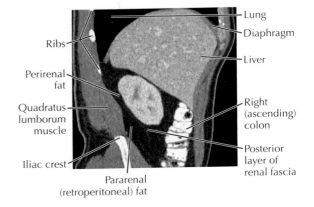

D. Sagittal CT through the kidneys

4.12 KIDNEY RELATIONSHIPS

The kidneys are embedded in a thick, fatty capsule containing a layer of renal fascia. They are retroperitoneal, with the top of the right kidney deep to the twelfth rib and the left kidney a bit higher under the eleventh and twelfth ribs. The quadratus lumborum muscles are posterior to the kidneys, and the psoas major muscles are medial. Sometimes the kidneys may have a lower position ("ptotic" or pelvic kidneys). If a kidney is not visible at its usual level, look lower down in the pelvis. In addition, a kidney may be agenic (did not develop) or atrophic (small), or the patient may have undergone nephrectomy (removal of a kidney). With the latter, bright surgical clips are usually seen in the retroperitoneum. CT without contrast is currently the best way to look for renal stones.

**A. Schematic cross section
of abdomen at L3-L4**

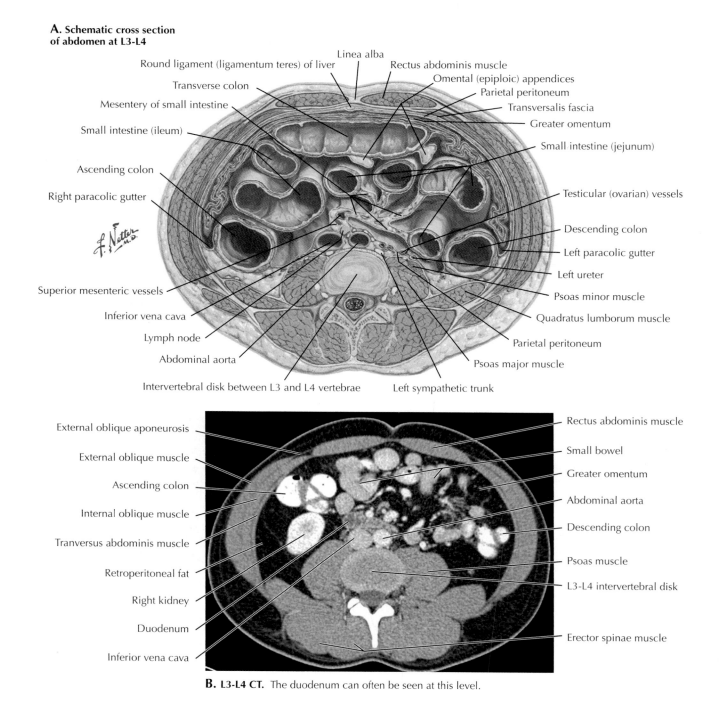

Round ligament (ligamentum teres) of liver

Transverse colon

Mesentery of small intestine

Small intestine (ileum)

Ascending colon

Right paracolic gutter

Superior mesenteric vessels

Inferior vena cava

Lymph node

Abdominal aorta

Intervertebral disk between L3 and L4 vertebrae

Linea alba

Rectus abdominis muscle

Omental (epiploic) appendices

Parietal peritoneum

Transversalis fascia

Greater omentum

Small intestine (jejunum)

Testicular (ovarian) vessels

Descending colon

Left paracolic gutter

Left ureter

Psoas minor muscle

Quadratus lumborum muscle

Parietal peritoneum

Psoas major muscle

Left sympathetic trunk

External oblique aponeurosis

External oblique muscle

Ascending colon

Internal oblique muscle

Tranversus abdominis muscle

Retroperitoneal fat

Right kidney

Duodenum

Inferior vena cava

Rectus abdominis muscle

Small bowel

Greater omentum

Abdominal aorta

Descending colon

Psoas muscle

L3-L4 intervertebral disk

Erector spinae muscle

B. L3-L4 CT. The duodenum can often be seen at this level.

4.13 L3-L4 CROSS SECTION WITH CT

Lower lumbar sections are below the level of the kidneys and large abdominal foregut organs. The small and large intestines fill the field and are covered anteriorly and laterally by the greater omentum. L3-L4 is below the termination of the spinal cord, and the cauda equina nerve roots are in the vertebral canal. This level is also just above the umbilicus, and the round ligament of the liver (the remnant of the umbilical vein) is in the plane of section. Below the umbilicus this would be the urachus (the remnant of the allantois) extending to the bladder. The round ligament and urachus are not well seen on a routine CT unless their embryonic primordia (the umbilical vein and allantois, respectively) persist as a cyst or sinus. Paraumbilical veins next to the round ligament may be visible if they are distended from portal hypertension.

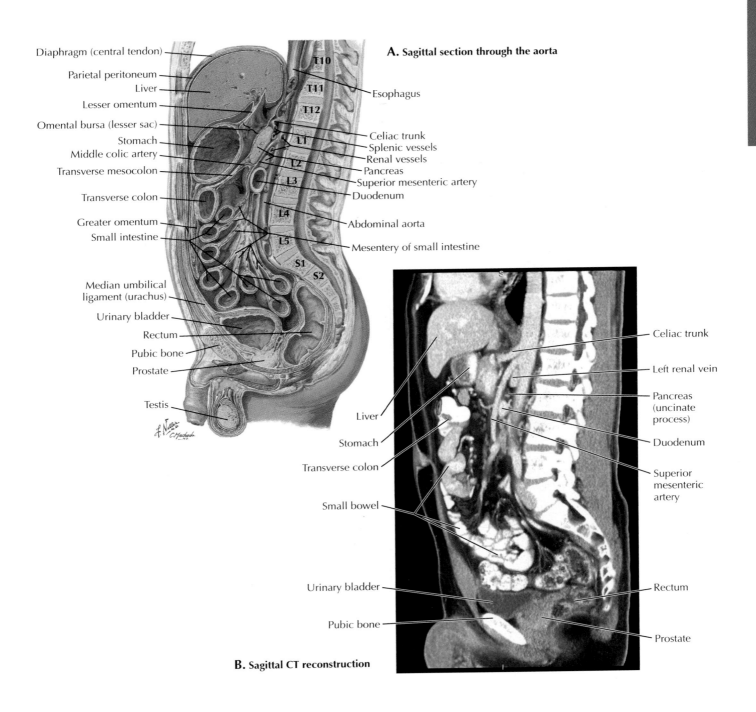

Diaphragm (central tendon)
Parietal peritoneum
Liver
Lesser omentum
Omental bursa (lesser sac)
Stomach
Middle colic artery
Transverse mesocolon
Transverse colon
Greater omentum
Small intestine
Median umbilical ligament (urachus)
Urinary bladder
Rectum
Pubic bone
Prostate
Testis

T10
T11
T12
L1
L2
L3
L4
L5
S1
S2

A. Sagittal section through the aorta

Esophagus
Celiac trunk
Splenic vessels
Renal vessels
Pancreas
Superior mesenteric artery
Duodenum
Abdominal aorta
Mesentery of small intestine

Liver
Stomach
Transverse colon
Small bowel
Urinary bladder
Pubic bone

Celiac trunk
Left renal vein
Pancreas (uncinate process)
Duodenum
Superior mesenteric artery
Rectum
Prostate

B. Sagittal CT reconstruction

4.14 SAGITTAL SECTION THROUGH AORTA WITH CT SAGITTAL RECONSTRUCTION

The aorta is just to the left of the midline in a paramedian (sagittal) section. The body of the pubic bone is sectioned rather than the pubic symphysis. T12 is the level of the aortic opening in the diaphragm and the origin of the celiac trunk above the pancreas. At L4-L5 the aorta and inferior vena cava bifurcate into the common iliac vessels. Other important anatomical relationships are the location of the stomach above the transverse colon and the pancreas above the inferior part of the duodenum in a retroperitoneal location. The superior mesenteric artery arises posterior to the pancreas. Sagittal reconstructions are helpful in looking for arterial stenosis (narrowing) that may be missed in an axial plane perpendicular to the more vertically oriented arteries.

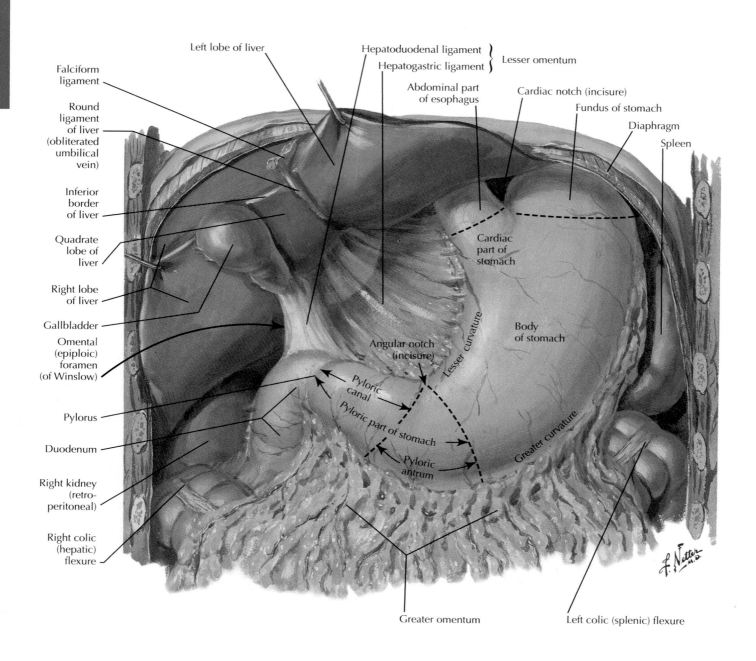

Falciform ligament

Round ligament of liver (obliterated umbilical vein)

Inferior border of liver

Quadrate lobe of liver

Right lobe of liver

Gallbladder

Omental (epiploic) foramen (of Winslow)

Pylorus

Duodenum

Right kidney (retro-peritoneal)

Right colic (hepatic) flexure

Left lobe of liver

Hepatoduodenal ligament
Hepatogastric ligament } Lesser omentum

Abdominal part of esophagus

Cardiac notch (incisure)

Fundus of stomach

Diaphragm

Spleen

Cardiac part of stomach

Angular notch (incisure)

Lesser curvature

Body of stomach

Pyloric canal

Pyloric part of stomach

Pyloric antrum

Greater curvature

Greater omentum

Left colic (splenic) flexure

4.15 STOMACH IN SITU

From the esophageal opening in the diaphragm the stomach extends anteriorly, inferiorly, and to the right, where it joins the duodenum at the pyloric sphincter. The lesser curvature of the stomach (ventral in the embryo) faces the liver; the greater curvature (dorsal in the embryo) faces the spleen to the left and gives off its dorsal mesentery, the greater omentum, inferiorly. The top curving part of the stomach is the fundus, the body is in the middle, and the pylorus tapers to the duodenum. Longitudinal folds of the mucosa and submucosa of the stomach are called *rugae*.

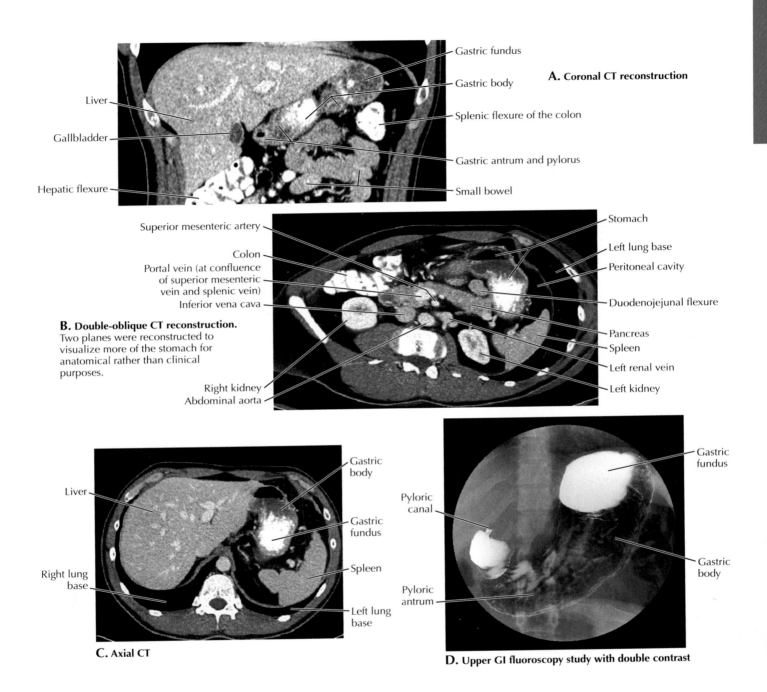

Liver

Gallbladder

Hepatic flexure

Gastric fundus

Gastric body

Splenic flexure of the colon

Gastric antrum and pylorus

Small bowel

A. Coronal CT reconstruction

Superior mesenteric artery

Colon

Portal vein (at confluence of superior mesenteric vein and splenic vein)

Inferior vena cava

B. Double-oblique CT reconstruction.
Two planes were reconstructed to visualize more of the stomach for anatomical rather than clinical purposes.

Right kidney
Abdominal aorta

Stomach

Left lung base

Peritoneal cavity

Duodenojejunal flexure

Pancreas
Spleen

Left renal vein

Left kidney

Liver

Right lung base

Gastric body

Gastric fundus

Spleen

Left lung base

C. Axial CT

Pyloric canal

Pyloric antrum

Gastric fundus

Gastric body

D. Upper GI fluoroscopy study with double contrast

4.16 UPPER GASTROINTESTINAL CT STUDIES

Because of the oblique orientation of the stomach, it expands over several axial CT cuts (one example in **C**). On the coronal plane (**A**), some of the organ relationships become easier to see. **B** is a double-oblique reconstructed image. The two combined planes make it look distorted. It is shown only to better profile the anatomical relationships. When interpreting a CT study, radiologists usually look at axial, coronal, and sagittal images. Reconstructions in the oblique plane are not usually done. **D** is a double-contrast upper gastrointestinal (GI) study that is a very good way to see the stomach in situ. It uses real-time x-ray to evaluate peristalsis as well. The patient drinks effervescent crystals that provide the air distention and oral barium that gives a white lining to the gastric mucosa.

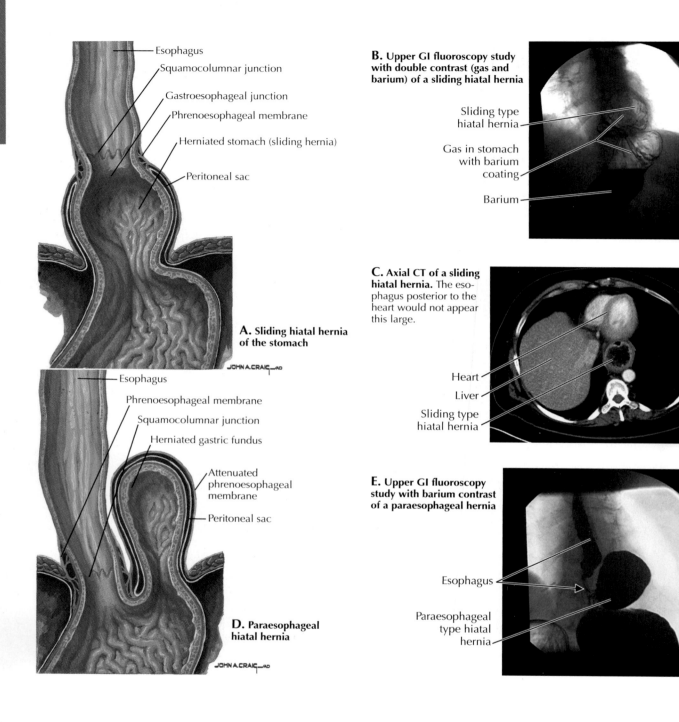

Esophagus
Squamocolumnar junction
Gastroesophageal junction
Phrenoesophageal membrane
Herniated stomach (sliding hernia)
Peritoneal sac

A. Sliding hiatal hernia of the stomach

JOHN A.CRAIG—AD

Esophagus
Phrenoesophageal membrane
Squamocolumnar junction
Herniated gastric fundus
Attenuated phrenoesophageal membrane
Peritoneal sac

D. Paraesophageal hiatal hernia

JOHN A.CRAIG—AD

B. Upper GI fluoroscopy study with double contrast (gas and barium) of a sliding hiatal hernia

Sliding type hiatal hernia
Gas in stomach with barium coating
Barium

C. Axial CT of a sliding hiatal hernia. The esophagus posterior to the heart would not appear this large.

Heart
Liver
Sliding type hiatal hernia

E. Upper GI fluoroscopy study with barium contrast of a paraesophageal hernia

Esophagus
Paraesophageal type hiatal hernia

4.17 HIATAL HERNIA

A double-contrast esophagram and an upper GI barium study can demonstrate hiatal hernias. In a hiatal hernia the stomach passes into the thoracic cavity through the esophageal hiatus in the diaphragm. Either the cardiac portion of the stomach extends through the diaphragm (a "sliding" hernia), or the fundus of the stomach passes upward alongside of the esophagus (a paraesophageal hernia). In both cases the herniated stomach is covered with a layer of parietal peritoneum. Larger hernias can also be seen on CT. In **B** and **E**, note the reversed images where bone and contrast are black. This is how they are displayed on the fluoroscopy monitor. They are reversed to white for interpretation.

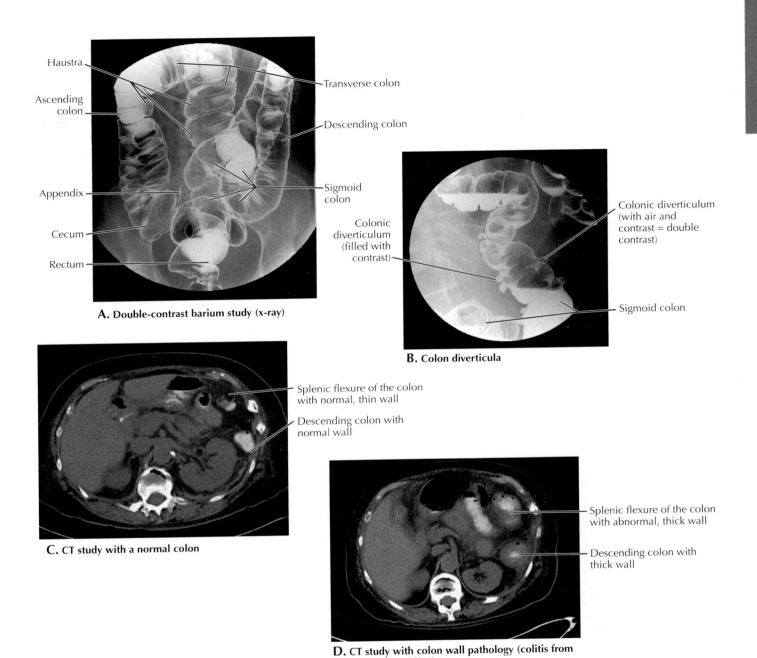

A. Double-contrast barium study (x-ray)

Haustra
Ascending colon
Appendix
Cecum
Rectum
Transverse colon
Descending colon
Sigmoid colon

B. Colon diverticula

Colonic diverticulum (filled with contrast)
Colonic diverticulum (with air and contrast = double contrast)
Sigmoid colon

C. CT study with a normal colon

Splenic flexure of the colon with normal, thin wall
Descending colon with normal wall

D. CT study with colon wall pathology (colitis from infection by *C. difficile*)

Splenic flexure of the colon with abnormal, thick wall
Descending colon with thick wall

4.18 LARGE INTESTINE IMAGING STUDIES

A shows a traditional lower GI study using both barium and air (double contrast) to add black and white definition to the contours of the colon. Barium is inserted via a rectal catheter, and the patient is rolled and moved so all the surfaces of the colon are coated. The excess barium is drained, air is introduced, and x-rays are then obtained. Lower GI studies are done less frequently as colonoscopies have become more widely available. Evaluation of the colonic wall is best done with CT (**C** and **D**), although polyps and cancer are better detected via colonoscopy or CT colonography (where available). Diverticulitis is also best evaluated with CT, which can demonstrate complications such as abscess and free air in the peritoneal cavity.

A. Gallbladder and extrahepatic bile ducts

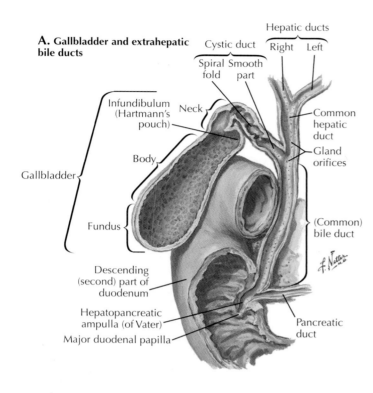

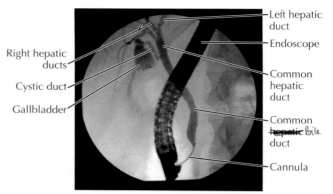

B. ERCP study of a normal biliary tree. Although there is no pathology, there is a double right hepatic duct. The pancreatic duct is not seen.

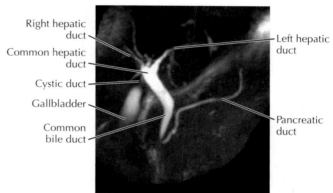

C. Anterior view of a biliary 3D reconstruction with T2 MRI that includes contrast in the pancreatic duct.

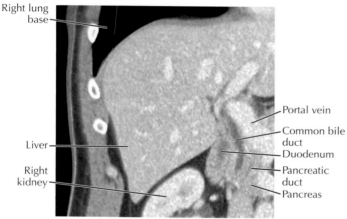

D. Coronal oblique CT. The bile and pancreatic ducts are darker than surrounding tissue.

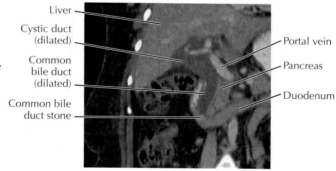

E. Choledocal ("bile duct") stone. Use of a positive *(white)* oral contrast makes it more difficult to see a stone near the ampulla. The best way is to distend the duodenum with water or any negative oral contrast.

4.19 GALLBLADDER, BILE DUCTS, AND PANCREATIC DUCT

The bile duct and pancreatic duct systems can be studied via endoscopic retrograde cholangiopancreatography (ERCP, **B**). Guided by an endoscope (black tube in the figure), the gastroenterologist passes a cannula through the upper GI tract to the greater duodenal papilla, where the common bile duct joins the pancreatic duct to form the ampulla (of Vater). Contrast is injected into the duct system and visualized with fluoroscopy (x-rays). Another good way of looking at the biliary tree is with magnetic resonance cholangiopancreatography (MRCP). No contrast is necessary. A T2 MRI sequence (where fluid is bright white) is used for 3D reconstructions of the duct system (**C**). Fluid in the small bowel is also seen as white. With CT the common bile duct is best seen in the coronal plane (**D**); it is also visualized over several axial images. Ultrasound is best for detecting gallstones since not all gallstones are radiopaque (therefore not seen with x-ray/ CT).

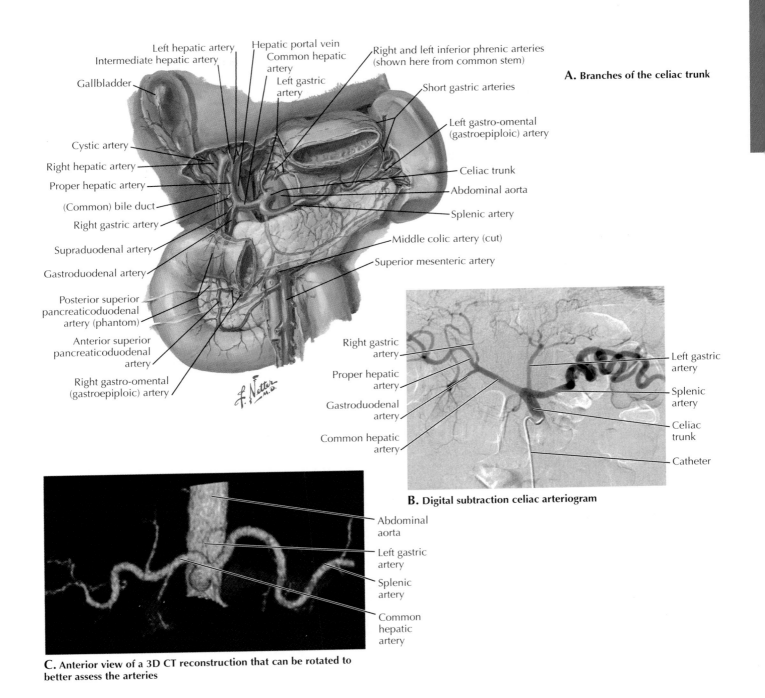

Left hepatic artery
Intermediate hepatic artery
Gallbladder
Cystic artery
Right hepatic artery
Proper hepatic artery
(Common) bile duct
Right gastric artery
Supraduodenal artery
Gastroduodenal artery
Posterior superior pancreaticoduodenal artery (phantom)
Anterior superior pancreaticoduodenal artery
Right gastro-omental (gastroepiploic) artery

Hepatic portal vein
Common hepatic artery
Left gastric artery

Right and left inferior phrenic arteries (shown here from common stem)
Short gastric arteries
Left gastro-omental (gastroepiploic) artery
Celiac trunk
Abdominal aorta
Splenic artery
Middle colic artery (cut)
Superior mesenteric artery

F. Netter, M.D.

A. Branches of the celiac trunk

Right gastric artery
Proper hepatic artery
Gastroduodenal artery
Common hepatic artery

Left gastric artery
Splenic artery
Celiac trunk
Catheter

B. Digital subtraction celiac arteriogram

Abdominal aorta
Left gastric artery
Splenic artery
Common hepatic artery

C. Anterior view of a 3D CT reconstruction that can be rotated to better assess the arteries

4.20 ABDOMINAL FOREGUT ARTERIES

The three branches of the celiac trunk, the common hepatic, splenic, and left gastric arteries, supply the organs of the abdominal foregut. The left gastric artery is in the lesser curvature of the stomach. The splenic artery is large and tortuous (curvy). It supplies the spleen and is the origin of short gastric arteries, the left gastroepiploic artery, and numerous branches to the pancreas. The common hepatic divides into the hepatic proper (the origin of the right gastric artery) and

the gastroduodenal artery, supplying the first half of the duodenum and head of the pancreas and giving origin to the right gastroepiploic artery. To create a traditional celiac angiogram (**B**), a catheter is inserted into the femoral artery and up the aorta just above the origin of the celiac trunk. Contrast is injected at a high rate into the aorta or its branches (**B**), and x-rays are rapidly taken (many frames per minute). The 3D rendering (**C**) is a computer reconstruction from CT, and different colors can be assigned to the arteries.

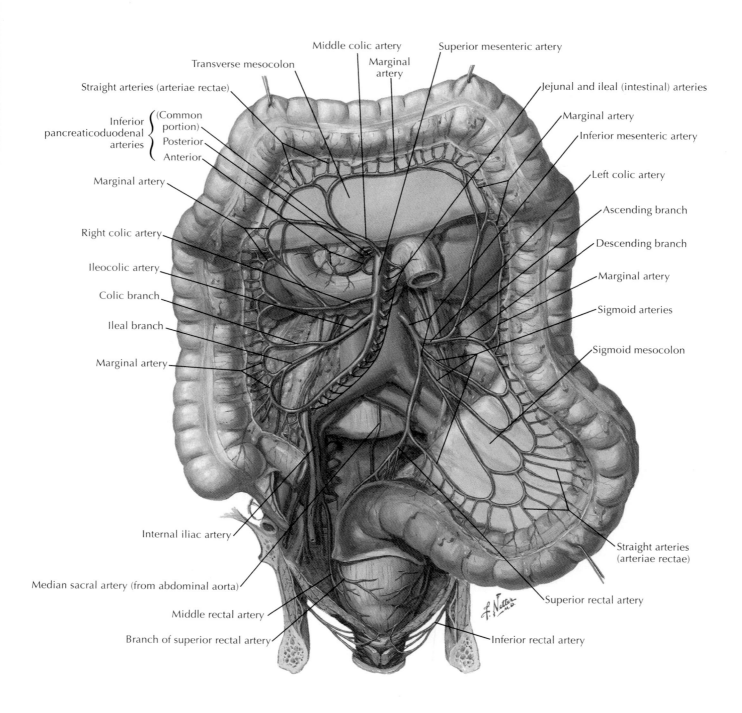

Middle colic artery

Transverse mesocolon

Marginal artery

Superior mesenteric artery

Straight arteries (arteriae rectae)

Jejunal and ileal (intestinal) arteries

Inferior pancreaticoduodenal arteries { (Common portion) Posterior Anterior

Marginal artery

Inferior mesenteric artery

Marginal artery

Left colic artery

Right colic artery

Ascending branch

Ileocolic artery

Descending branch

Colic branch

Marginal artery

Ileal branch

Sigmoid arteries

Marginal artery

Sigmoid mesocolon

Internal iliac artery

Straight arteries (arteriae rectae)

Median sacral artery (from abdominal aorta)

Superior rectal artery

Middle rectal artery

Branch of superior rectal artery

Inferior rectal artery

4.21 MIDGUT AND HINDGUT ARTERIES

The superior mesenteric artery arises behind the pancreas and supplies the midgut, which consists of the second half of the duodenum, as well as the jejunum, ileum, ascending colon, and two thirds of the transverse colon. Its branches are the right and middle colic arteries, the ileocolic artery, and numerous intestinal branches to the small bowel. The inferior mesenteric artery, with its left colic branch, supplies the hindgut, which consists of the last third of the transverse colon, the descending colon, the sigmoid colon, and the upper part of the rectum. It ends by becoming the superior rectal artery. Arcades are anastomosing loops of intestinal branches. Close to the colon they form a continuous marginal artery that gives rise to the vasa recta ("straight vessels") that enter the mesenteric surface of the intestine.

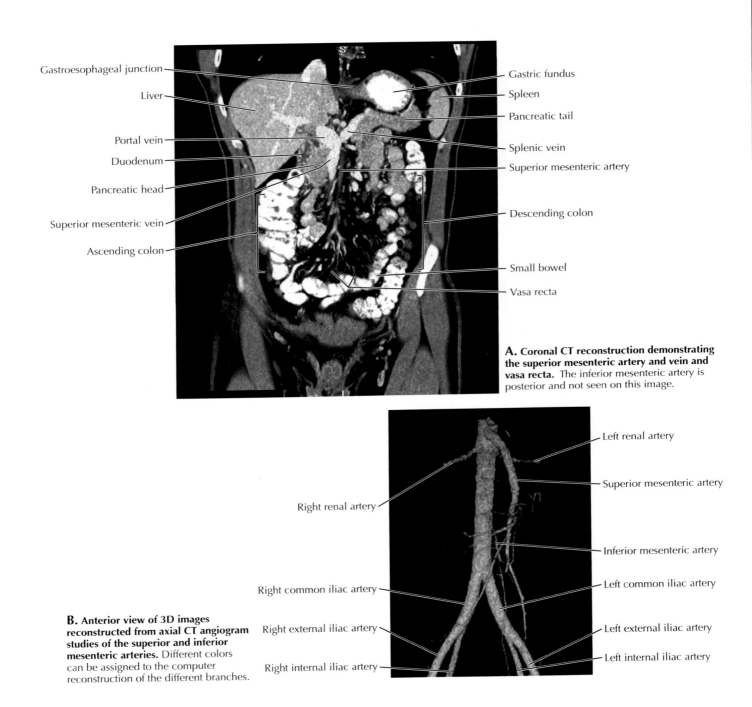

A. Coronal CT reconstruction demonstrating the superior mesenteric artery and vein and vasa recta. The inferior mesenteric artery is posterior and not seen on this image.

B. Anterior view of 3D images reconstructed from axial CT angiogram studies of the superior and inferior mesenteric arteries. Different colors can be assigned to the computer reconstruction of the different branches.

4.22 ANGIOGRAMS OF THE SUPERIOR AND INFERIOR MESENTERIC VESSELS

In a CT angiogram (CTA), IV contrast is used, and vessels are studied by scrolling through thin CT images (0.6 to 1.5 mm) in all three planes (**A** has one example in the coronal plane) during the arterial phase of contrast enhancement. The 3D reconstruction (**B**) includes the superior and inferior mesenteric arteries. The more distal branches are best seen with CTA. A CTA is a less invasive way to look at the vessels compared to a conventional angiogram because it uses IV rather than arterial contrast. The advantage of a traditional angiogram is that procedures such as balloon dilation and stent placement for stenosis can be performed. With CT the stenosis can be diagnosed, but intervention is not performed. However, it can be a very good road map before intervention. Be aware of the radiation exposure and amount of contrast the patient will receive in CT and conventional angiograms. The kidneys may also be damaged from filtering the contrast.

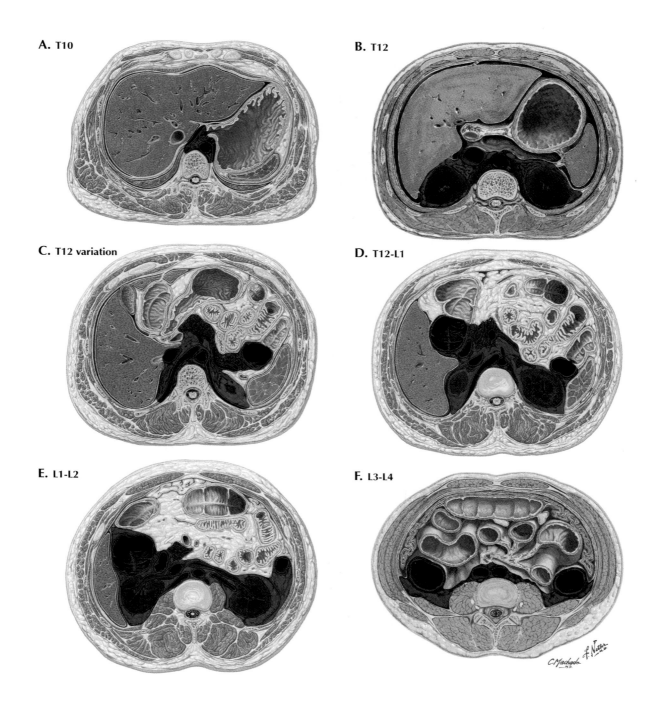

A. T10

B. T12

C. T12 variation

D. T12-L1

E. L1-L2

F. L3-L4

4.23 PERITONEAL/RETROPERITONEAL RELATIONSHIPS

The retroperitoneal compartment (retroperitoneum) of the abdomen is shaded in these figures. The stomach, liver and gallbladder, spleen, jejunum, ileum, and transverse and sigmoid colon are suspended by mesenteries of visceral peritoneum in the abdominal cavity (greater peritoneal sac of parietal peritoneum). The aorta, inferior vena cava, kidneys, and suprarenal glands are outside the abdominal cavity in a retroperitoneal location (in the body wall superficial to parietal peritoneum). The pancreas, duodenum, and ascending and descending colon were suspended by mesenteries in the embryo but become secondarily retroperitoneal as they are pressed against and fuse to parietal peritoneum as a result of the rotation and tremendous growth of the midgut loop of intestines.

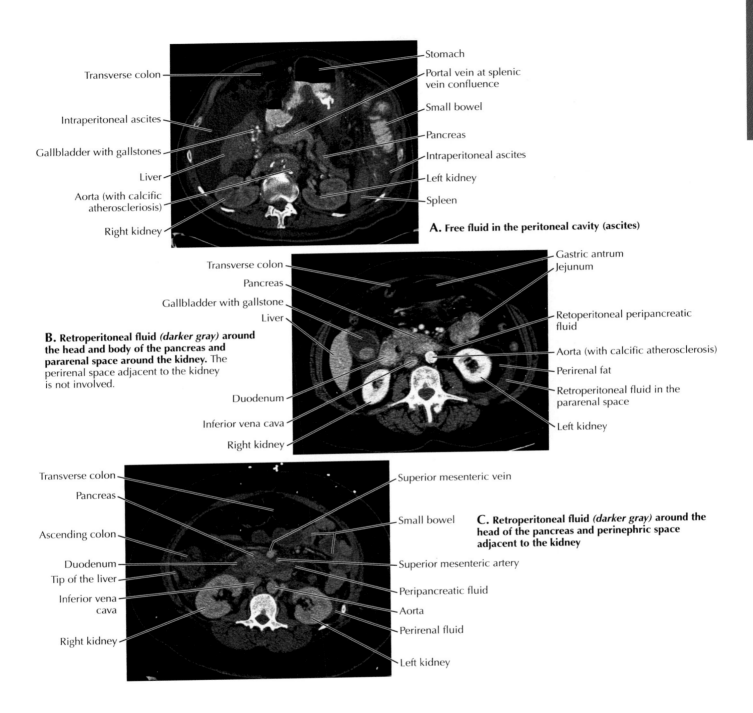

Transverse colon

Intraperitoneal ascites

Gallbladder with gallstones

Liver

Aorta (with calcific atheroscleriosis)

Right kidney

Stomach

Portal vein at splenic vein confluence

Small bowel

Pancreas

Intraperitoneal ascites

Left kidney

Spleen

A. Free fluid in the peritoneal cavity (ascites)

Transverse colon

Pancreas

Gallbladder with gallstone

Liver

B. Retroperitoneal fluid *(darker gray)* **around the head and body of the pancreas and pararenal space around the kidney.** The perirenal space adjacent to the kidney is not involved.

Duodenum

Inferior vena cava

Right kidney

Gastric antrum
Jejunum

Retoperitoneal peripancreatic fluid

Aorta (with calcific atherosclerosis)

Perirenal fat

Retroperitoneal fluid in the pararenal space

Left kidney

Transverse colon

Pancreas

Ascending colon

Duodenum

Tip of the liver

Inferior vena cava

Right kidney

Superior mesenteric vein

Small bowel

Superior mesenteric artery

Peripancreatic fluid

Aorta

Perirenal fluid

Left kidney

C. Retroperitoneal fluid *(darker gray)* **around the head of the pancreas and perinephric space adjacent to the kidney**

4.24 GASTROINTESTINAL PATHOLOGY

The abdominal cavity is a potential space surrounding the abdominal organs. Visceral and parietal peritoneum has a thin film of serous fluid coating it to reduce friction from the movement of organs against the body wall and the retroperitoneal compartment (retroperitoneum) and against each other. "Free fluid" (ascites) is an abnormal accumulation of fluid in the abdominal cavity (**A**) from peritonitis or other pathological processes. Note how the fluid does not extend around the retroperitoneal organs (the fat around the kidneys and pancreas is black). The same concept applies to "free air" in the abdominal cavity. In contrast, note the fluid surrounding the kidneys and pancreas (**B** and **C**). It is contained within the retroperitoneal compartment.

5

PELVIS AND PERINEUM

5.1 BONY FRAMEWORK: MEDIAL AND LATERAL VIEWS

5.2 BONY FRAMEWORK: ANTERIOR AND POSTERIOR VIEWS

5.3 FEMALE AND MALE PELVIC X-RAYS

5.4 FEMALE MIDSAGITTAL SECTION AND CT

5.5 CT VS. MRI IN THE PELVIS

5.6 FEMALE PELVIC CONTENTS

5.7 SEARCH STRATEGY: UPPER FEMALE PELVIS

5.8 SEARCH STRATEGY: LOWER FEMALE PELVIS

5.9 UTERUS, ADNEXA, AND HYSTEROSALPINGOGRAM

5.10 MALE PELVIC CONTENTS

5.11 MALE MIDSAGITTAL SECTION AND CT

5.12 MALE AXIAL CT AND MRI

5.13 CROSS SECTION AT BLADDER-PROSTATE JUNCTION AND CT

5.14 MALE AND FEMALE CORONAL SECTIONS THROUGH THE URINARY BLADDER

5.15 BLADDER RELATIONSHIPS IN AXIAL AND CORONAL CT

5.16 CYSTOGRAM

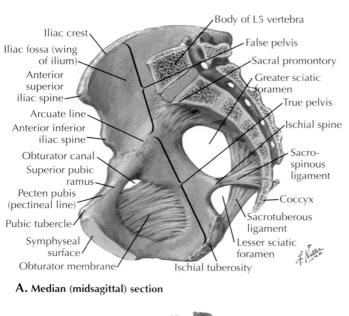

A. Median (midsagittal) section

Iliac crest
Iliac fossa (wing of ilium)
Anterior superior iliac spine
Arcuate line
Anterior inferior iliac spine
Obturator canal
Superior pubic ramus
Pecten pubis (pectineal line)
Pubic tubercle
Symphyseal surface
Obturator membrane
Body of L5 vertebra
False pelvis
Sacral promontory
Greater sciatic foramen
True pelvis
Ischial spine
Sacro-spinous ligament
Coccyx
Sacrotuberous ligament
Lesser sciatic foramen
Ischial tuberosity

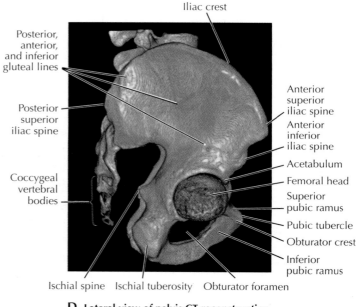

B. Medial view of pelvis CT reconstruction

Body of L5 vertebra
Iliac crest
Iliac fossa
Anterior superior iliac spine
Arcuate line
Anterior inferior iliac spine
Symphyseal surface
Obturator foramen
Inferior pubic ramus
False pelvis
Sacral promontory
True pelvis
Ischial spine
Ischial tuberosity

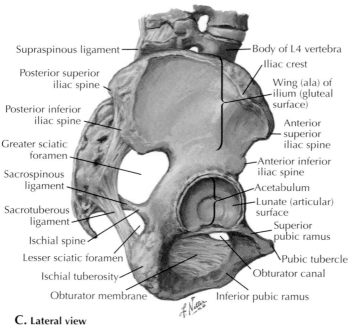

C. Lateral view

Supraspinous ligament
Posterior superior iliac spine
Posterior inferior iliac spine
Greater sciatic foramen
Sacrospinous ligament
Sacrotuberous ligament
Ischial spine
Lesser sciatic foramen
Ischial tuberosity
Obturator membrane
Body of L4 vertebra
Iliac crest
Wing (ala) of ilium (gluteal surface)
Anterior superior iliac spine
Anterior inferior iliac spine
Acetabulum
Lunate (articular) surface
Superior pubic ramus
Pubic tubercle
Obturator canal
Inferior pubic ramus

D. Lateral view of pelvis CT reconstruction with femoral head

Iliac crest
Posterior, anterior, and inferior gluteal lines
Posterior superior iliac spine
Coccygeal vertebral bodies
Ischial spine Ischial tuberosity Obturator foramen
Anterior superior iliac spine
Anterior inferior iliac spine
Acetabulum
Femoral head
Superior pubic ramus
Pubic tubercle
Obturator crest
Inferior pubic ramus

5.1 BONY FRAMEWORK: MEDIAL AND LATERAL VIEWS

The pelvis consists of the left and right innominate bones and the sacrum. The ilium, pubis, and ischium are fused with one another at the acetabulum of the hip joint to comprise each innominate bone. The pubic bones articulate with each other anteriorly in the midline at the pubic symphysis. We sit on our ischial tuberosity, and the ischial spine separates the greater and lesser sciatic notches posteriorly. The greater or false

pelvis consists of the lateral curve of the iliac blades that help support the abdominal viscera. The pubis and ischium make up the lesser or true pelvis that surrounds the birth canal and pelvic viscera.

Three-dimensional (3D) computer reconstructions from computed tomography (CT) scans (**B** and **D**) are most often used to plan surgical reconstructions in patients with fractures.

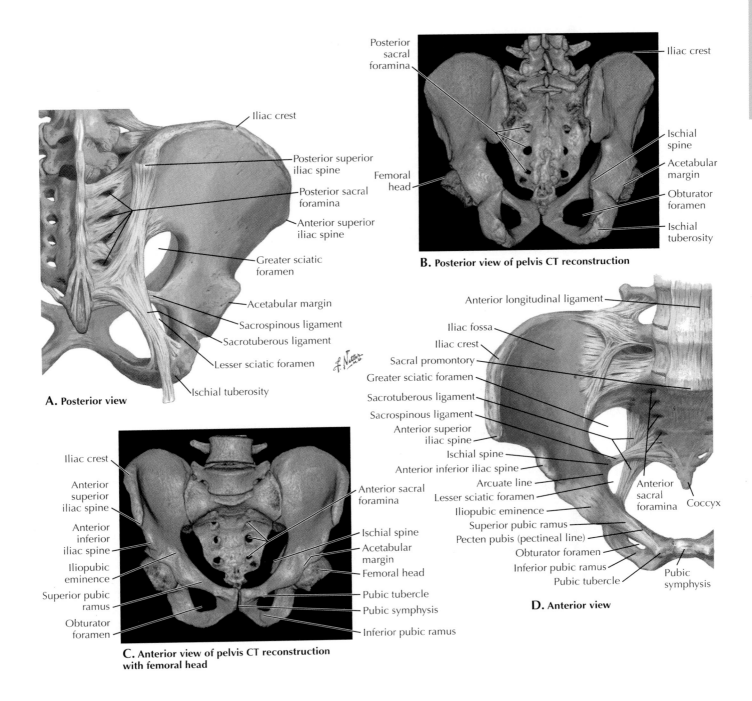

Iliac crest

Posterior superior iliac spine

Posterior sacral foramina

Anterior superior iliac spine

Greater sciatic foramen

Acetabular margin

Sacrospinous ligament

Sacrotuberous ligament

Lesser sciatic foramen

Ischial tuberosity

A. Posterior view

Posterior sacral foramina

Femoral head

Iliac crest

Ischial spine

Acetabular margin

Obturator foramen

Ischial tuberosity

B. Posterior view of pelvis CT reconstruction

Iliac crest

Anterior superior iliac spine

Anterior inferior iliac spine

Iliopubic eminence

Superior pubic ramus

Obturator foramen

Anterior sacral foramina

Ischial spine

Acetabular margin

Femoral head

Pubic tubercle

Pubic symphysis

Inferior pubic ramus

C. Anterior view of pelvis CT reconstruction with femoral head

Anterior longitudinal ligament

Iliac fossa

Iliac crest

Sacral promontory

Greater sciatic foramen

Sacrotuberous ligament

Sacrospinous ligament

Anterior superior iliac spine

Ischial spine

Anterior inferior iliac spine

Arcuate line

Lesser sciatic foramen

Iliopubic eminence

Superior pubic ramus

Pecten pubis (pectineal line)

Obturator foramen

Inferior pubic ramus

Pubic tubercle

Anterior sacral foramina

Coccyx

Pubic symphysis

D. Anterior view

5.2 BONY FRAMEWORK: ANTERIOR AND POSTERIOR VIEWS

The pelvic brim encircles the pelvic inlet to the birth canal that includes, from front to back, the pubic tubercle, pectin pubis, arcuate line of the ilium, and ala and promontory of the sacrum. The pelvic outlet is bounded by the ischial spines and tip of the coccyx. Laterally are the obturator foramina that are closed off in life by obturator membranes. The sacrospinous and sacrotuberous ligaments convert the sciatic notches into greater and lesser sciatic foramina.

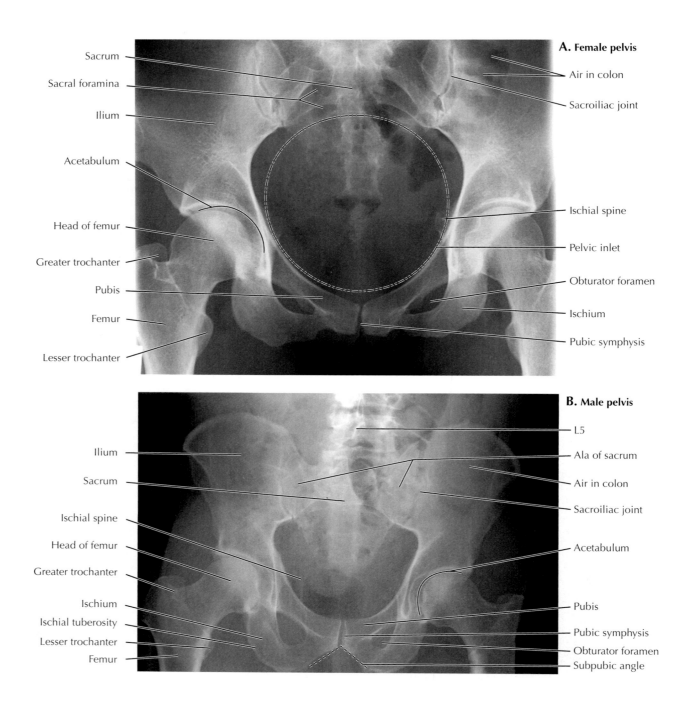

A. Female pelvis

Sacrum

Sacral foramina

Ilium

Acetabulum

Head of femur

Greater trochanter

Pubis

Femur

Lesser trochanter

Air in colon

Sacroiliac joint

Ischial spine

Pelvic inlet

Obturator foramen

Ischium

Pubic symphysis

B. Male pelvis

Ilium

Sacrum

Ischial spine

Head of femur

Greater trochanter

Ischium

Ischial tuberosity

Lesser trochanter

Femur

L5

Ala of sacrum

Air in colon

Sacroiliac joint

Acetabulum

Pubis

Pubic symphysis

Obturator foramen

Subpubic angle

5.3 FEMALE AND MALE PELVIC X-RAYS

A plain film (x-ray) of the pelvis is a good initial way to look for fractures. CT is sometimes needed to better evaluate fractures or to look for nondisplaced fractures that may be missed on the plain film. Magnetic resonance imaging (MRI) is very sensitive for bone marrow edema and displays bone contusions not seen with plain film or CT. It is also best for tendon, ligament, and other soft tissue injuries. In the x-rays, note the sacroiliac joints, acetabulum of the hip joint, sacral foramina, and pubic symphysis. The obturator foramina appear narrow because of their oblique angle of view. The darker contours over the sacrum and ilium represent air in the colon. A female pelvis has a relatively larger birth canal than a male pelvis. It is wider because of relatively wider ala of the sacrum and relatively wider superior pubic rami and ischiopubic rami. The longer rami result in a wider subpubic angle in the female pelvis compared to that of the male. The sacrum is also angled more posteriorly in the female to enlarge the pelvic outlet. This accounts for the larger greater sciatic notch in the female.

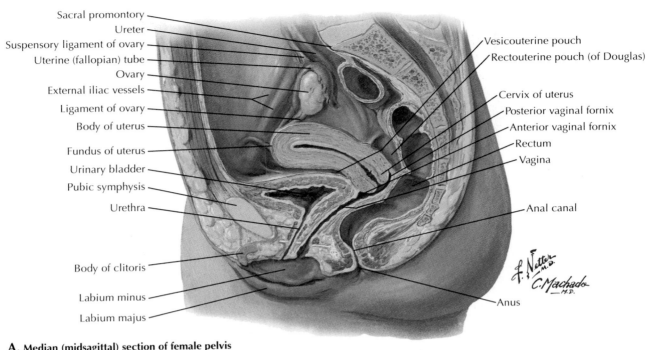

Sacral promontory
Ureter
Suspensory ligament of ovary
Uterine (fallopian) tube
Ovary
External iliac vessels
Ligament of ovary
Body of uterus
Fundus of uterus
Urinary bladder
Pubic symphysis
Urethra

Body of clitoris

Labium minus
Labium majus

Vesicouterine pouch
Rectouterine pouch (of Douglas)

Cervix of uterus
Posterior vaginal fornix
Anterior vaginal fornix
Rectum
Vagina

Anal canal

Anus

A. Median (midsagittal) section of female pelvis

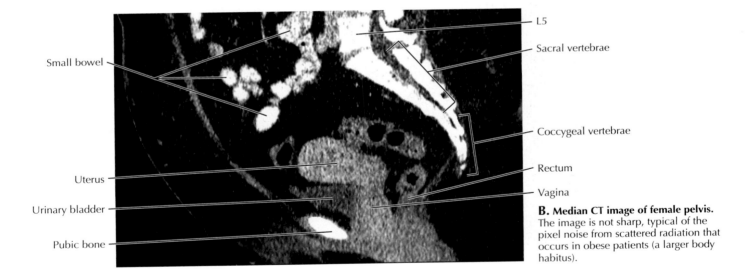

Small bowel

Uterus

Urinary bladder

Pubic bone

L5

Sacral vertebrae

Coccygeal vertebrae

Rectum

Vagina

B. Median CT image of female pelvis.
The image is not sharp, typical of the pixel noise from scattered radiation that occurs in obese patients (a larger body habitus).

5.4 FEMALE MIDSAGITTAL SECTION AND CT

From anterior to posterior in a midsagittal section of the female pelvis are the pubic symphysis, urinary bladder and urethra, vagina, and rectum and anal canal. The uterus extends anteriorly over the bladder at a sharp angle to the axis of the vagina. The anterior and posterior (and lateral) fornices of the vagina are recesses around the cervix. The bladder, vagina, and rectum are retroperitoneal. The rectouterine pouch (of Douglas) is a peritoneal fold adjacent to the posterior fornix of the vagina. The urogenital diaphragm extends from the pubic symphysis to the perineal body (central tendon of the perineum) just anterior to the anal canal. The CT image depicts the uterus and underdistended urinary bladder. The ovaries are usually off midline and therefore not seen.

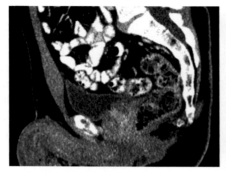

A. Median CT of male pelvis

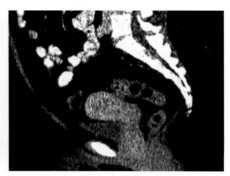

B. Median CT of female pelvis

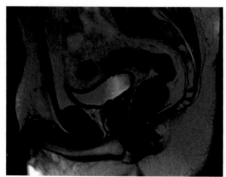

C. Median T2-weighted MRI of male pelvis

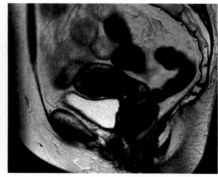

D. Median T2-weighted MRI of female pelvis

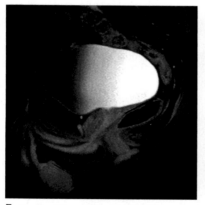

E. Median T1-weighted MRI with contrast of male pelvis with a full bladder

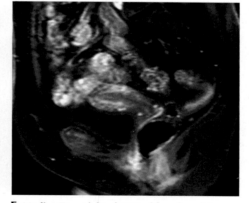

F. Median T1-weighted MRI of female pelvis with contrast that has not yet reached the bladder

5.5 CT VS. MRI IN THE PELVIS

For the evaluation of the reproductive organs, MRI is preferred because it can best display the anatomy of the uterus, cervix, vagina, and adnexa (accessory structures) in the female patient and prostate, seminal vesicles, penis, and testes in the male patient. CT is currently the preferred method for the bowel, with a few exceptions, because it is faster and less affected by peristaltic motion. CT is a great method to look for lymphadenopathy and to start the search for an unknown pelvic pathology.

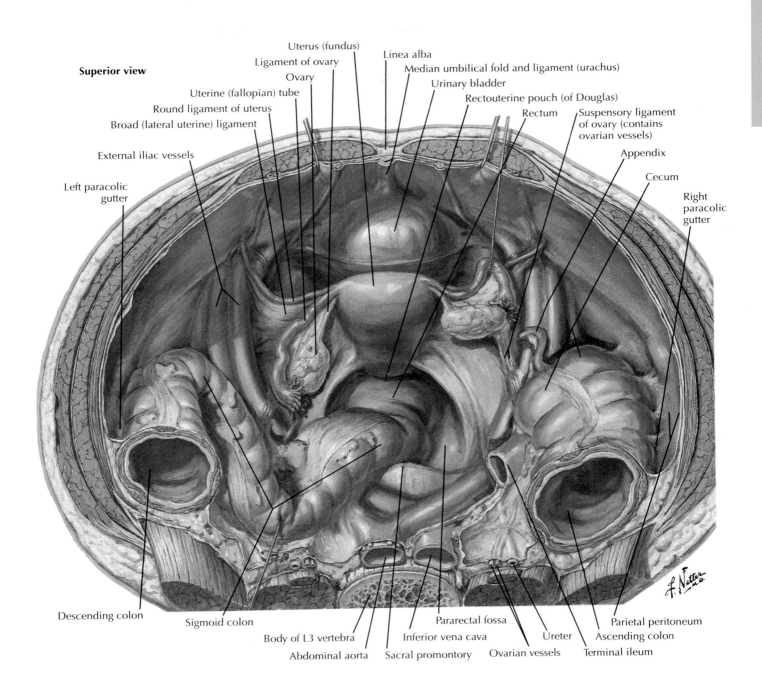

Superior view

Uterus (fundus)
Ligament of ovary
Ovary
Uterine (fallopian) tube
Round ligament of uterus
Broad (lateral uterine) ligament
External iliac vessels
Left paracolic gutter

Linea alba
Median umbilical fold and ligament (urachus)
Urinary bladder
Rectouterine pouch (of Douglas)
Rectum
Suspensory ligament of ovary (contains ovarian vessels)
Appendix
Cecum
Right paracolic gutter

Descending colon
Sigmoid colon
Body of L3 vertebra
Abdominal aorta
Sacral promontory
Inferior vena cava
Pararectal fossa
Ovarian vessels
Ureter
Terminal ileum
Ascending colon
Parietal peritoneum

5.6 FEMALE PELVIC CONTENTS

This is the 3D view looking down into the female pelvis from above. Keep in mind that radiologic convention orients an axial image as seen from below, where left and right are "reversed." Here the iliocecal junction, appendix, and ascending colon are on the right, and the descending and sigmoid colons are on the left. The uterine tubes are in the upper free edge of the broad ligament of the uterus, and the ovaries are posterior. The ovarian ligaments attach to the uterus, where they continue anteriorly to the inguinal canal as the round ligaments of the uterus.

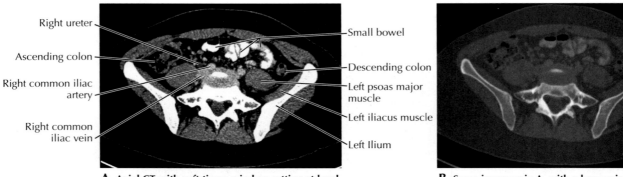

Right ureter
Ascending colon
Right common iliac artery
Right common iliac vein

Small bowel
Descending colon
Left psoas major muscle
Left iliacus muscle
Left Ilium

A. Axial CT with soft tissue window setting at level of L5-S1

B. Same image as in A, with a bone window setting

Terminal ileum
Ileocecal valve
Ascending colon/cecal junction
Right common iliac artery
Right common iliac vein
Sacral alae

Small bowel
Descending colon
Left psoas muscle
Left iliacus muscle
Left gluteus medius muscle
Left ilium
Left gluteus maximus muscle

C. Axial CT with soft tissue setting at level of S1-S2

D. Same image as in C, with bone window setting

Search Strategy for Image Interpretation in the Pelvis
- Lymph node chains (along iliac vessels and obturator internus region, inguinal region)
- Vessels
- Uterus/adnexa (female patient); prostate and seminal vesicles (male)
- Bowel
- Fat planes
- Pelvic wall
- Bones

5.7 SEARCH STRATEGY: UPPER FEMALE PELVIS

The table in this figure has a useful search strategy for the systematic study of pelvic images. The pelvic contents cannot all be seen on a single image of the pelvis. In the upper pelvis the small bowel, colon, appendix, ureters, vessels, and lymph node chains are evaluated together with the body wall. To better evaluate the bones, the radiologist changes the window (the amount of gray shades to be displayed) and level (the center of the gray scale) of the images so the bones are not so white and more bone detail is seen (**B** and **D**).

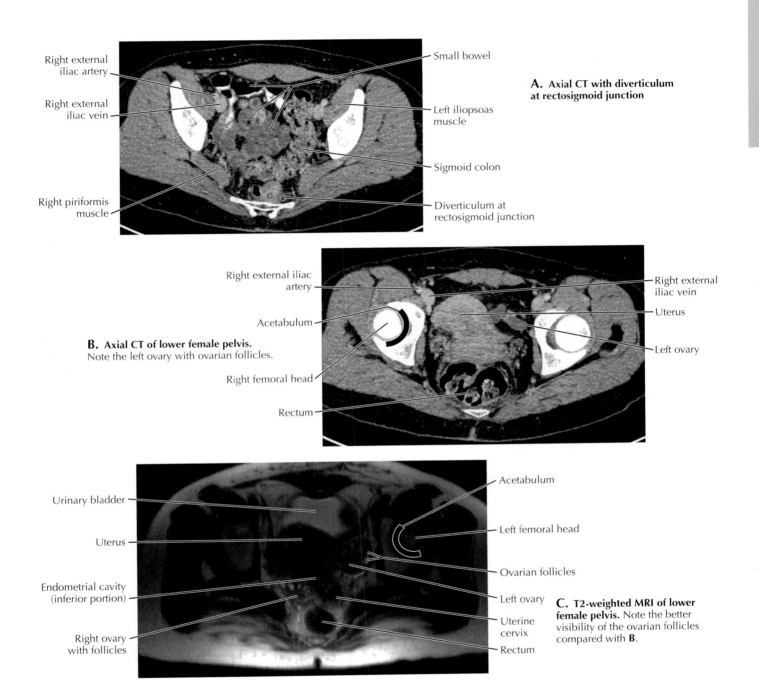

A. Axial CT with diverticulum at rectosigmoid junction

Right external iliac artery

Right external iliac vein

Right piriformis muscle

Small bowel

Left iliopsoas muscle

Sigmoid colon

Diverticulum at rectosigmoid junction

B. Axial CT of lower female pelvis.
Note the left ovary with ovarian follicles.

Right external iliac artery

Acetabulum

Right femoral head

Rectum

Right external iliac vein

Uterus

Left ovary

Urinary bladder

Uterus

Endometrial cavity (inferior portion)

Right ovary with follicles

Acetabulum

Left femoral head

Ovarian follicles

Left ovary

Uterine cervix

Rectum

C. T2-weighted MRI of lower female pelvis. Note the better visibility of the ovarian follicles compared with **B**.

5.8 SEARCH STRATEGY: LOWER FEMALE PELVIS

In the lower pelvis are the uterus and adnexa, sigmoid colon, rectum, small bowel, vessels, lymph node chains, bony framework, and pelvic wall. **A** shows how a small diverticulum at the junction of the sigmoid colon and rectum looks on CT. The uterus and adnexa are better evaluated with ultrasound (US) and MRI. Compare the appearance of the ovaries in CT (**B**) with MRI (**C**). On the CT (**B**), the left ovary is an oval gray (soft tissue density) structure; ovarian follicles appear as a few dots of a lower shade of gray. **C** is a T2-weighted MRI, in which the fluid in the follicles has a much brighter *(white)* signal compared to the ovarian stroma. The follicles appear as small white dots, and they help to localize the ovaries on the MRI.

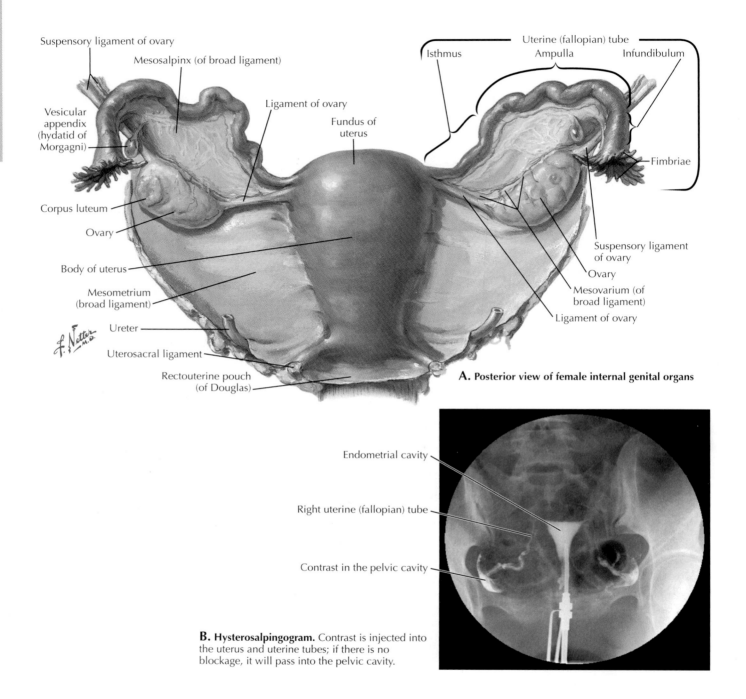

A. Posterior view of female internal genital organs

Endometrial cavity

Right uterine (fallopian) tube

Contrast in the pelvic cavity

B. Hysterosalpingogram. Contrast is injected into the uterus and uterine tubes; if there is no blockage, it will pass into the pelvic cavity.

5.9 UTERUS, ADNEXA, AND HYSTEROSALPINGOGRAM

The uterine tubes are in a fold of mesosalpinx, the upper portion of the broad ligament of the uterus. The uterine tubes are not physically connected to the ovaries; their lumen is open to the peritoneal cavity. At the time of ovulation the fimbriae of the uterine tubes envelop the ovaries to facilitate movement of an ovulated oocyte into a uterine tube. **B** shows a hysterosalpingogram (HSG) to evaluate the lumen of the uterus ("hystera," which is Greek for "womb") and uterine

tube ("salpinx" means "trumpet" or "tube"). The uterine cervix is cannulated, contrast is injected, and x-rays are obtained. Contrast fills the cavity of the uterus and extends into the uterine tubes; its presence in the peritoneal cavity indicates that the uterine tubes are free of blockage (e.g., from infection or scar tissue).

The procedure has to be under sterile conditions, or the patient may get an infection in the endometrium (endometritis) or peritoneal cavity (peritonitis). The contrast used is water soluble and is absorbed.

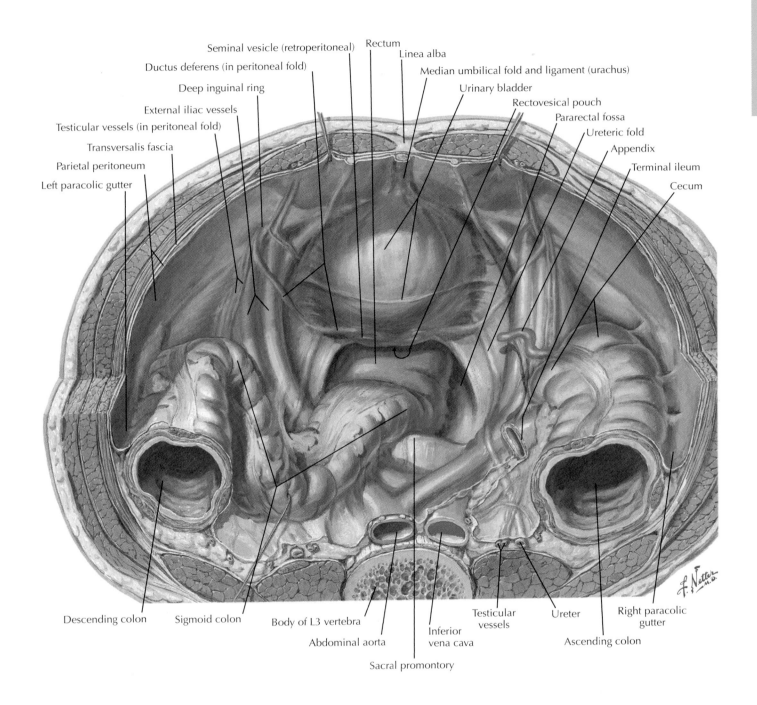

Seminal vesicle (retroperitoneal)

Ductus deferens (in peritoneal fold)

Deep inguinal ring

External iliac vessels

Testicular vessels (in peritoneal fold)

Transversalis fascia

Parietal peritoneum

Left paracolic gutter

Rectum

Linea alba

Median umbilical fold and ligament (urachus)

Urinary bladder

Rectovesical pouch

Pararectal fossa

Ureteric fold

Appendix

Terminal ileum

Cecum

Descending colon

Sigmoid colon

Body of L3 vertebra

Abdominal aorta

Sacral promontory

Inferior vena cava

Testicular vessels

Ureter

Ascending colon

Right paracolic gutter

5.10 MALE PELVIC CONTENTS

The most notable difference between the male and female pelvic organs as seen from above is the absence of the uterus, uterine tubes, ovaries, and vagina in the male. The rectouterine pouch of peritoneum in the female corresponds to the rectovesical pouch in the male, between the rectum and urinary bladder.

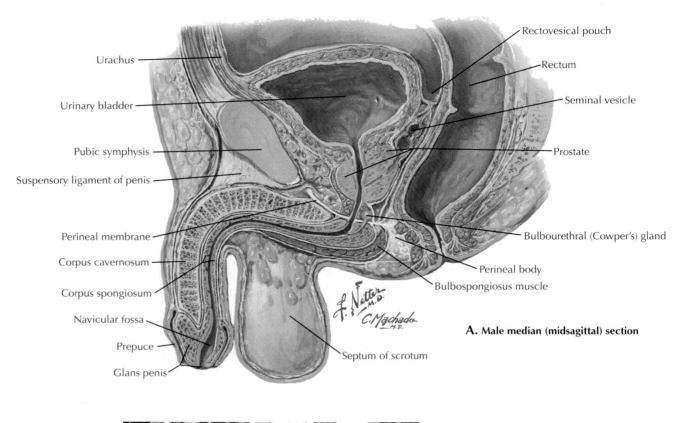

Urachus

Urinary bladder

Pubic symphysis

Suspensory ligament of penis

Perineal membrane

Corpus cavernosum

Corpus spongiosum

Navicular fossa

Prepuce

Glans penis

Septum of scrotum

Rectovesical pouch

Rectum

Seminal vesicle

Prostate

Bulbourethral (Cowper's) gland

Perineal body

Bulbospongiosus muscle

A. Male median (midsagittal) section

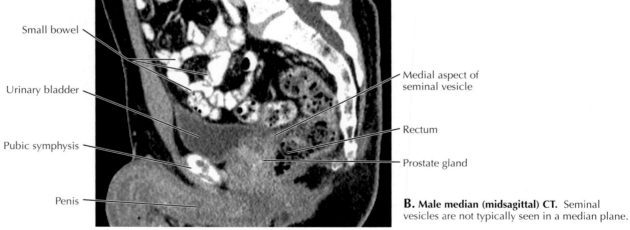

Small bowel

Urinary bladder

Pubic symphysis

Penis

Medial aspect of seminal vesicle

Rectum

Prostate gland

B. Male median (midsagittal) CT. Seminal vesicles are not typically seen in a median plane.

5.11 MALE MIDSAGITTAL SECTION AND CT

A midsagittal section in the male contains the prostate gland inferior to the urinary bladder but not the bilateral seminal vesicles. All of these structures are retroperitoneal.

On a routine pelvic CT, the entire penis and the scrotal sacs are usually not included. The best way to evaluate the testes is ultrasound (US), and the penis can be evaluated with MRI and/or US, depending on the type of pathology that is suspected. If a process extends beyond the penis and scrotum to involve the perineum/pelvis, CT is a good way to look at the extent of disease, whereas MRI can give more detailed information. Recognizing that the space anterior to the bladder is retroperitoneal is important since treatments of bladder rupture, for example, differ, depending on the location (intraperitoneal vs. retroperitoneal).

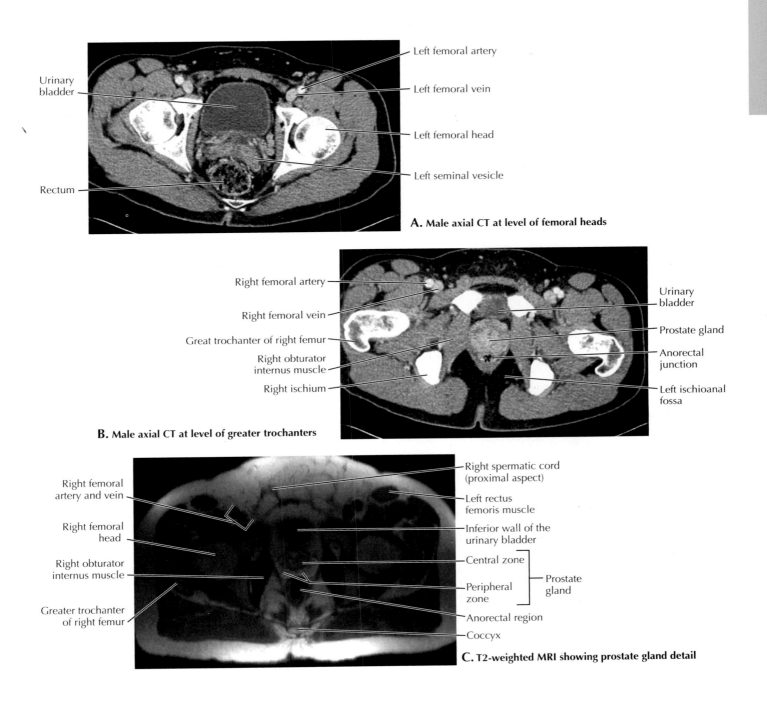

Urinary bladder

Left femoral artery

Left femoral vein

Left femoral head

Left seminal vesicle

Rectum

A. Male axial CT at level of femoral heads

Right femoral artery

Right femoral vein

Great trochanter of right femur

Right obturator internus muscle

Right ischium

Urinary bladder

Prostate gland

Anorectal junction

Left ischioanal fossa

B. Male axial CT at level of greater trochanters

Right femoral artery and vein

Right femoral head

Right obturator internus muscle

Greater trochanter of right femur

Right spermatic cord (proximal aspect)

Left rectus femoris muscle

Inferior wall of the urinary bladder

Central zone

Peripheral zone

Anorectal region

Coccyx

Prostate gland

C. T2-weighted MRI showing prostate gland detail

5.12 MALE AXIAL CT AND MRI

The seminal vesicles and prostate gland are in the lower male pelvis. The urinary bladder is superior and anterior to the prostate gland; the rectum is posterior to the seminal vesicles. CT can be used to evaluate the size of the prostate gland, but it cannot detect prostate cancer well. CT can be used to look for lymphadenopathy. Tissue detail of the prostate gland is best seen with MRI (with or without an endorectal coil) and endorectal US. The same is true for the seminal vesicles. On the MR image the peripheral and central zones of the prostate gland can be distinguished from one another because the peripheral zone has a whiter T2 signal.

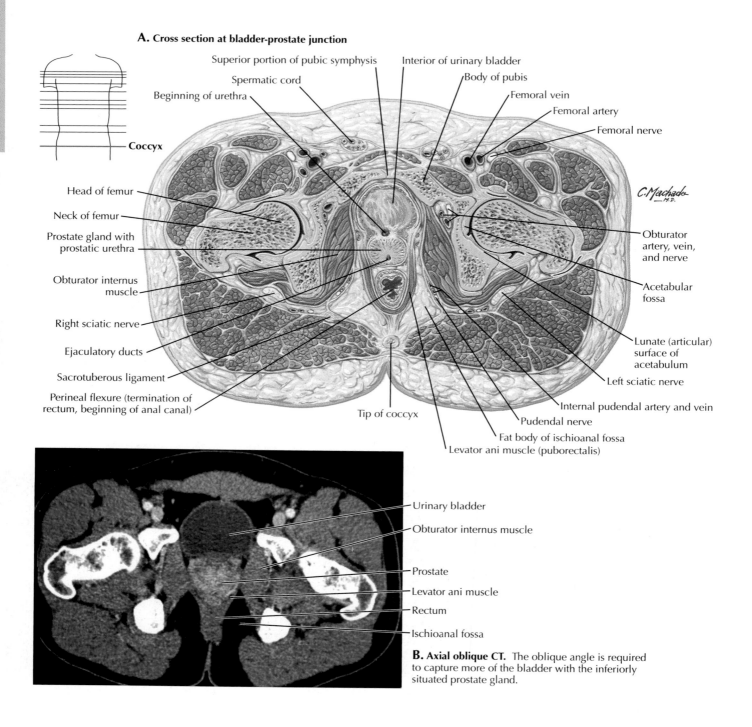

A. Cross section at bladder-prostate junction

Superior portion of pubic symphysis

Spermatic cord

Beginning of urethra

Head of femur

Neck of femur

Prostate gland with prostatic urethra

Obturator internus muscle

Right sciatic nerve

Ejaculatory ducts

Sacrotuberous ligament

Perineal flexure (termination of rectum, beginning of anal canal)

Coccyx

Interior of urinary bladder

Body of pubis

Femoral vein

Femoral artery

Femoral nerve

Obturator artery, vein, and nerve

Acetabular fossa

Lunate (articular) surface of acetabulum

Left sciatic nerve

Internal pudendal artery and vein

Pudendal nerve

Fat body of ischioanal fossa

Levator ani muscle (puborectalis)

Tip of coccyx

Urinary bladder

Obturator internus muscle

Prostate

Levator ani muscle

Rectum

Ischioanal fossa

B. Axial oblique CT. The oblique angle is required to capture more of the bladder with the inferiorly situated prostate gland.

5.13 CROSS SECTION AT BLADDER-PROSTATE JUNCTION AND CT

This section in **A** is through the middle of the hip joint and the prostate gland at the most inferior end of the urinary bladder. Just posterior is the junction of rectum and anal canal. The pelvic viscera are supported by the levator ani muscles of the pelvic diaphragm. The muscle fibers are sweeping around the bladder, prostate, and rectum and will end inferiorly at the external anal sphincter. On the lateral walls of the pelvic cavity are the obturator internus muscles attaching to the pubis, ischium, and obturator membrane. Between the lateral wall and pelvic viscera is the fat-filled ischioanal fossa. The axial oblique CT image (**B**) demonstrates the relationship of the bladder base and prostate gland. The male urethra travels through the prostate but cannot be visualized on a routine CT study.

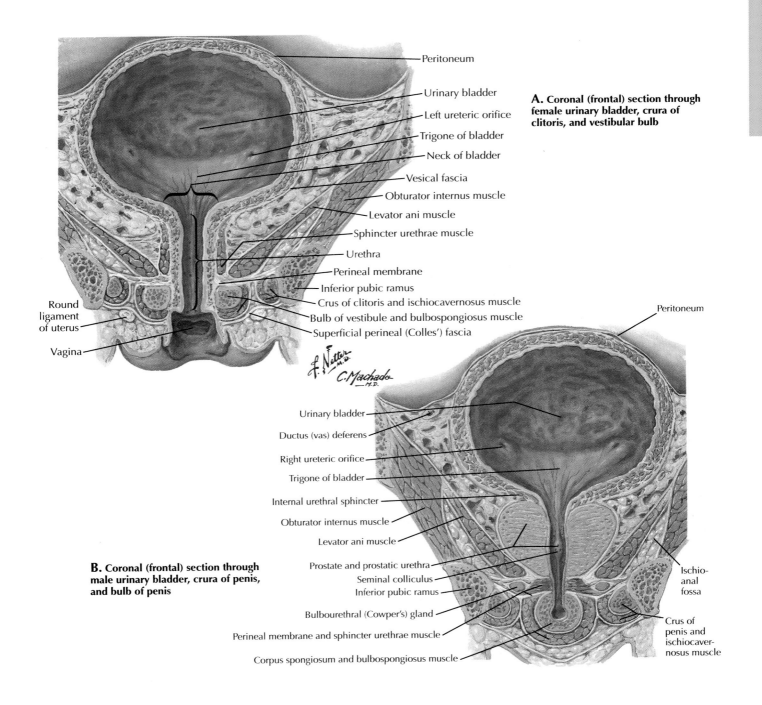

A. Coronal (frontal) section through female urinary bladder, crura of clitoris, and vestibular bulb

Peritoneum

Urinary bladder

Left ureteric orifice

Trigone of bladder

Neck of bladder

Vesical fascia

Obturator internus muscle

Levator ani muscle

Sphincter urethrae muscle

Urethra

Perineal membrane

Inferior pubic ramus

Crus of clitoris and ischiocavernosus muscle

Bulb of vestibule and bulbospongiosus muscle

Superficial perineal (Colles') fascia

Round ligament of uterus

Vagina

Peritoneum

Urinary bladder

Ductus (vas) deferens

Right ureteric orifice

Trigone of bladder

Internal urethral sphincter

Obturator internus muscle

Levator ani muscle

Prostate and prostatic urethra

Seminal colliculus

Inferior pubic ramus

Bulbourethral (Cowper's) gland

Perineal membrane and sphincter urethrae muscle

Corpus spongiosum and bulbospongiosus muscle

Ischio-anal fossa

Crus of penis and ischiocaver-nosus muscle

B. Coronal (frontal) section through male urinary bladder, crura of penis, and bulb of penis

5.14 MALE AND FEMALE CORONAL SECTIONS THROUGH THE URINARY BLADDER

The trigone of the urinary bladder in both genders is the triangular area at the base of the bladder between the openings of the two ureters and the urethra. Females have a short urethra that passes through the urogenital diaphragm. Males have a prostatic urethra, a membranous urethra (through the urogenital diaphragm), and a penile urethra. Note in both genders the levator ani muscles, obturator internus muscles, and ischioanal fossa. The external genital organs in both genders are attached to the ischiopubic rami and urogenital diaphragm.

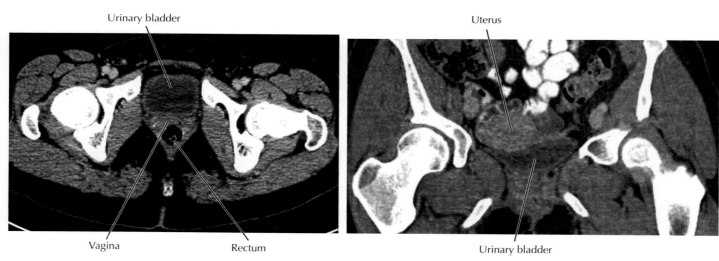

Urinary bladder

Vagina   Rectum

A. Axial CT through female urinary bladder

Uterus

Urinary bladder

B. Coronal CT through female urinary bladder

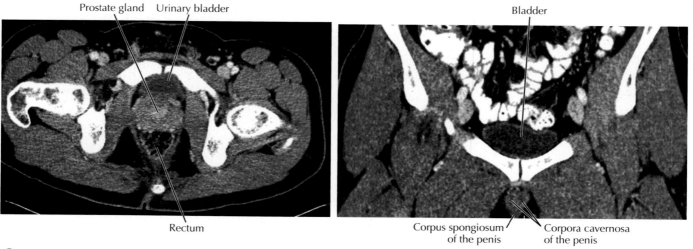

Prostate gland   Urinary bladder

Rectum

C. Axial CT through male urinary bladder

Bladder

Corpus spongiosum   Corpora cavernosa
of the penis   of the penis

D. Coronal CT through male urinary bladder

5.15 BLADDER RELATIONSHIPS IN AXIAL AND CORONAL CT

A and **B** demonstrate the relationships of the urinary bladder, uterus, and vagina. The labia, clitoris, and lower vagina are not discretely identified on the CT. **C** and **D** demonstrate male bladder relationships. The prostate is posterior and inferior to the bladder and is often difficult to be displayed on the same plane in a coronal image. The corpora cavernosa and corpus spongiosum of the penis are visualized inferior to the pubic symphysis.

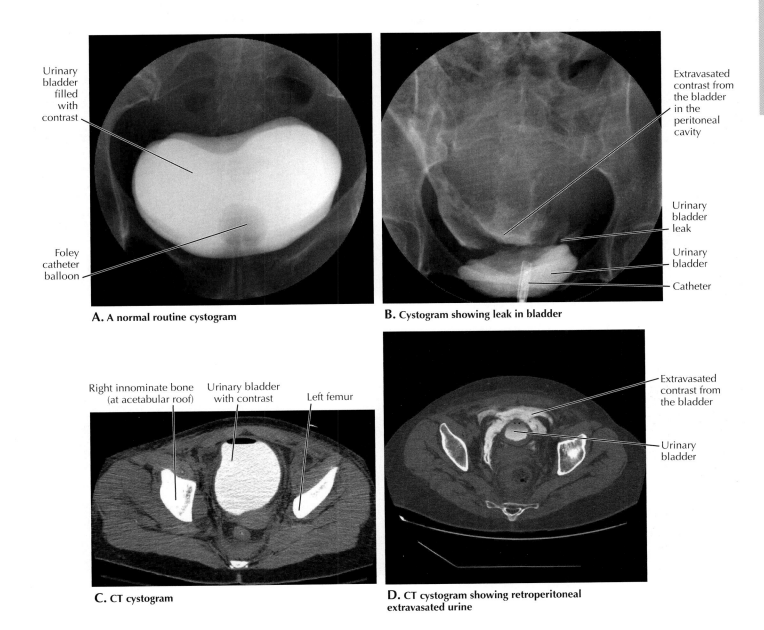

Urinary
bladder
filled
with
contrast

Foley
catheter
balloon

A. **A normal routine cystogram**

Extravasated
contrast from
the bladder
in the
peritoneal
cavity

Urinary
bladder
leak

Urinary
bladder

Catheter

B. **Cystogram showing leak in bladder**

Right innominate bone   Urinary bladder
(at acetabular roof)   with contrast   Left femur

C. **CT cystogram**

Extravasated
contrast from
the bladder

Urinary
bladder

D. **CT cystogram showing retroperitoneal
extravasated urine**

5.16 CYSTOGRAM

In a routine cystogram (**A**) a Foley catheter is placed in the bladder, contrast is instilled by gravity to outline the urinary bladder lumen, and x-rays are taken. It is a good way to look for a leak, as seen in **B.** An even better way to identify the location of a urinary leak (intraperitoneal vs. retroperitoneal) is a CT cystogram (**C** and **D**). A lower concentration of the contrast is instilled by the Foley catheter, and a CT of the pelvis is performed. A CT before the instillation of contrast is also obtained. This helps distinguish leaks from preexisting areas of high density such as calcifications. In addition, after drainage a CT is again performed to look for contrast outside the bladder. This may help differentiate a leak from irregularity in the urinary bladder contour. The urine in the pelvic cavity in **D** is retroperitoneal. It does not extend over the posterior peritoneal surface of the bladder.

6

UPPER LIMBS

6.1   HUMERUS AND SCAPULA

6.2   ANTEROPOSTERIOR SHOULDER X-RAY

6.3   AXILLARY AND Y VIEW X-RAYS OF THE SHOULDER JOINT

6.4   SHOULDER JOINT ANATOMY

6.5   CORONAL T2 MRI OF THE SHOULDER JOINT

6.6   AXIAL T1 ARTHROGRAM OF THE SHOULDER JOINT

6.7   AXILLARY, BRACHIAL, AND ELBOW ARTERIES

6.8   VASCULAR STUDIES OF THE UPPER EXTREMITY

6.9   ARM MUSCLES

6.10   ARM SERIAL CROSS SECTIONS

6.11   ARM MRI

6.12   BONES OF THE ELBOW

6.13   JOINTS OF THE ELBOW

6.14   ELBOW X-RAYS

6.15   ELBOW IMAGING STUDIES

6.16   MUSCLES OF THE FOREARM: ANTERIOR VIEW

6.17   MUSCLES OF THE FOREARM: POSTERIOR VIEW

6.18   FOREARM SERIAL CROSS SECTIONS

6.19   UPPER AND MIDDLE FOREARM MRI

6.20   BONES OF THE HAND AND WRIST

6.21   ANTEROPOSTERIOR X-RAY OF THE WRIST AND HAND

6.22   CARPAL BONES AND WRIST JOINT

6.23   T1 AND T2 MRI OF THE WRIST JOINT

6.24   DISTAL RADIOCARPAL JOINT AND WRIST

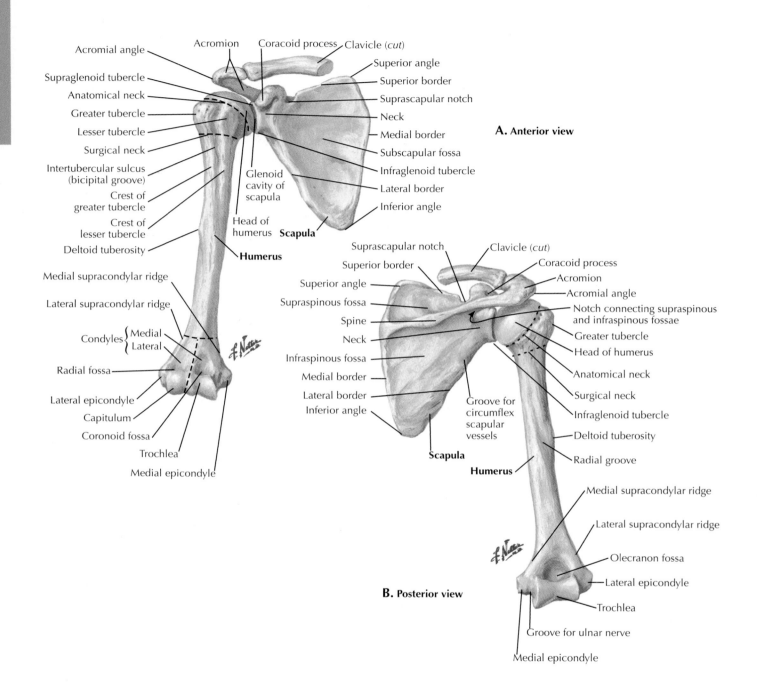

Acromial angle
Acromion
Coracoid process
Clavicle (cut)
Supraglenoid tubercle
Anatomical neck
Greater tubercle
Lesser tubercle
Surgical neck
Intertubercular sulcus (bicipital groove)
Crest of greater tubercle
Crest of lesser tubercle
Deltoid tuberosity
Medial supracondylar ridge
Lateral supracondylar ridge
Condyles { Medial / Lateral }
Radial fossa
Lateral epicondyle
Capitulum
Coronoid fossa
Trochlea
Medial epicondyle
Superior angle
Superior border
Suprascapular notch
Neck
Medial border
Subscapular fossa
Infraglenoid tubercle
Lateral border
Inferior angle
Glenoid cavity of scapula
Head of humerus
Scapula
Humerus

A. Anterior view

Suprascapular notch
Superior border
Superior angle
Supraspinous fossa
Spine
Neck
Infraspinous fossa
Medial border
Lateral border
Inferior angle
Groove for circumflex scapular vessels
Scapula
Clavicle (cut)
Coracoid process
Acromion
Acromial angle
Notch connecting supraspinous and infraspinous fossae
Greater tubercle
Head of humerus
Anatomical neck
Surgical neck
Infraglenoid tubercle
Deltoid tuberosity
Radial groove
Humerus
Medial supracondylar ridge
Lateral supracondylar ridge
Olecranon fossa
Lateral epicondyle
Trochlea
Groove for ulnar nerve
Medial epicondyle

B. Posterior view

6.1 HUMERUS AND SCAPULA

The coracoid ("shaped like a crow's beak") process is the most prominent feature on the anterior of the scapula. Three muscles attach to it: pectoralis minor, coracobrachialis, and the short head of the biceps brachii muscle. On the humerus the bicipital groove separates the lesser tubercle of the humerus anteriorly from the greater tubercle laterally. The tendon of the long head of the biceps brachii muscle lies in the groove as it enters the joint cavity to attach to the supraglenoid tubercle of the scapula. The infraglenoid tubercle is the attachment of the long head of the triceps brachii muscle. Posteriorly the scapular spine divides the scapula into supraspinatus and infraspinatus fossae that contain muscles of the same name. The acromion is the termination of the scapular spine; it articulates anteriorly with the clavicle.

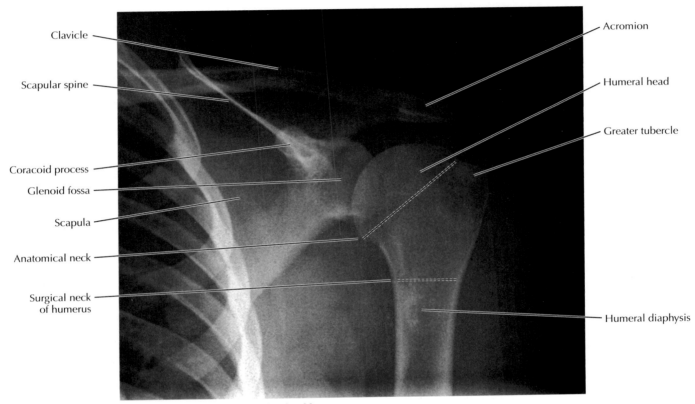

Clavicle

Scapular spine

Coracoid process

Glenoid fossa

Scapula

Anatomical neck

Surgical neck
of humerus

Acromion

Humeral head

Greater tubercle

Humeral diaphysis

Anteroposterior radiograph of the shoulder

6.2 ANTEROPOSTERIOR SHOULDER X-RAY

Plain films of the shoulder can be good for assessing the bony anatomy for abnormalities that may be a result of such conditions as osteoarthritis or trauma. Three views that are commonly done include the anteroposterior (AP) view, the axillary view, and the Y view. The humeral head should appear as a smooth hemisphere. In the AP view seen here, the medial portion of the humeral head overlaps with the lateral aspect of the glenoid fossa. If a patient has a history of chronic anterior dislocations, there may be a Hill-Sachs deformity, which appears as an indented groove in the upper outer portion of the humeral head. The acromion and acromioclavicular joint should be evaluated for osteophytes (bony projections) that can impinge on the supraspinatus muscle. All the bones should be assessed for fractures, and whatever portion of the lung is visible should be evaluated as well. A radiologist is responsible for everything visualized on a study, and lung cancers have been found incidentally on shoulder films!

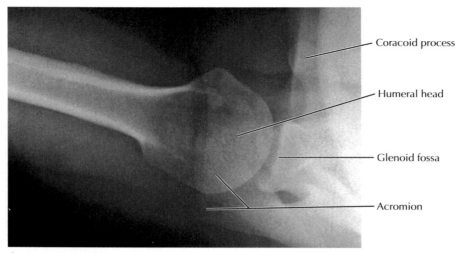

Coracoid process

Humeral head

Glenoid fossa

Acromion

A. Axillary view from above

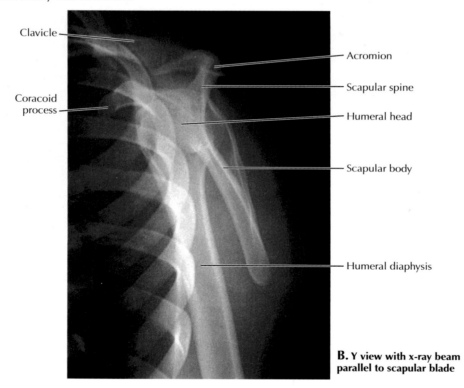

Clavicle

Coracoid process

Acromion

Scapular spine

Humeral head

Scapular body

Humeral diaphysis

B. Y view with x-ray beam parallel to scapular blade

6.3 AXILLARY AND Y VIEW X-RAYS OF THE SHOULDER JOINT

In the axillary view of the shoulder shown in **A,** the arm is abducted 90 degrees, and the beam is projected down through the shoulder. This allows clear visualization of the relation of the glenoid fossa with the humeral head; the fossa should be adjacent to the humeral head. This view is helpful for identifying dislocation of the humeral head and anterior or posterior glenoid rim fractures. On this projection, the acromion is seen overlapping with the humeral head. In the upper right corner of this image is the coracoid process of the scapula. In the Y view x-ray of the scapula (**B),** the x-ray beam is directed along the scapular spine, and the body of the scapula (stem of the Y) is viewed on edge. The upper limbs of the Y are the coracoid process and scapular spine. This projection aids in evaluation for a shoulder dislocation or a fracture of the scapula.

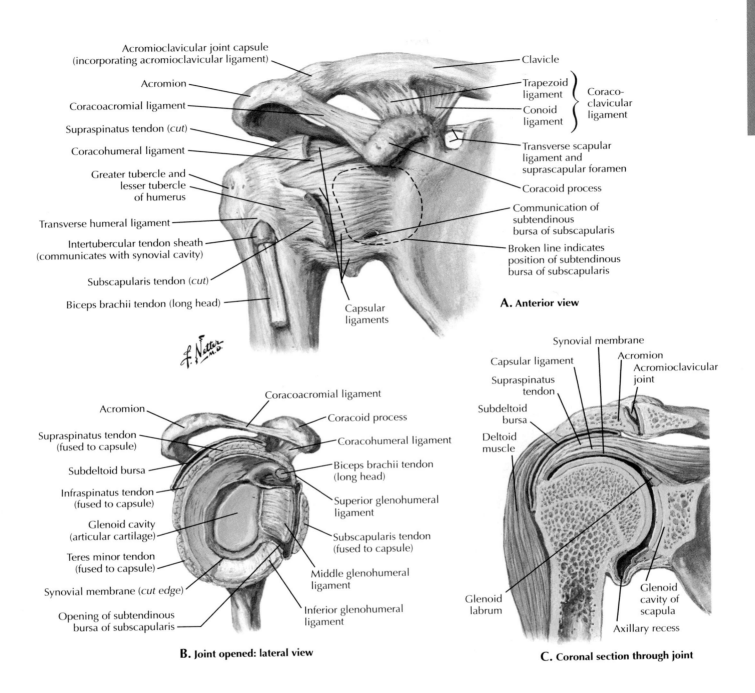

Acromioclavicular joint capsule
(incorporating acromioclavicular ligament)

Acromion

Coracoacromial ligament

Supraspinatus tendon (cut)

Coracohumeral ligament

Greater tubercle and
lesser tubercle
of humerus

Transverse humeral ligament

Intertubercular tendon sheath
(communicates with synovial cavity)

Subscapularis tendon (cut)

Biceps brachii tendon (long head)

Capsular
ligaments

Clavicle

Trapezoid
ligament

Conoid
ligament

} Coraco-
clavicular
ligament

Transverse scapular
ligament and
suprascapular foramen

Coracoid process

Communication of
subtendinous
bursa of subscapularis

Broken line indicates
position of subtendinous
bursa of subscapularis

A. Anterior view

Coracoacromial ligament

Acromion

Supraspinatus tendon
(fused to capsule)

Subdeltoid bursa

Infraspinatus tendon
(fused to capsule)

Glenoid cavity
(articular cartilage)

Teres minor tendon
(fused to capsule)

Synovial membrane (cut edge)

Opening of subtendinous
bursa of subscapularis

Coracoid process

Coracohumeral ligament

Biceps brachii tendon
(long head)

Superior glenohumeral
ligament

Subscapularis tendon
(fused to capsule)

Middle glenohumeral
ligament

Inferior glenohumeral
ligament

B. Joint opened: lateral view

Synovial membrane

Capsular ligament

Supraspinatus
tendon

Subdeltoid
bursa

Deltoid
muscle

Glenoid
labrum

Acromion

Acromioclavicular
joint

Glenoid
cavity of
scapula

Axillary recess

C. Coronal section through joint

6.4 SHOULDER JOINT ANATOMY

The interior of the shoulder (glenohumeral) joint is lined with a synovial membrane that attaches to the periphery of the articular cartilages. The fibrous joint capsule covers the joint. The three glenohumeral ligaments are thickenings of the anterior half of the joint capsule. The synovial membrane (red) is cut in **B** to show the capsule and capsular ligaments. There is a bursa under the deltoid muscle and tendon of the subscapularis muscle. The latter communicates with the synovial joint cavity between the middle and inferior glenohumeral ligaments. The subdeltoid bursa can communicate with the joint cavity through a tear in the supraspinatus tendon from trauma or as the tendon thins with age.

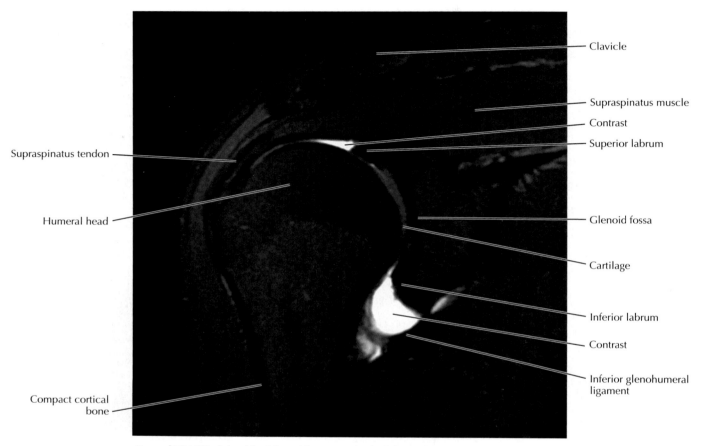

Clavicle

Supraspinatus muscle

Contrast

Superior labrum

Supraspinatus tendon

Humeral head

Glenoid fossa

Cartilage

Inferior labrum

Contrast

Inferior glenohumeral ligament

Compact cortical bone

Coronal T2 MRI of shoulder joint with contrast in the joint cavity

6.5 CORONAL T2 MRI OF THE SHOULDER JOINT

Most of the clinically significant problems of the four rotator cuff muscles involve the supraspinatus. It may be impinged between the acromion and the greater tubercle or under the acromioclavicular joint if there are downward-pointing osteophytes. It may also be torn. Because MRI provides good soft tissue contrast, it is often the modality of choice for evaluation of the rotator cuff and labrum. This is a T2, fat-saturated, coronal MRI arthrogram of the right shoulder. Note the rim of black surrounding the bones. This is cortex, which is mineral rich and low in water content and thus appears black (absent signal) on both T1- and T2-weighted sequences. The superior and inferior labra also have a low signal and are triangular shaped. Note the low signal of the tendons in this image. Because of their collagenous tissue, tendons are normally uniformly hypointense on all sequences (both T1 and T2). A tendon that is bright on a T2 sequence is often indicative of edema.

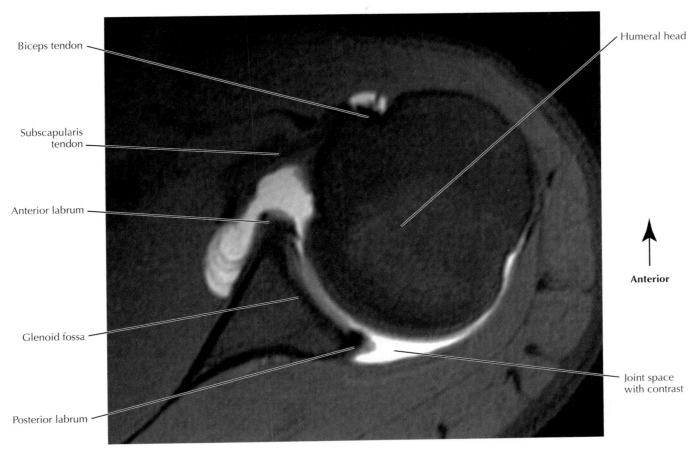

Biceps tendon

Subscapularis tendon

Anterior labrum

Glenoid fossa

Posterior labrum

Humeral head

Anterior

Joint space with contrast

Left axial T1 arthrogram

6.6 AXIAL T1 ARTHROGRAM OF THE SHOULDER JOINT

Note the high signal within the joint space. Normally on T1, synovial fluid should have a low-intermediate signal. The bright signal on this T1 image comes from contrast injected into the joint space using fluoroscopic guidance, which aids in assessment of the labrum. Normal anterior and posterior labra are seen here as triangular shaped, low-signal structures at the periphery of the glenoid fossa. The anterior labrum is typically larger than the posterior labrum and is more commonly involved in tears. A tear or detachment of the labrum would be indicated by the presence of fluid extending between the glenoid and labrum. The long head of the biceps tendon can be seen in the bicipital groove partly surrounded by contrast. It inserts onto the superior labrum, which is above the plane of this section. In athletes who throw a lot, the pull of the biceps tendon onto the superior labrum can cause it to tear in what is referred to as a *SLAP lesion* (superior labrum anterior to posterior). The superior glenoid is best visualized on an oblique coronal view.

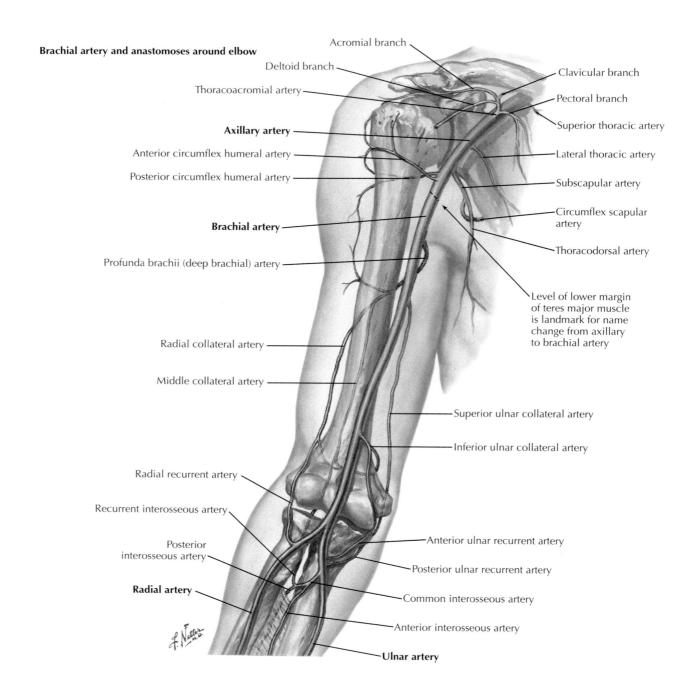

Brachial artery and anastomoses around elbow

Acromial branch

Deltoid branch

Thoracoacromial artery

Clavicular branch

Pectoral branch

Superior thoracic artery

Axillary artery

Anterior circumflex humeral artery

Posterior circumflex humeral artery

Lateral thoracic artery

Subscapular artery

Circumflex scapular artery

Brachial artery

Thoracodorsal artery

Profunda brachii (deep brachial) artery

Level of lower margin of teres major muscle is landmark for name change from axillary to brachial artery

Radial collateral artery

Middle collateral artery

Superior ulnar collateral artery

Inferior ulnar collateral artery

Radial recurrent artery

Recurrent interosseous artery

Posterior interosseous artery

Anterior ulnar recurrent artery

Posterior ulnar recurrent artery

Radial artery

Common interosseous artery

Anterior interosseous artery

Ulnar artery

6.7 AXILLARY, BRACHIAL, AND ELBOW ARTERIES

The brachial artery, a continuation of the axillary artery, divides just past the elbow into the radial and ulnar arteries. The common interosseus artery is the largest branch of the ulnar artery. The subclavian artery becomes the axillary artery at the lateral border of the first rib; the three largest branches of the latter are (1) the thoracoacromial artery to the pectoralis muscles and anterior part of the deltoid muscle, (2) the subscapular artery to scapular muscles and latissimus dorsi muscle, and (3) the posterior humeral circumflex artery to the larger, more posterior part of the deltoid muscle. The main branch of the brachial artery is the profunda brachii artery passing behind the humerus with the radial nerve to the triceps muscle. There are numerous anastomoses of arteries around the scapula and at the elbow via radial and ulnar collateral arteries.

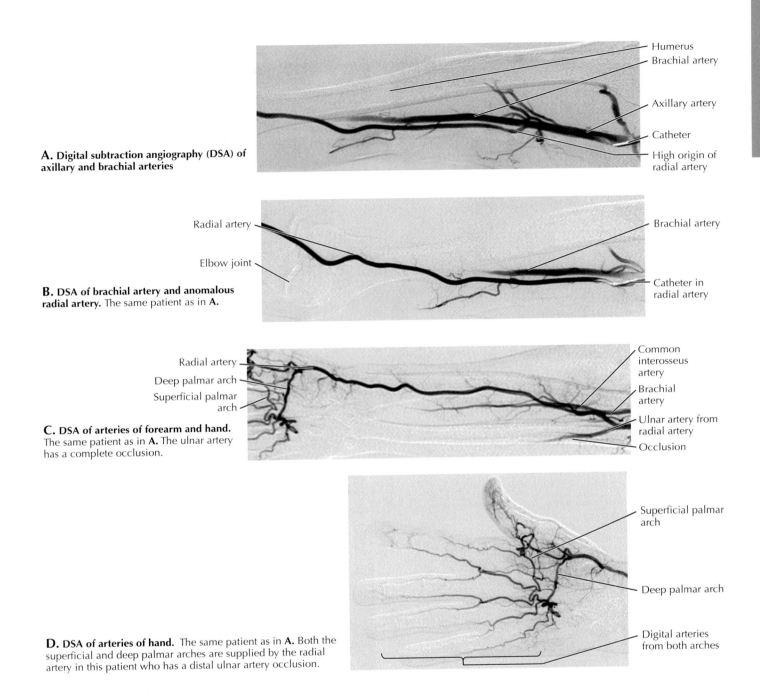

A. Digital subtraction angiography (DSA) of axillary and brachial arteries

Humerus
Brachial artery
Axillary artery
Catheter
High origin of radial artery

Radial artery
Elbow joint

Brachial artery
Catheter in radial artery

B. DSA of brachial artery and anomalous radial artery. The same patient as in **A.**

Radial artery
Deep palmar arch
Superficial palmar arch

Common interosseus artery
Brachial artery
Ulnar artery from radial artery
Occlusion

C. DSA of arteries of forearm and hand. The same patient as in **A.** The ulnar artery has a complete occlusion.

Superficial palmar arch
Deep palmar arch
Digital arteries from both arches

D. DSA of arteries of hand. The same patient as in **A.** Both the superficial and deep palmar arches are supplied by the radial artery in this patient who has a distal ulnar artery occlusion.

6.8 VASCULAR STUDIES OF THE UPPER EXTREMITY

Digital subtraction angiography (DSA), computed tomography angiography (CTA), and magnetic resonance angiography (MRA) all are used to detect vascular pathology such as arterial occlusions, stenoses, aneurysms, fistulas, and trauma. They are also useful for detecting anatomical variations. This particular patient (**A** to **D**) had symptoms consistent with intermittent hand ischemia. DSA confirmed ulnar artery occlusion and revealed anatomy amenable to vascular bypass of the occlusion. Findings from this DSA include: (1) a high origin of the radial artery from the brachial artery (**A** and **B**); (2) the ulnar artery arising from the radial artery (**C**) but completely occluded in the forearm; and (3) both the superficial and deep palmar arches in the hand supplied by the radial artery (the superficial palmar arch is typically supplied by the ulnar artery).

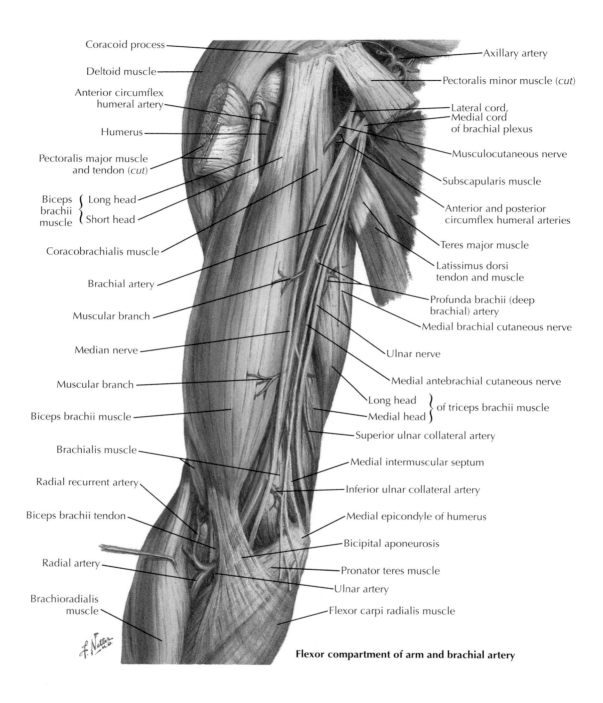

Coracoid process

Deltoid muscle

Anterior circumflex humeral artery

Humerus

Pectoralis major muscle and tendon (*cut*)

Biceps brachii muscle { Long head / Short head }

Coracobrachialis muscle

Brachial artery

Muscular branch

Median nerve

Muscular branch

Biceps brachii muscle

Brachialis muscle

Radial recurrent artery

Biceps brachii tendon

Radial artery

Brachioradialis muscle

Axillary artery

Pectoralis minor muscle (*cut*)

Lateral cord, Medial cord of brachial plexus

Musculocutaneous nerve

Subscapularis muscle

Anterior and posterior circumflex humeral arteries

Teres major muscle

Latissimus dorsi tendon and muscle

Profunda brachii (deep brachial) artery

Medial brachial cutaneous nerve

Ulnar nerve

Medial antebrachial cutaneous nerve

Long head / Medial head } of triceps brachii muscle

Superior ulnar collateral artery

Medial intermuscular septum

Inferior ulnar collateral artery

Medial epicondyle of humerus

Bicipital aponeurosis

Pronator teres muscle

Ulnar artery

Flexor carpi radialis muscle

Flexor compartment of arm and brachial artery

6.9 ARM MUSCLES

The flexor compartment of the arm contains the coracobrachialis muscle and the biceps brachii muscle overlying the brachialis muscle. At the shoulder the biceps brachii muscle has long and short heads. The short head runs with the coracobrachialis muscle; both attach to the coracoid process of the scapula and flex the shoulder joint. The tendon of the long head enters the cavity of the glenohumeral joint to attach to the supraglenoid tubercle. The two heads of the biceps brachii and the coracobrachialis muscle are covered by pectoralis major. The large neurovascular bundle containing the median nerve, ulnar nerve, brachial artery and veins, and basilic vein is medial to the biceps brachii muscle.

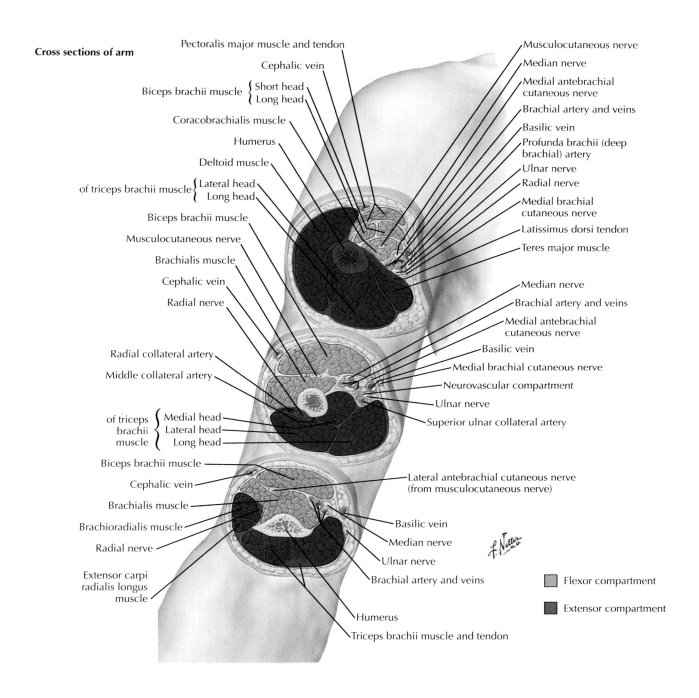

Cross sections of arm

Pectoralis major muscle and tendon
Cephalic vein
Biceps brachii muscle { Short head / Long head
Coracobrachialis muscle
Humerus
Deltoid muscle
of triceps brachii muscle { Lateral head / Long head
Biceps brachii muscle
Musculocutaneous nerve
Brachialis muscle
Cephalic vein
Radial nerve
Radial collateral artery
Middle collateral artery
of triceps brachii muscle { Medial head / Lateral head / Long head
Biceps brachii muscle
Cephalic vein
Brachialis muscle
Brachioradialis muscle
Radial nerve
Extensor carpi radialis longus muscle

Musculocutaneous nerve
Median nerve
Medial antebrachial cutaneous nerve
Brachial artery and veins
Basilic vein
Profunda brachii (deep brachial) artery
Ulnar nerve
Radial nerve
Medial brachial cutaneous nerve
Latissimus dorsi tendon
Teres major muscle
Median nerve
Brachial artery and veins
Medial antebrachial cutaneous nerve
Basilic vein
Medial brachial cutaneous nerve
Neurovascular compartment
Ulnar nerve
Superior ulnar collateral artery
Lateral antebrachial cutaneous nerve (from musculocutaneous nerve)
Basilic vein
Median nerve
Ulnar nerve
Brachial artery and veins
Humerus
Triceps brachii muscle and tendon

Flexor compartment
Extensor compartment

6.10 ARM SERIAL CROSS SECTIONS

A useful approach to cross sections is to first identify the flexor and extensor muscle compartments. The middle of the arm has the biceps brachii and brachialis flexor muscles anteriorly and the triceps (an extensor) posteriorly. At the shoulder the deltoid (extensor compartment) and pectoralis major (flexor compartment) are prominent superficial muscles. Near the elbow two additional forearm extensor compartment muscles are seen: brachioradialis and extensor carpi radialis longus. The large neurovascular bundle supplying much of the upper extremity is medial and deep to the biceps brachii muscle. The radial nerve and profunda brachii artery pass posterior to the humerus to enter the extensor compartment.

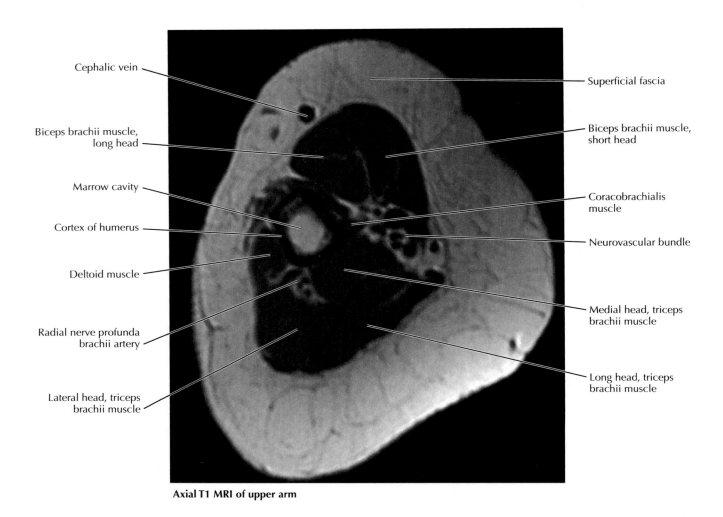

Cephalic vein

Biceps brachii muscle,
long head

Marrow cavity

Cortex of humerus

Deltoid muscle

Radial nerve profunda
brachii artery

Lateral head, triceps
brachii muscle

Superficial fascia

Biceps brachii muscle,
short head

Coracobrachialis
muscle

Neurovascular bundle

Medial head, triceps
brachii muscle

Long head, triceps
brachii muscle

Axial T1 MRI of upper arm

6.11 ARM MRI

This is a T1-weighted axial image of the left upper arm. MRI in musculoskeletal radiology is good for evaluation of soft tissues (muscles, tendons, and ligaments), pathology affecting the bone marrow such as neoplasms or osteomyelitis, and occult fractures that are suspected but not seen on conventional x-rays. In this T1-weighted MR image, what appears to be white bone of the humerus is actually the fatty marrow within the bone. The black ring is the cortex. The biceps and the long and lateral heads of the triceps are seen here. The black "space" between the two heads of the triceps in this image is an area of absent signal coming from the triceps tendon. Tendons appear black on MRI because they have little water content and thus lack the mobile protons necessary to create a signal. This is also why bone cortex, fibrocartilage, collagenous tissues, and tissue fibrosis do not produce a signal on MRI. Also seen in this image are the brachial vessels, the ulnar and median nerve, and the cephalic vein. The cephalic vein is located within the high signal–producing fatty subcutaneous tissue.

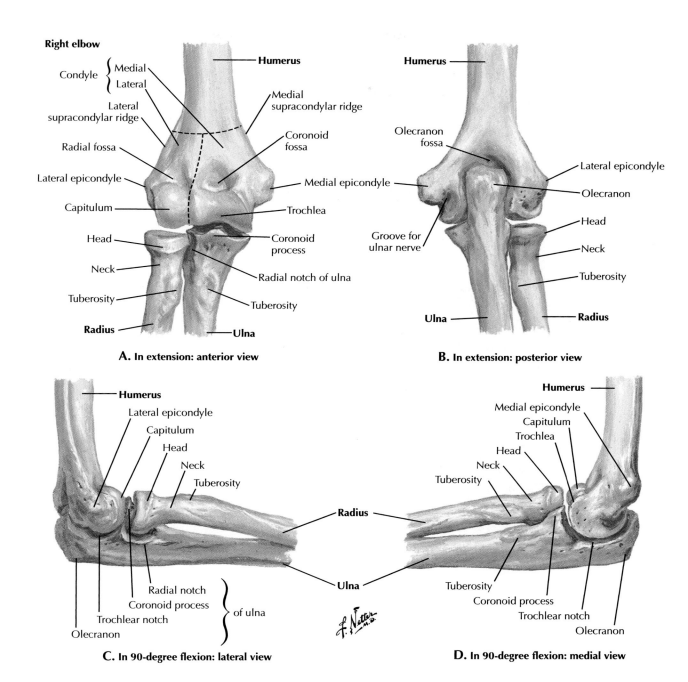

Right elbow

Condyle { Medial, Lateral

Humerus

Medial supracondylar ridge

Lateral supracondylar ridge

Coronoid fossa

Radial fossa

Lateral epicondyle

Medial epicondyle

Capitulum

Trochlea

Head

Coronoid process

Neck

Radial notch of ulna

Tuberosity

Tuberosity

Radius

Ulna

A. In extension: anterior view

Humerus

Olecranon fossa

Lateral epicondyle

Olecranon

Groove for ulnar nerve

Head

Neck

Tuberosity

Ulna

Radius

B. In extension: posterior view

Humerus

Lateral epicondyle

Capitulum

Head

Neck

Tuberosity

Radius

Radial notch

Coronoid process } of ulna

Trochlear notch

Olecranon

Ulna

C. In 90-degree flexion: lateral view

Humerus

Medial epicondyle

Capitulum

Trochlea

Head

Neck

Tuberosity

Tuberosity

Coronoid process

Trochlear notch

Olecranon

D. In 90-degree flexion: medial view

6.12 BONES OF THE ELBOW

The elbow joint is a uniaxial hinge joint between the ulna and the trochlea of the humerus where flexion and extension occur. The head of the radius pivots on the capitulum for pronation and supination of the forearm. The medial epicondyle is larger than the lateral epicondyle because the stronger flexor muscles of the forearm and hand originate from it. It is called the *funny bone* because the ulnar nerve passes behind it, and tingling (or more severe symptoms) can occur when it is compressed. The extensor muscles originate from the lateral epicondyle. Extension is checked as the olecranon process of the ulna encounters the olecranon fossa of the humerus.

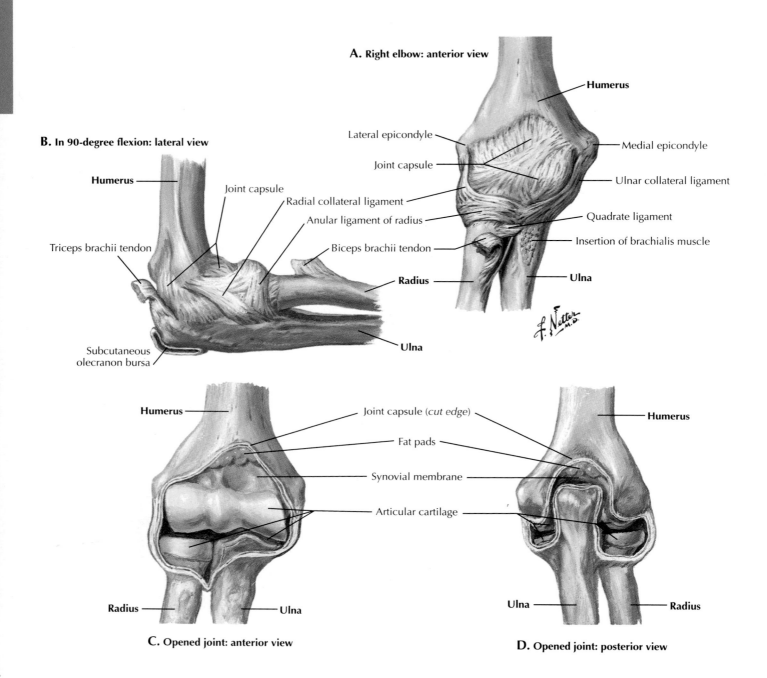

A. Right elbow: anterior view

Humerus

Lateral epicondyle

Joint capsule

Medial epicondyle

Ulnar collateral ligament

Quadrate ligament

Insertion of brachialis muscle

Radius

Ulna

B. In 90-degree flexion: lateral view

Humerus

Joint capsule

Radial collateral ligament

Anular ligament of radius

Triceps brachii tendon

Biceps brachii tendon

Radius

Subcutaneous olecranon bursa

Ulna

Humerus

Joint capsule (*cut edge*)

Fat pads

Synovial membrane

Articular cartilage

Humerus

Radius

Ulna

Ulna

Radius

C. Opened joint: anterior view

D. Opened joint: posterior view

6.13 JOINTS OF THE ELBOW

There is one common joint cavity for the articulation of the radius and ulna with the humerus in flexion/extension and with the head of the radius against the ulna in pronation/supination. Strong ulnar (medial) and radial (lateral) collateral ligaments prevent abduction and adduction of the elbow joint. The annular ligament holds the head of the radius against the ulna. The olecranon bursa reduces friction as the skin moves over the olecranon process of the ulna during flexion and extension.

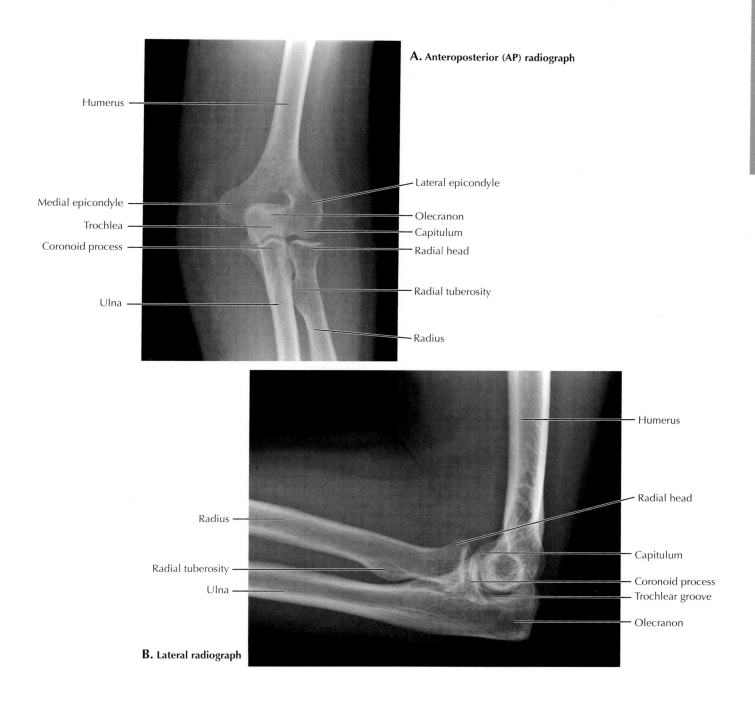

A. Anteroposterior (AP) radiograph

Humerus

Medial epicondyle

Trochlea

Coronoid process

Ulna

Lateral epicondyle

Olecranon

Capitulum

Radial head

Radial tuberosity

Radius

Radius

Radial tuberosity

Ulna

Humerus

Radial head

Capitulum

Coronoid process

Trochlear groove

Olecranon

B. Lateral radiograph

6.14 ELBOW X-RAYS

Most of the elbow imaging is done for the evaluation of trauma. The two views normally taken are an AP with the arm extended and a lateral with the arm flexed 90 degrees. In the lateral image, one should check the alignment of the anterior cortex of the humerus with the capitulum. This is called the *anterior humeral line*. If it does not pass through the middle third of the capitulum, a supracondylar fracture should be suspected. In addition, the radial head should be aligned with the capitulum on every view. In the lateral view, one should evaluate for the presence and location of the fat pads inside the elbow joint anterior and posterior to the distal humerus. If the anterior fat pad is visible, it should appear as a thin lucent line adjacent to the distal anterior humerus. A posterior fat pad should never be visible. If trauma has occurred, intra-articular accumulation of blood may push the fat pads away from the bone. In such cases the fat pad appears anteriorly as a radiolucent "sail" on a sailboat (the "sail" sign), and the posterior fat pad may become visible. These signs should raise suspicion for a fracture, most often of the radial head in adults and of the distal humerus in children.

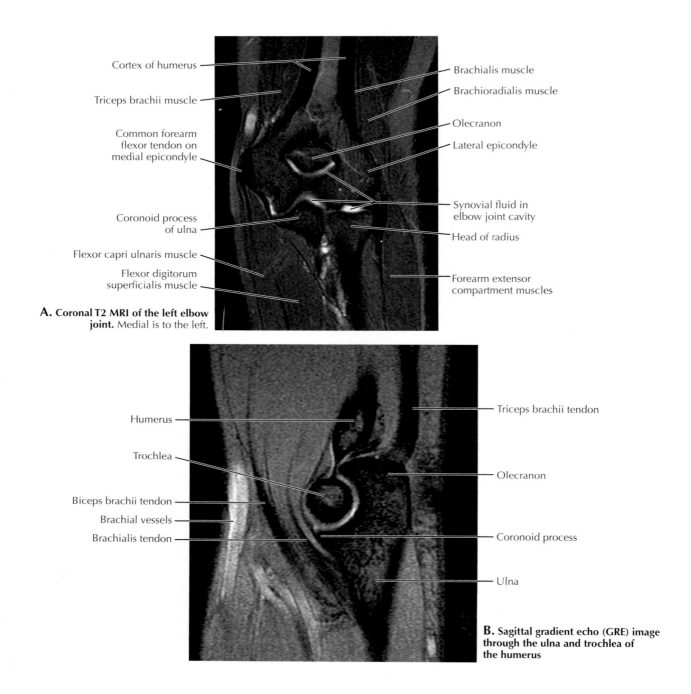

Cortex of humerus

Triceps brachii muscle

Common forearm flexor tendon on medial epicondyle

Coronoid process of ulna

Flexor capri ulnaris muscle

Flexor digitorum superficialis muscle

Brachialis muscle

Brachioradialis muscle

Olecranon

Lateral epicondyle

Synovial fluid in elbow joint cavity

Head of radius

Forearm extensor compartment muscles

A. Coronal T2 MRI of the left elbow joint. Medial is to the left.

Humerus

Trochlea

Biceps brachii tendon

Brachial vessels

Brachialis tendon

Triceps brachii tendon

Olecranon

Coronoid process

Ulna

B. Sagittal gradient echo (GRE) image through the ulna and trochlea of the humerus

6.15 ELBOW IMAGING STUDIES

A is a coronal T2 image of the left arm. Superior to the joint one can see the triceps brachii medially and the brachioradialis and brachialis muscles laterally. On the medial epicondyle there is an area void of signal. This is the origin of the common flexor tendon, which is usually shorter and broader than the common extensor tendon seen originating from the lateral epicondyle. A high signal coming from these tendons may be seen in someone who has medial epicondylitis (golfer) or lateral epicondylitis (tennis player), respectively. The areas of high signal within the joint are from the intraarticular fluid, which is bright in T2 images. **B** was taken using a gradient echo (GRE) sequence, which can be completed faster than most sequences but with lower image contrast. Flowing blood has a high signal on GRE sequences, as seen here in the brachial artery and veins located anteriorly. The hypointense triceps tendon is seen inserting onto the olecranon process posteriorly, and the distal aspects of the biceps brachii and brachialis muscles can be seen anteriorly.

Muscles of forearm (superficial layer): anterior view

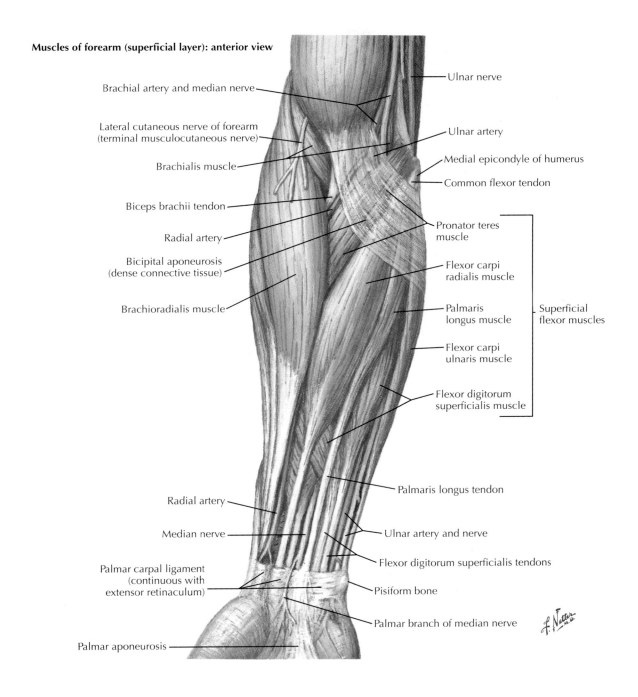

Brachial artery and median nerve

Lateral cutaneous nerve of forearm
(terminal musculocutaneous nerve)

Brachialis muscle

Biceps brachii tendon

Radial artery

Bicipital aponeurosis
(dense connective tissue)

Brachioradialis muscle

Radial artery

Median nerve

Palmar carpal ligament
(continuous with
extensor retinaculum)

Palmar aponeurosis

Ulnar nerve

Ulnar artery

Medial epicondyle of humerus

Common flexor tendon

Pronator teres
muscle

Flexor carpi
radialis muscle

Palmaris
longus muscle

Flexor carpi
ulnaris muscle

Flexor digitorum
superficialis muscle

Superficial
flexor muscles

Palmaris longus tendon

Ulnar artery and nerve

Flexor digitorum superficialis tendons

Pisiform bone

Palmar branch of median nerve

6.16 MUSCLES OF THE FOREARM: ANTERIOR VIEW

The flexor compartment of the forearm originates from the medial epicondyle of the humerus. The extensor compartment originates from the lateral epicondyle. Although the brachioradialis muscle flexes the elbow joint, it is part of the extensor compartment and innervated by the radial nerve (a posterior division nerve). The pronator teres is the most proximal flexor compartment muscle. The superficial muscles abduct and adduct the wrist joint and flex the wrist and medial four digits. The deep flexor compartment muscles are flexor pollicis longus, flexor digitorum longus, and pronator quadratus.

Muscles of forearm (superficial layer): posterior view

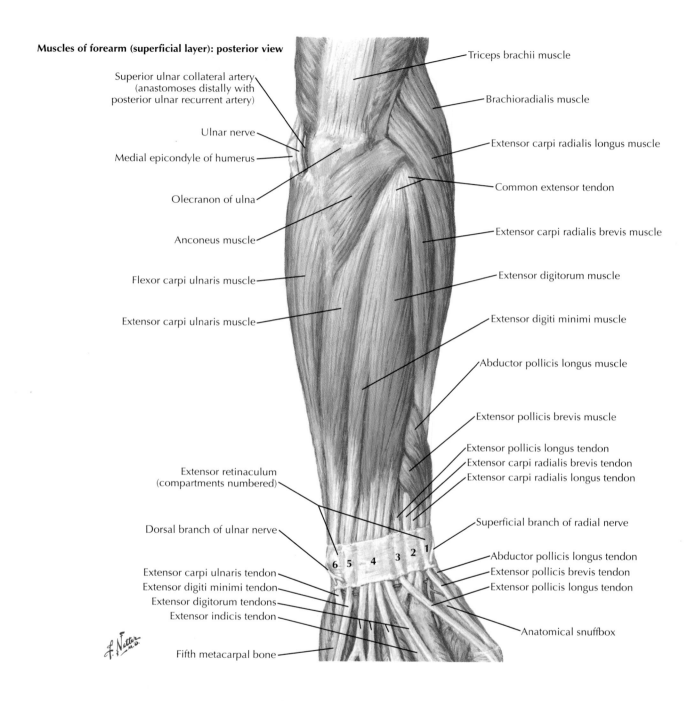

Superior ulnar collateral artery (anastomoses distally with posterior ulnar recurrent artery)

Ulnar nerve

Medial epicondyle of humerus

Olecranon of ulna

Anconeus muscle

Flexor carpi ulnaris muscle

Extensor carpi ulnaris muscle

Extensor retinaculum (compartments numbered)

Dorsal branch of ulnar nerve

Extensor carpi ulnaris tendon

Extensor digiti minimi tendon

Extensor digitorum tendons

Extensor indicis tendon

Fifth metacarpal bone

Triceps brachii muscle

Brachioradialis muscle

Extensor carpi radialis longus muscle

Common extensor tendon

Extensor carpi radialis brevis muscle

Extensor digitorum muscle

Extensor digiti minimi muscle

Abductor pollicis longus muscle

Extensor pollicis brevis muscle

Extensor pollicis longus tendon
Extensor carpi radialis brevis tendon
Extensor carpi radialis longus tendon

Superficial branch of radial nerve

Abductor pollicis longus tendon
Extensor pollicis brevis tendon
Extensor pollicis longus tendon

Anatomical snuffbox

6 5 4 3 2 1

6.17 MUSCLES OF THE FOREARM: POSTERIOR VIEW

Here we can see the extensor compartment originating from the lateral epicondyle and lateral supracondylar ridge. A bit of the flexor compartment (flexor carpi ulnaris) is seen medially.

As the name implies, the extensor compartment muscles extend the wrist and digits. They join flexor compartment muscles in abducting and adducting the wrist. They also extend and abduct the thumb.

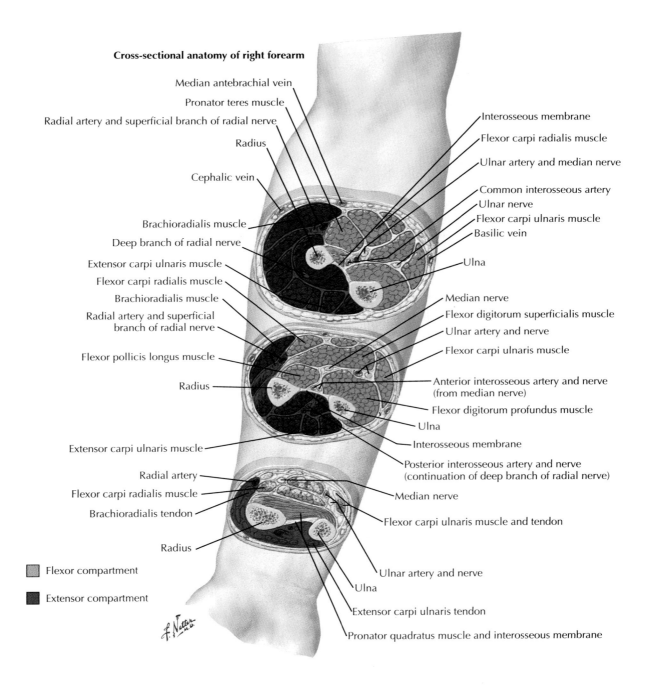

Cross-sectional anatomy of right forearm

Median antebrachial vein

Pronator teres muscle

Radial artery and superficial branch of radial nerve

Radius

Cephalic vein

Brachioradialis muscle

Deep branch of radial nerve

Extensor carpi ulnaris muscle

Flexor carpi radialis muscle

Brachioradialis muscle

Radial artery and superficial branch of radial nerve

Flexor pollicis longus muscle

Radius

Extensor carpi ulnaris muscle

Radial artery

Flexor carpi radialis muscle

Brachioradialis tendon

Radius

Interosseous membrane

Flexor carpi radialis muscle

Ulnar artery and median nerve

Common interosseous artery

Ulnar nerve

Flexor carpi ulnaris muscle

Basilic vein

Ulna

Median nerve

Flexor digitorum superficialis muscle

Ulnar artery and nerve

Flexor carpi ulnaris muscle

Anterior interosseous artery and nerve (from median nerve)

Flexor digitorum profundus muscle

Ulna

Interosseous membrane

Posterior interosseous artery and nerve (continuation of deep branch of radial nerve)

Median nerve

Flexor carpi ulnaris muscle and tendon

Ulnar artery and nerve

Ulna

Extensor carpi ulnaris tendon

Pronator quadratus muscle and interosseous membrane

☐ Flexor compartment

■ Extensor compartment

f. Netter M.D.

6.18 FOREARM SERIAL CROSS SECTIONS

The interosseus membrane between the radius and ulna separates the flexor and extensor compartments, although the extensors are also lateral on the forearm and the flexors are medial because of their origins from the humerus. The median nerve is in the middle of the flexor compartment that it supplies; the ulnar nerve is medial to it, innervating flexor carpi ulnaris, the ulnar half of flexor digitorum profundus, and intrinsic hand muscles. The radial nerve supplies the extensor muscles.

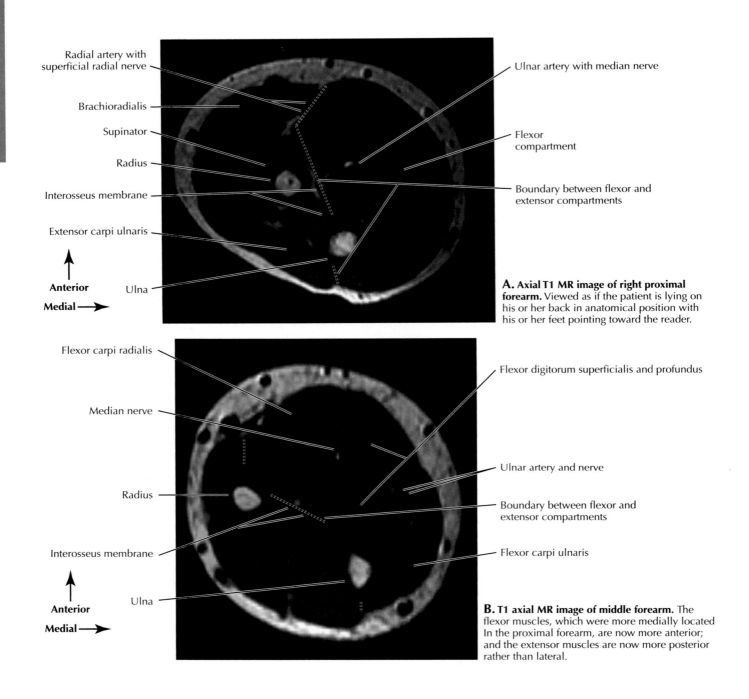

Radial artery with superficial radial nerve

Brachioradialis

Supinator

Radius

Interosseus membrane

Extensor carpi ulnaris

Anterior

Medial →

Ulna

Ulnar artery with median nerve

Flexor compartment

Boundary between flexor and extensor compartments

A. Axial T1 MR image of right proximal forearm. Viewed as if the patient is lying on his or her back in anatomical position with his or her feet pointing toward the reader.

Flexor carpi radialis

Median nerve

Radius

Interosseus membrane

Anterior

Medial →

Ulna

Flexor digitorum superficialis and profundus

Ulnar artery and nerve

Boundary between flexor and extensor compartments

Flexor carpi ulnaris

B. T1 axial MR image of middle forearm. The flexor muscles, which were more medially located in the proximal forearm, are now more anterior; and the extensor muscles are now more posterior rather than lateral.

6.19 UPPER AND MIDDLE FOREARM MRI

MRI in general is very sensitive but nonspecific for muscle abnormalities. T1-weighted sequences are good for assessment of muscle architecture and identification of muscle atrophy. On MR images muscles generally have a marbled appearance because of the presence of fat interposed between fibers within the muscle and between adjacent muscles. In areas where there is little intermuscular fat, individual muscle groups blend together and are difficult to identify, as is the case in this image with the flexor muscles that are located medially. The extensor muscles are a little easier to make out individually. Superior to the radius is an area of increased signal. This area contains the radial artery and the superficial branch of the radial nerve that lie within the intermuscular fat between the extensor and flexor compartments. A muscle that atrophies, which is not present in this image, is replaced with fat and therefore appears as an area of increased signal in T1-weighted images. A loss of the normal fatty marbling within muscle or distortion of the intermuscular fascial planes may suggest a tumor.

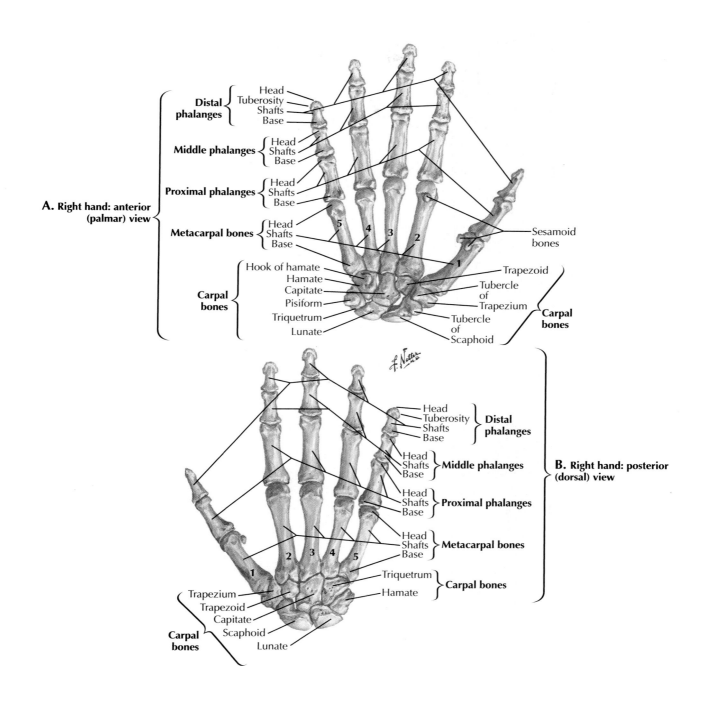

A. Right hand: anterior (palmar) view

Distal phalanges
- Head
- Tuberosity
- Shafts
- Base

Middle phalanges
- Head
- Shafts
- Base

Proximal phalanges
- Head
- Shafts
- Base

Metacarpal bones
- Head
- Shafts
- Base

Carpal bones
- Hook of hamate
- Hamate
- Capitate
- Pisiform
- Triquetrum
- Lunate

Trapezoid
Tubercle of Trapezium
Tubercle of Scaphoid

Sesamoid bones

Carpal bones

B. Right hand: posterior (dorsal) view

Distal phalanges
- Head
- Tuberosity
- Shafts
- Base

Middle phalanges
- Head
- Shafts
- Base

Proximal phalanges
- Head
- Shafts
- Base

Metacarpal bones
- Head
- Shafts
- Base

Carpal bones
- Triquetrum
- Hamate

Carpal bones
- Trapezium
- Trapezoid
- Capitate
- Scaphoid
- Lunate

6.20 BONES OF THE HAND AND WRIST

The radiocarpal joint is the wrist joint, a biaxial joint where flexion/extension and abduction/adduction occur but no rotation. The radius articulates with the scaphoid and lunate bones. The digital rays have a metacarpal bone and three phalanges (proximal, middle, and distal), although the thumb has only two phalanges (proximal and distal). The metacarpophalangeal joints ("knuckles") of digits 2 to 5 are biaxial joints like the wrist joint; ligaments prevent rotation.

Carpometacarpal joints for digits 2 to 4 have little movement, whereas the joint between the trapezium and first metacarpal of the thumb is a multiaxial joint. Because of the naturally rotated position of the thumb, flexion/extension is in a coronal plane, and abduction/adduction is in a sagittal plane. The saddle-shaped joint with the trapezium allows the rotation that is required in opposition of the thumb with the other digits.

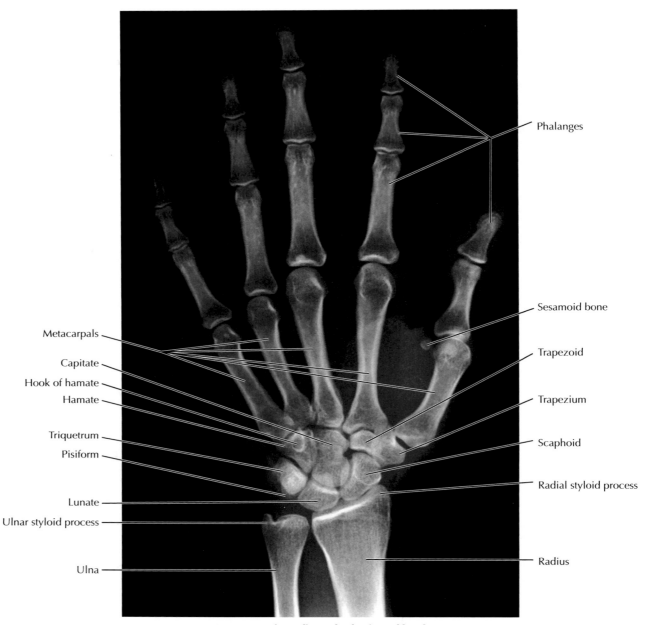

Metacarpals

Capitate

Hook of hamate

Hamate

Triquetrum

Pisiform

Lunate

Ulnar styloid process

Ulna

Phalanges

Sesamoid bone

Trapezoid

Trapezium

Scaphoid

Radial styloid process

Radius

Anteroposterior radiograph of wrist and hand

6.21 ANTEROPOSTERIOR X-RAY OF THE WRIST AND HAND

When evaluating an AP radiograph of the wrist, examine the distal radius and ulna, including the styloid processes. Note the angle of inclination (called *radial tilt)* of the distal radius articular surface should be 16 to 28 degrees to a line perpendicular to the long axis of the radius. A common injury is a fracture to the distal radius (Colles and Smith fractures). Angulation of the distal fragment should be assessed in a lateral film if such a fracture is seen or suspected. Next evaluate the carpal bones. The space between the carpal bones should be uniform and similar to that at the radiocarpal joint.

One should also be able to clearly make out the crescent-shaped proximal row (scaphoid, lunate, triquetrum, pisiform) and the distal row (trapezium, trapezoid, capitate, hamate) row. The most common carpal bone to be fractured is the scaphoid. This should be considered in a patient complaining of pain in the snuffbox region following a fall on an outstretched arm. Because the blood supply to the scaphoid flows distally to proximally, a fracture can disrupt the blood supply to the proximal part of the bone, leading to avascular necrosis (tissue death). If the fracture is occult on plain film, the patient can be casted and reimaged in 7 to 10 days, or they can get a CT or MRI, which readily identifies a fracture if it is present.

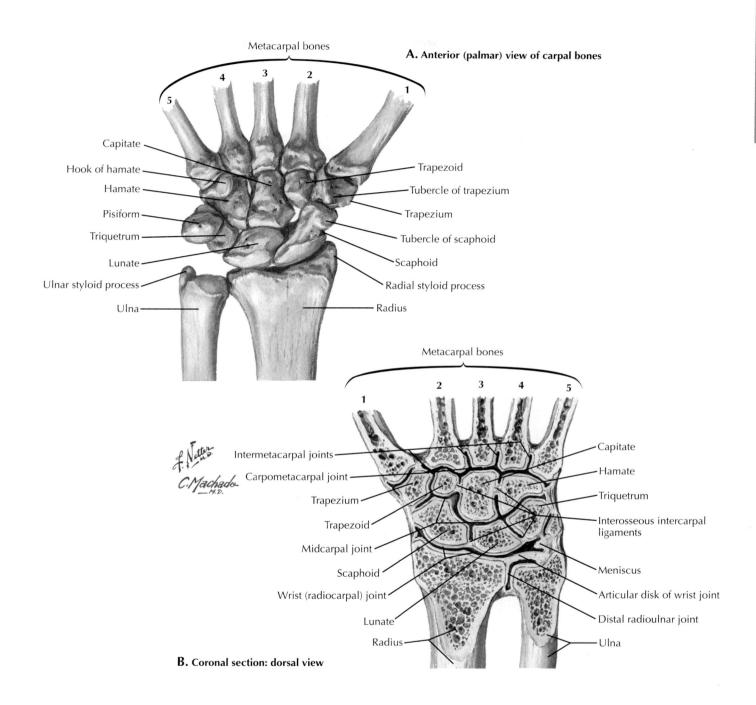

A. Anterior (palmar) view of carpal bones

Metacarpal bones

Capitate
Hook of hamate
Hamate
Pisiform
Triquetrum
Lunate
Ulnar styloid process
Ulna

Trapezoid
Tubercle of trapezium
Trapezium
Tubercle of scaphoid
Scaphoid
Radial styloid process
Radius

Metacarpal bones

Intermetacarpal joints
Carpometacarpal joint
Trapezium
Trapezoid
Midcarpal joint
Scaphoid
Wrist (radiocarpal) joint
Lunate
Radius

Capitate
Hamate
Triquetrum
Interosseous intercarpal ligaments
Meniscus
Articular disk of wrist joint
Distal radioulnar joint
Ulna

B. Coronal section: dorsal view

6.22 CARPAL BONES AND WRIST JOINT

There are two rows of carpal bones between the radius and metacarpal bones. The radius articulates mostly with the scaphoid ("boat-shaped") and a bit of the lunate bone to form the wrist joint. The head of the capitate ("head-shaped") bone articulates in the midcarpal joint between the two rows of bones, although little movement occurs here. The trapezium articulates with the first metacarpal of the thumb. The flexor retinaculum attaches to the hook of the hamate ("hooklike") bone, pisiform bone, and tubercles of the trapezium and scaphoid bones to enclose the carpal tunnel, which contains the long flexor tendons to the digits, the flexor pollicis longus tendon, and the median nerve. The ulnar artery and nerve pass into the hand superficial to the flexor retinaculum.

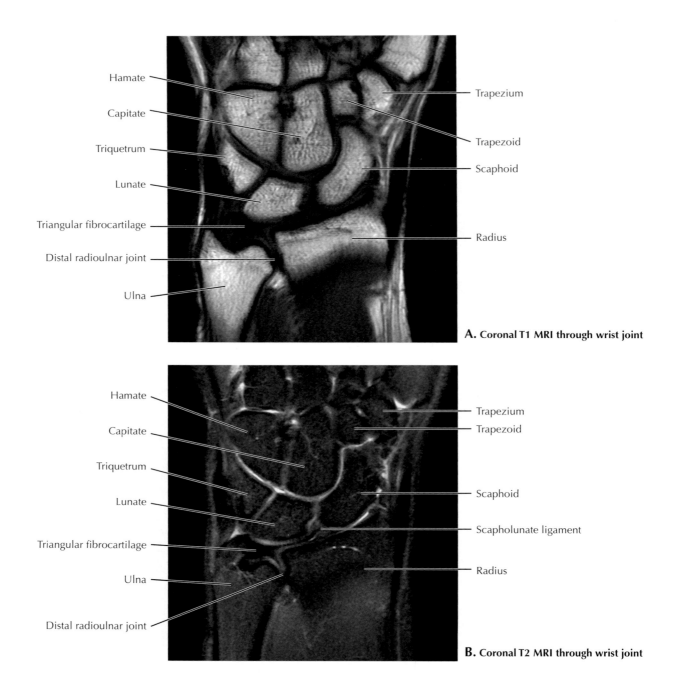

Hamate — Capitate — Triquetrum — Lunate — Triangular fibrocartilage — Distal radioulnar joint — Ulna

Trapezium — Trapezoid — Scaphoid — Radius

A. Coronal T1 MRI through wrist joint

Hamate — Capitate — Triquetrum — Lunate — Triangular fibrocartilage — Ulna — Distal radioulnar joint

Trapezium — Trapezoid — Scaphoid — Scapholunate ligament — Radius

B. Coronal T2 MRI through wrist joint

6.23 T1 AND T2 MRI OF THE WRIST JOINT

A and **B** are coronal slices of the wrist in a T1-weighted and T2-weighted MR sequence, respectively. If a fracture is present, it would appear as a linear area of low signal intensity. On a T2-weighted sequence, an acute fracture has a surrounding area of high signal representing bone marrow edema. The interosseous areas of high signal on the T2-weighted MR sequence represent normal synovial fluid. Osteoneonecrosis would appear as an area of low signal within the bone on both T1-weighted and T2-weighted sequences. On both sequences,

the areas of lowest signals come from tendons and other connective tissues such as the triangular fibrocartilage just distal to the ulna. A T2-weighted coronal slice of the wrist is particularly good for evaluation of the ligaments in the wrist and hand. The scapholunate and lunotriquetral ligaments are the most important intrinsic ligaments because they help maintain the alignment of the carpal bones. As in an AP x-ray, the spaces between the carpal bones should be uniform and similar to that of the radiocarpal joint.

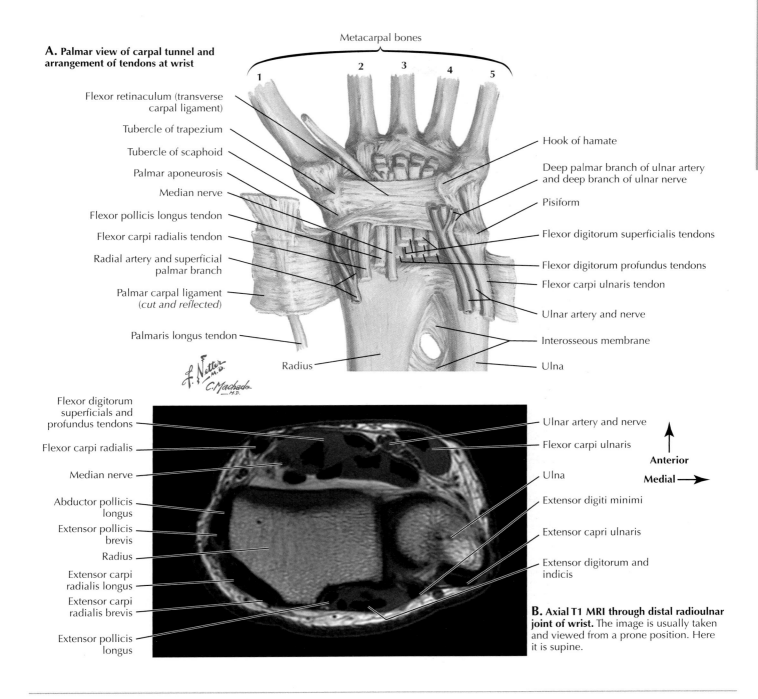

A. Palmar view of carpal tunnel and arrangement of tendons at wrist

Metacarpal bones

1 2 3 4 5

Flexor retinaculum (transverse carpal ligament)

Tubercle of trapezium

Tubercle of scaphoid

Palmar aponeurosis

Median nerve

Flexor pollicis longus tendon

Flexor carpi radialis tendon

Radial artery and superficial palmar branch

Palmar carpal ligament (*cut and reflected*)

Palmaris longus tendon

Radius

Hook of hamate

Deep palmar branch of ulnar artery and deep branch of ulnar nerve

Pisiform

Flexor digitorum superficialis tendons

Flexor digitorum profundus tendons

Flexor carpi ulnaris tendon

Ulnar artery and nerve

Interosseous membrane

Ulna

Flexor digitorum superficials and profundus tendons

Flexor carpi radialis

Median nerve

Abductor pollicis longus

Extensor pollicis brevis

Radius

Extensor carpi radialis longus

Extensor carpi radialis brevis

Extensor pollicis longus

Ulnar artery and nerve

Flexor carpi ulnaris

Anterior

Medial →

Ulna

Extensor digiti minimi

Extensor capri ulnaris

Extensor digitorum and indicis

B. Axial T1 MRI through distal radioulnar joint of wrist. The image is usually taken and viewed from a prone position. Here it is supine.

6.24 DISTAL RADIOCARPAL JOINT AND WRIST

The tendons of the wrist are best assessed in an axial image such as in **B,** taken at the distal radioulnar joint. This is a T1-weighted image, as indicated by the high signal coming from the fat located in the subcutaneous tissue and the bone marrow. The tendons should appear as oval-round areas of low signal intensity, as they do in this image. The extensor tendons are located dorsal to the ulna and radius. They are divided into six compartments (I to VI). Compartment number I is located just lateral to the radius and contains the extensor pollicis brevis tendon and the abductor pollicis longus tendon. In this image they are adjacent to one another and appear as one tendon. Compartment VI is located just dorsal to the ulna and contains the extensor carpi ulnaris. Note the relative sizes of the tendons and the signal surrounding them. Abnormally large tendons may indicate tendon fibrosis (e.g., De Quervain's syndrome), whereas a relatively enlarged tendon surrounded by fluid may indicate tenosynovitis. Located on the ventral side of the radioulnar joint are the flexor tendons, the palmaris longus tendon, and the median and ulnar nerves. The median nerve can be differentiated from the surrounding lower-intensity tendons.

7

LOWER LIMBS

7.1   HIP (COXAL OR INNOMINATE) BONE

7.2   HIP JOINT

7.3   HIP JOINT X-RAY

7.4   IMAGING STUDIES OF THE HIP JOINT

7.5   FEMUR

7.6   MUSCLES OF THE THIGH: ANTERIOR VIEW

7.7   MUSCLES OF THE THIGH: POSTERIOR VIEW

7.8   THIGH SERIAL CROSS SECTIONS

7.9   UPPER RIGHT THIGH T1 MRI

7.10   MIDDLE RIGHT THIGH T1 MRI

7.11   LOWER RIGHT THIGH T1 MRI

7.12   KNEE AND KNEE JOINT OVERVIEW

7.13   KNEE JOINT INTERIOR

7.14   KNEE JOINT LIGAMENTS

7.15   KNEE JOINT X-RAY

7.16   SAGITTAL SECTION OF THE KNEE JOINT AND T2 MRI

7.17   CORONAL AND AXIAL T2 MRI STUDIES OF THE KNEE

7.18   ARTERIES OF THE THIGH AND KNEE

7.19   MAGNETIC RESONANCE ANGIOGRAPHY OF THE THIGH

7.20   TIBIA AND FIBULA

7.21   MUSCLES OF THE LEG: ANTERIOR VIEW

7.22   MUSCLES OF THE LEG: POSTERIOR VIEW

7.23   MUSCLES OF THE LEG: LATERAL VIEW

7.24   LEG CROSS SECTION AND FASCIAL COMPARTMENTS

7.25 AXIAL T1 MRI THROUGH THE LEG

7.26 VASCULAR STUDIES OF THE LOWER EXTREMITY: CTA/MRA OF THE LEG AND LOWER EXTREMITIES

7.27 DIGITAL SUBTRACTION ANGIOGRAPHY OF THE RIGHT LOWER EXTREMITY

7.28 BONES OF THE FOOT: SUPERIOR AND INFERIOR VIEWS

7.29 BONES OF THE FOOT: MEDIAL AND LATERAL VIEWS

7.30 ANKLE X-RAYS

7.31 CORONAL T1 AND T2 MRI OF THE ANKLE

7.32 SAGITTAL T1 AND T2 MRI OF THE ANKLE

7.33 X-RAYS OF THE FOOT

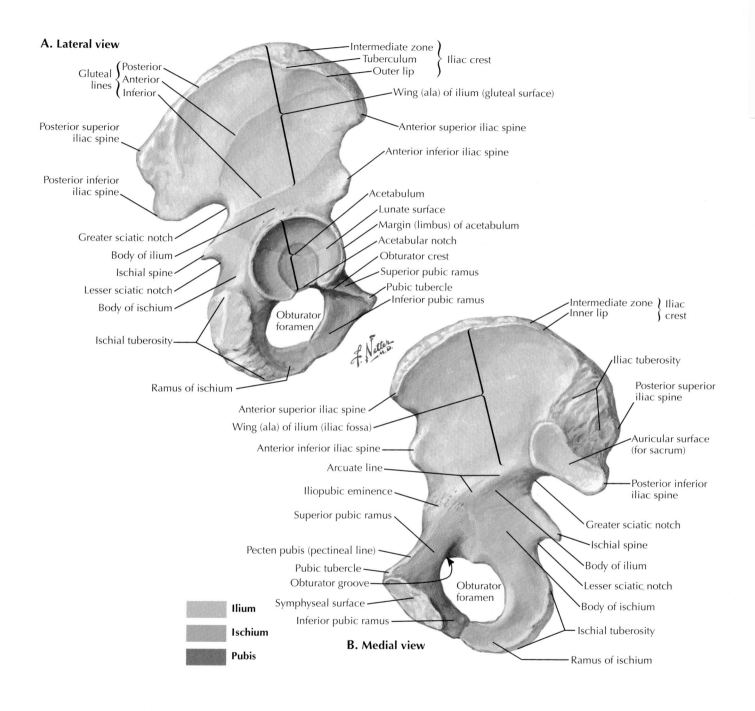

A. Lateral view

Gluteal lines { Posterior / Anterior / Inferior }

Intermediate zone ⎫
Tuberculum ⎬ Iliac crest
Outer lip ⎭

Wing (ala) of ilium (gluteal surface)

Posterior superior iliac spine

Anterior superior iliac spine

Anterior inferior iliac spine

Posterior inferior iliac spine

Acetabulum
Lunate surface
Margin (limbus) of acetabulum
Acetabular notch
Obturator crest
Superior pubic ramus
Pubic tubercle
Inferior pubic ramus

Greater sciatic notch
Body of ilium
Ischial spine
Lesser sciatic notch
Body of ischium

Obturator foramen

Ischial tuberosity

f. Netter M.D.

Ramus of ischium

Anterior superior iliac spine
Wing (ala) of ilium (iliac fossa)
Anterior inferior iliac spine
Arcuate line
Iliopubic eminence
Superior pubic ramus
Pecten pubis (pectineal line)
Pubic tubercle
Obturator groove
Symphyseal surface
Inferior pubic ramus

Intermediate zone ⎫ Iliac
Inner lip ⎬ crest

Iliac tuberosity

Posterior superior iliac spine

Auricular surface (for sacrum)

Posterior inferior iliac spine

Greater sciatic notch
Ischial spine
Body of ilium
Lesser sciatic notch
Body of ischium

Obturator foramen

Ischial tuberosity

Ramus of ischium

B. Medial view

Ilium
Ischium
Pubis

7.1 HIP (COXAL OR INNOMINATE) BONE

The hip bone is an innominate bone consisting of fused ilium, ischium, and pubic bones. Each has its own ossification center. Cartilage is replaced by bone by age 10, and complete fusion in the acetabulum occurs around puberty. Left and right innominate bones articulate with the sacrum at the auricular ("ear-shaped") surfaces to comprise the pelvis.

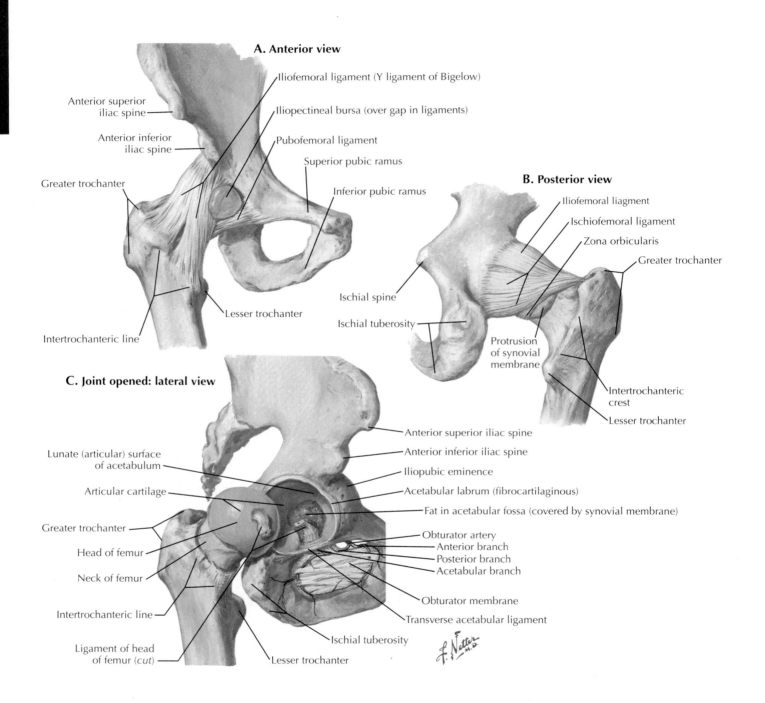

A. Anterior view

Iliofemoral ligament (Y ligament of Bigelow)

Anterior superior iliac spine

Iliopectineal bursa (over gap in ligaments)

Anterior inferior iliac spine

Pubofemoral ligament

Greater trochanter

Superior pubic ramus

Inferior pubic ramus

Intertrochanteric line

Lesser trochanter

B. Posterior view

Iliofemoral liagment

Ischiofemoral ligament

Zona orbicularis

Greater trochanter

Ischial spine

Ischial tuberosity

Protrusion of synovial membrane

Intertrochanteric crest

Lesser trochanter

C. Joint opened: lateral view

Lunate (articular) surface of acetabulum

Articular cartilage

Greater trochanter

Head of femur

Neck of femur

Intertrochanteric line

Ligament of head of femur (*cut*)

Lesser trochanter

Anterior superior iliac spine

Anterior inferior iliac spine

Iliopubic eminence

Acetabular labrum (fibrocartilaginous)

Fat in acetabular fossa (covered by synovial membrane)

Obturator artery

Anterior branch

Posterior branch

Acetabular branch

Obturator membrane

Transverse acetabular ligament

Ischial tuberosity

7.2 HIP JOINT

The head of the femur articulates with the lunate surface of the acetabulum of the innominate bone. The fibrous joint capsule has thickenings that form the iliofemoral, ischiofemoral, and pubofemoral ligaments. The iliofemoral ligament, called the *Y ligament* because it is shaped like an inverted Y,

has an anterior location that restricts extension at the hip joint. The ligament of the head of the femur inside the hip joint cavity provides a route for a small artery to the head of the femur. It has no supportive role in maintaining the integrity of the joint.

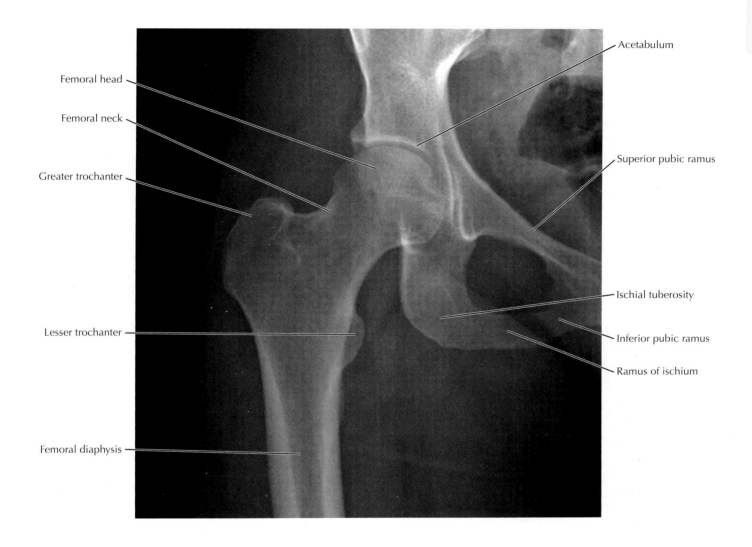

Femoral head

Femoral neck

Greater trochanter

Lesser trochanter

Femoral diaphysis

Acetabulum

Superior pubic ramus

Ischial tuberosity

Inferior pubic ramus

Ramus of ischium

7.3 HIP JOINT X-RAY

A conventional x-ray should be the initial form of imaging when evaluating joint complaints. Causes of acute hip pain include inflammatory arthritis, septic arthritis, trauma, and tumors. The most common cause of chronic hip pain is degenerative arthritis, which may present as groin pain, thigh pain, or a loss of mobility. Radiographic signs of osteoarthritis are similar, regardless of the joint in which they occur, and include joint-space narrowing, subchondral cyst formation, and outgrowths of bone at the bone ends known as osteophytes. Subchondral cysts appear as well-defined lytic lesions at the articular surface.

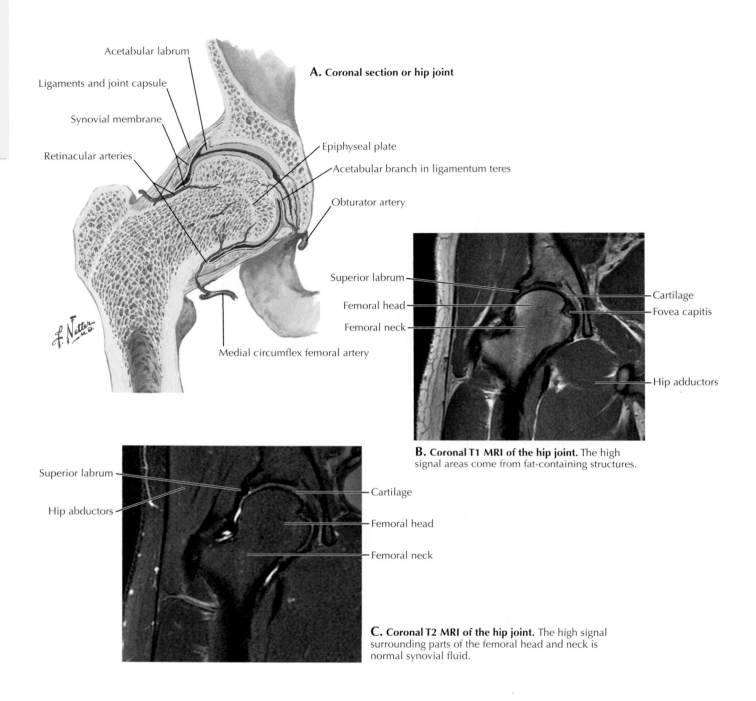

A. Coronal section or hip joint

Acetabular labrum

Ligaments and joint capsule

Synovial membrane

Retinacular arteries

Epiphyseal plate

Acetabular branch in ligamentum teres

Obturator artery

Medial circumflex femoral artery

Superior labrum

Femoral head

Femoral neck

Cartilage

Fovea capitis

Hip adductors

B. Coronal T1 MRI of the hip joint. The high signal areas come from fat-containing structures.

Superior labrum

Hip abductors

Cartilage

Femoral head

Femoral neck

C. Coronal T2 MRI of the hip joint. The high signal surrounding parts of the femoral head and neck is normal synovial fluid.

7.4 IMAGING STUDIES OF THE HIP JOINT

If an initial hip x-ray is normal or inconclusive, magnetic resonance imaging (MRI) is usually the next modality of choice. MRI is advantageous over other imaging modalities in its soft tissue contrast and high resolution. It can often detect pathophysiological changes before they are seen on conventional radiography. It is the most sensitive imaging modality for stress fractures, which appear as a low-signal line on both T1-weighted and T2-weighted images, with a surrounding high-signal area on T2-weighted images representing edema.

Fractures of the hip most often occur in the femoral neck or the intertrochanteric region. A potential complication of femoral neck fractures is avascular necrosis (AVN), which can lead to total joint destruction requiring a hip replacement if not caught early. In these two coronal images, there is an area of depression in the otherwise spherical femoral head. This is the fovea capitis, which is the attachment site of the ligamentum teres. It is the only part of the femoral head not covered by articular cartilage.

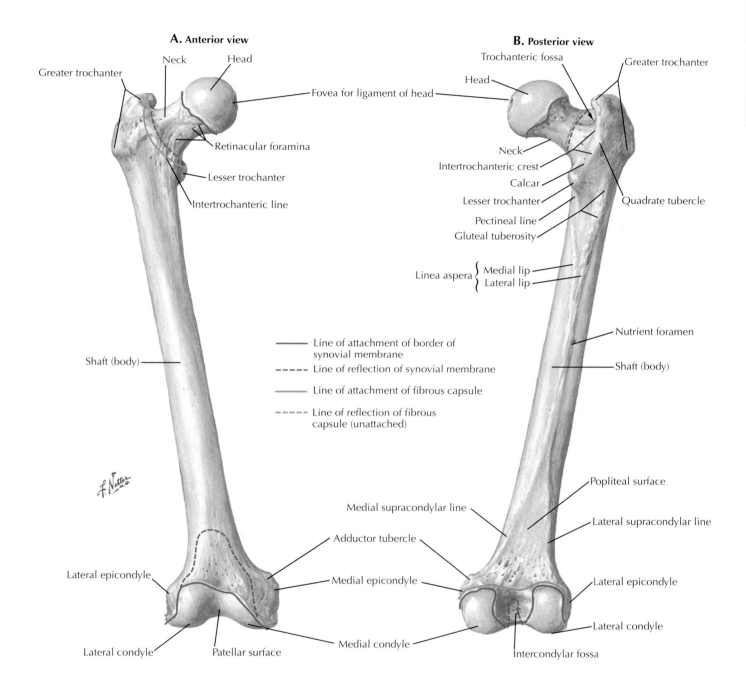

A. Anterior view

Greater trochanter

Neck

Head

Fovea for ligament of head

Retinacular foramina

Lesser trochanter

Intertrochanteric line

Shaft (body)

Lateral epicondyle

Lateral condyle

Patellar surface

Adductor tubercle

Medial epicondyle

Medial condyle

B. Posterior view

Trochanteric fossa

Head

Greater trochanter

Neck

Intertrochanteric crest

Calcar

Lesser trochanter

Pectineal line

Gluteal tuberosity

Quadrate tubercle

Linea aspera { Medial lip / Lateral lip

Nutrient foramen

Shaft (body)

Popliteal surface

Medial supracondylar line

Lateral supracondylar line

Lateral epicondyle

Lateral condyle

Intercondylar fossa

——— Line of attachment of border of synovial membrane

----- Line of reflection of synovial membrane

——— Line of attachment of fibrous capsule

----- Line of reflection of fibrous capsule (unattached)

7.5 FEMUR

The femur articulates with the acetabulum of the hip bone in a multiaxial ball-and-socket joint and with the tibia in a modified hinge joint at the knee (where flexion/extension is the primary movement; a little rotation is possible when the knee is flexed). The greater trochanter is the attachment of the abductor muscles of the hip joint and lateral rotators. The iliopsoas muscle, a powerful flexor, inserts on the lesser trochanter. The adductor muscle group inserts on the linea aspera on the back of the femur. The adductor magnus muscle also inserts on the adductor tubercle at the top of the medial condyle.

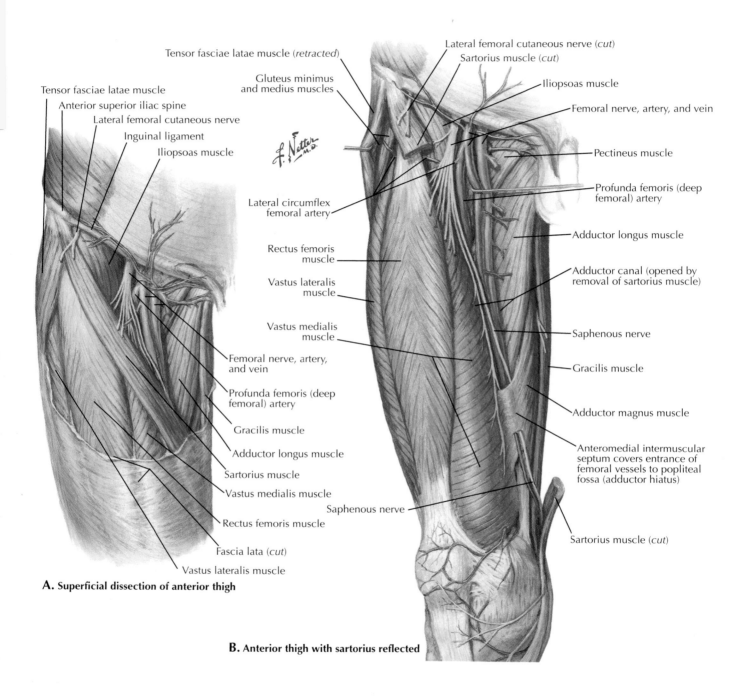

Tensor fasciae latae muscle (*retracted*)

Gluteus minimus and medius muscles

Tensor fasciae latae muscle

Anterior superior iliac spine

Lateral femoral cutaneous nerve

Inguinal ligament

Iliopsoas muscle

Lateral circumflex femoral artery

Rectus femoris muscle

Vastus lateralis muscle

Vastus medialis muscle

Femoral nerve, artery, and vein

Profunda femoris (deep femoral) artery

Gracilis muscle

Adductor longus muscle

Sartorius muscle

Vastus medialis muscle

Rectus femoris muscle

Fascia lata (*cut*)

Vastus lateralis muscle

Lateral femoral cutaneous nerve (*cut*)

Sartorius muscle (*cut*)

Iliopsoas muscle

Femoral nerve, artery, and vein

Pectineus muscle

Profunda femoris (deep femoral) artery

Adductor longus muscle

Adductor canal (opened by removal of sartorius muscle)

Saphenous nerve

Gracilis muscle

Adductor magnus muscle

Anteromedial intermuscular septum covers entrance of femoral vessels to popliteal fossa (adductor hiatus)

Sartorius muscle (*cut*)

Saphenous nerve

A. Superficial dissection of anterior thigh

B. Anterior thigh with sartorius reflected

7.6 MUSCLES OF THE THIGH: ANTERIOR VIEW

This right lower limb is rotated laterally a bit to show the adductor compartment to better advantage. The extensor compartment of the thigh (quadriceps, sartorius), innervated by the femoral nerve, is anterior; the adductors are medial.

The obturator nerve (an anterior division nerve) and artery supply the latter. The femoral nerve (a posterior division nerve) supplies the extensor compartment, and the femoral artery supplies the entire lower extremity with the exception of the adductors.

A. Superficial dissection

B. Deeper dissection

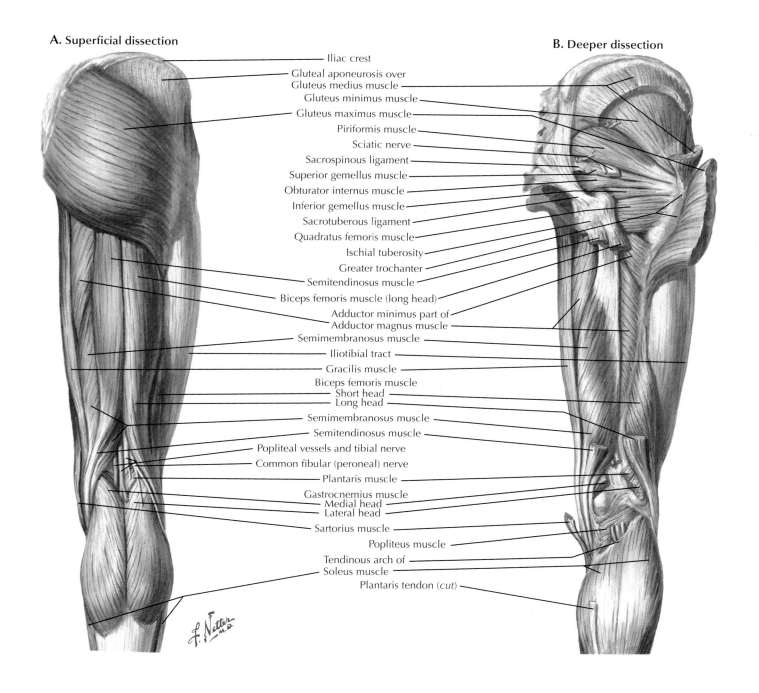

Iliac crest

Gluteal aponeurosis over
Gluteus medius muscle

Gluteus minimus muscle

Gluteus maximus muscle

Piriformis muscle

Sciatic nerve

Sacrospinous ligament

Superior gemellus muscle

Obturator internus muscle

Inferior gemellus muscle

Sacrotuberous ligament

Quadratus femoris muscle

Ischial tuberosity

Greater trochanter

Semitendinosus muscle

Biceps femoris muscle (long head)

Adductor minimus part of
Adductor magnus muscle

Semimembranosus muscle

Iliotibial tract

Gracilis muscle

Biceps femoris muscle
Short head
Long head

Semimembranosus muscle

Semitendinosus muscle

Popliteal vessels and tibial nerve

Common fibular (peroneal) nerve

Plantaris muscle

Gastrocnemius muscle
Medial head
Lateral head

Sartorius muscle

Popliteus muscle

Tendinous arch of
Soleus muscle

Plantaris tendon (*cut*)

f. Netter
M.D.

7.7 MUSCLES OF THE THIGH: POSTERIOR VIEW

The gluteal muscles are posterior and lateral to the hip joint. Posterior on the thigh are the hamstring muscles that extend the hip and flex the knee. The sciatic nerve, with tibial and common fibular nerve components, supplies the flexor compartment of the thigh and all of the muscles of the leg and foot. It is not accompanied by an artery and vein. The hamstring muscles receive their blood supply from the profunda femoris branch of the femoral artery. After supplying the anterior muscles of the thigh, the femoral vessels course medially to the back of the knee, where they become the popliteal vessels after passing through the hiatus of the adductor magnus tendon.

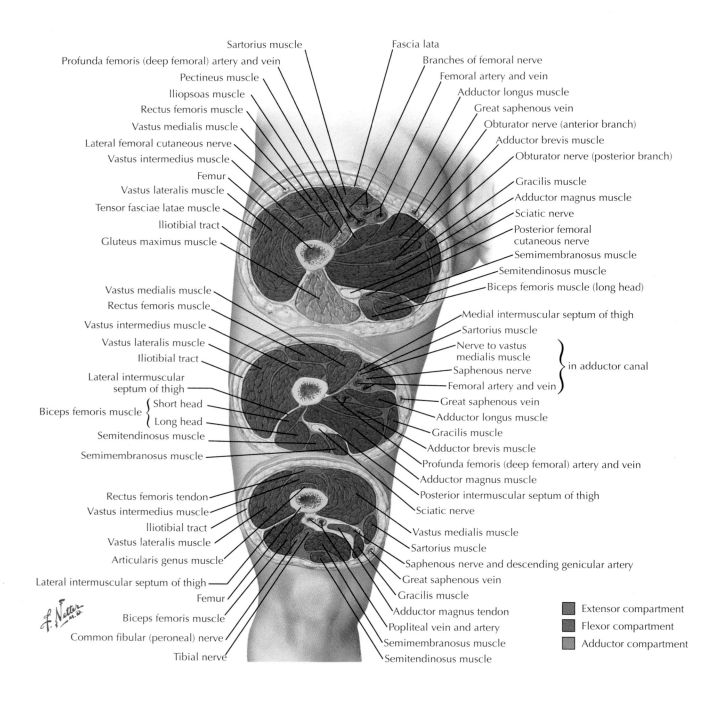

Sartorius muscle

Profunda femoris (deep femoral) artery and vein

Pectineus muscle

Iliopsoas muscle

Rectus femoris muscle

Vastus medialis muscle

Lateral femoral cutaneous nerve

Vastus intermedius muscle

Femur

Vastus lateralis muscle

Tensor fasciae latae muscle

Iliotibial tract

Gluteus maximus muscle

Fascia lata

Branches of femoral nerve

Femoral artery and vein

Adductor longus muscle

Great saphenous vein

Obturator nerve (anterior branch)

Adductor brevis muscle

Obturator nerve (posterior branch)

Gracilis muscle

Adductor magnus muscle

Sciatic nerve

Posterior femoral cutaneous nerve

Semimembranosus muscle

Semitendinosus muscle

Biceps femoris muscle (long head)

Vastus medialis muscle

Rectus femoris muscle

Vastus intermedius muscle

Vastus lateralis muscle

Iliotibial tract

Lateral intermuscular septum of thigh

Biceps femoris muscle { Short head / Long head }

Semitendinosus muscle

Semimembranosus muscle

Medial intermuscular septum of thigh

Sartorius muscle

Nerve to vastus medialis muscle

Saphenous nerve } in adductor canal

Femoral artery and vein }

Great saphenous vein

Adductor longus muscle

Gracilis muscle

Adductor brevis muscle

Profunda femoris (deep femoral) artery and vein

Adductor magnus muscle

Posterior intermuscular septum of thigh

Sciatic nerve

Rectus femoris tendon

Vastus intermedius muscle

Iliotibial tract

Vastus lateralis muscle

Articularis genus muscle

Lateral intermuscular septum of thigh

Femur

Biceps femoris muscle

Common fibular (peroneal) nerve

Tibial nerve

Vastus medialis muscle

Sartorius muscle

Saphenous nerve and descending genicular artery

Great saphenous vein

Gracilis muscle

Adductor magnus tendon

Popliteal vein and artery

Semimembranosus muscle

Semitendinosus muscle

Extensor compartment

Flexor compartment

Adductor compartment

7.8 THIGH SERIAL CROSS SECTIONS

The anterior extensor compartment *(red)* is supplied by the femoral nerve and (superficial) femoral artery. The posterior flexor compartment *(gray)* is supplied by the tibial component of the sciatic nerve and profunda femoris branch of the (common) femoral artery. The medial adductor compartment *(purple)* is supplied by the obturator nerve and artery.

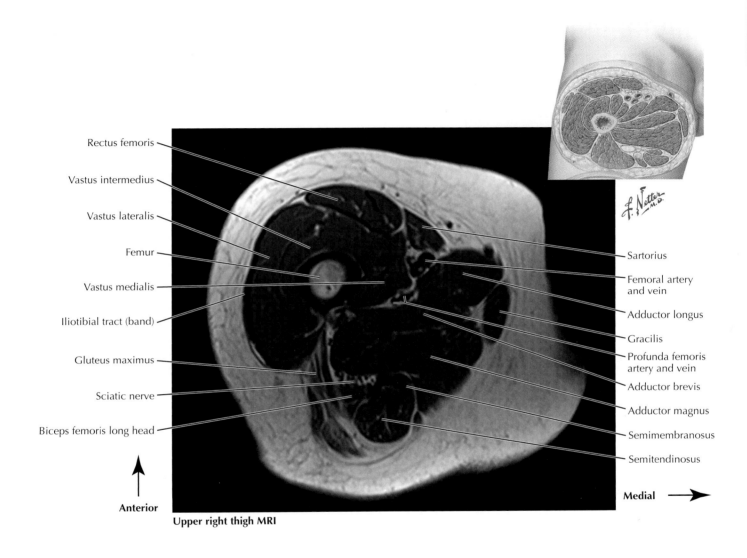

Rectus femoris

Vastus intermedius

Vastus lateralis

Femur

Vastus medialis

Iliotibial tract (band)

Gluteus maximus

Sciatic nerve

Biceps femoris long head

Sartorius

Femoral artery and vein

Adductor longus

Gracilis

Profunda femoris artery and vein

Adductor brevis

Adductor magnus

Semimembranosus

Semitendinosus

Anterior

Medial →

Upper right thigh MRI

7.9 UPPER RIGHT THIGH T1 MRI

On T1 images fat produces a high signal, as seen here in the bone marrow, the subcutaneous tissue, and between muscle fibers and muscle groups. The cortex of the femur is a low-signal area *(black)*. Compare the muscles of the anterior, posterior, and medial compartments with Fig. 7.8. Surrounded by fatty tissue between the anterior and medial compartments are the (superficial) femoral and deep femoral artery and vein.

Within the posterior compartment in this image are the semi-tendinosus muscle, the semimembranosus tendon (low-signal area), the biceps femoris muscle, and the sciatic nerve. Also visualized is the inferior part of the gluteus maximus muscle and the iliotibial tract (area of low signal located lateral to the vastus lateralis). The inferiormost insertion of the gluteus maximus muscle is onto the gluteal tuberosity and the upper extent of the linea aspera.

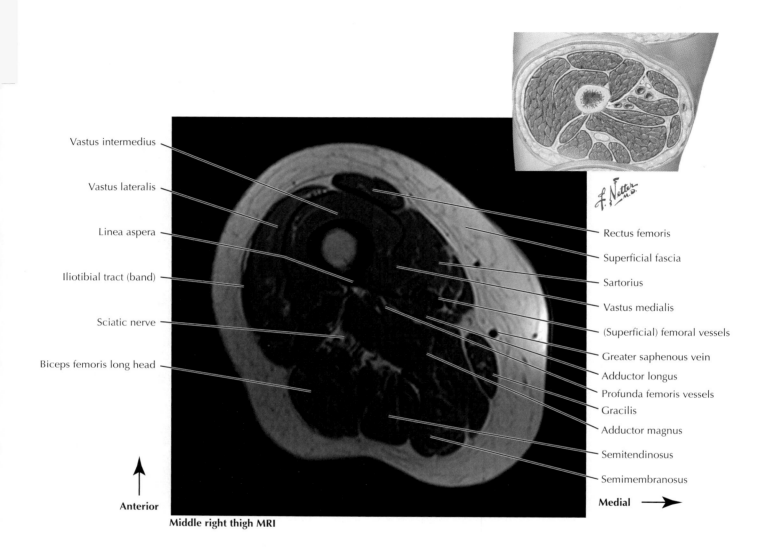

Vastus intermedius

Vastus lateralis

Linea aspera

Iliotibial tract (band)

Sciatic nerve

Biceps femoris long head

Rectus femoris

Superficial fascia

Sartorius

Vastus medialis

(Superficial) femoral vessels

Greater saphenous vein

Adductor longus

Profunda femoris vessels

Gracilis

Adductor magnus

Semitendinosus

Semimembranosus

Anterior

Medial →

Middle right thigh MRI

7.10 MIDDLE RIGHT THIGH T1 MRI

In this axial T1 MRI of the midthigh, all three hamstring muscles can be seen posteriorly. As one moves distally down the thigh, the semimembranosus muscle belly increases in size while the semitendinosus muscle belly decreases in size; in the more proximal cross section, only the tendon of the semimembranosus was visible. Embedded within the fatty tissue between the gracilis and the sartorius muscles on the medial side of the thigh is the greater saphenous vein. All four of the quadriceps muscles can be differentiated in the anterior compartment. It is difficult to differentiate the planes of the adductor muscles medially. Throughout the thigh the adductor longus muscle lies anterior to the adductor magnus muscle. The adductor canal is formed by the adductus longus muscle posteriorly, the vastus medialis muscle laterally, and the sartorius muscle anteriorly. Within the canal are the (superficial) femoral vessels.

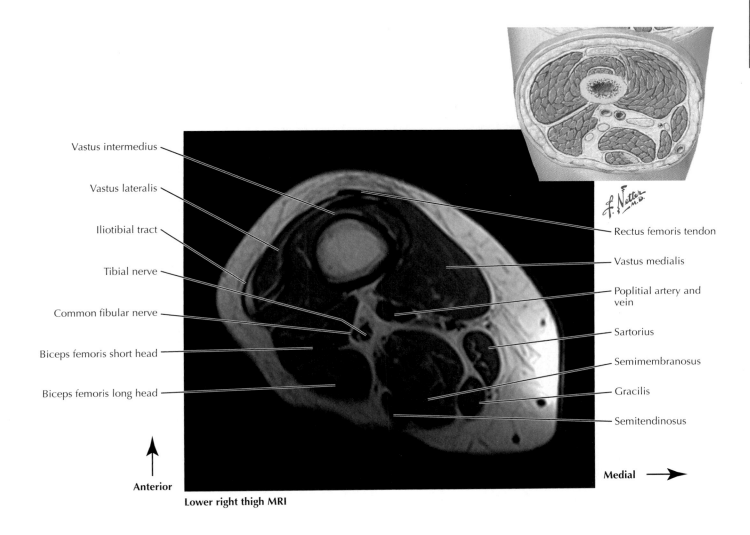

Vastus intermedius

Vastus lateralis

Iliotibial tract

Tibial nerve

Common fibular nerve

Biceps femoris short head

Biceps femoris long head

Rectus femoris tendon

Vastus medialis

Poplitial artery and vein

Sartorius

Semimembranosus

Gracilis

Semitendinosus

Anterior

Medial

Lower right thigh MRI

7.11 LOWER RIGHT THIGH T1 MRI

This cross section is just proximal to the knee. Located most anteriorly is a thin rectangular area of low signal. This is the rectus femoris tendon. The muscle bellies of vastus lateralis, vastus intermedius, and vastus medialis are clearly defined, and the tendon of vastus intermedius is the area of low signal just deep to the rectus femoris tendon. The sartorius muscle passes from the anterior to the medial aspect of the thigh, and at this level it is adjacent to the gracilis muscle within the posterior half of the medial aspect of the thigh. In the distal thigh seen here, the small muscle belly of the semitendinosus muscle has decreased in size, and the short head of the biceps femoris muscle, located deep to the long head, is more prominent. The sciatic nerve here begins to separate into the tibial and common fibular (peroneal) nerves. The femoral vessels have just emerged from the adductor hiatus in the adductor magnus tendon to become the popliteal vein and artery.

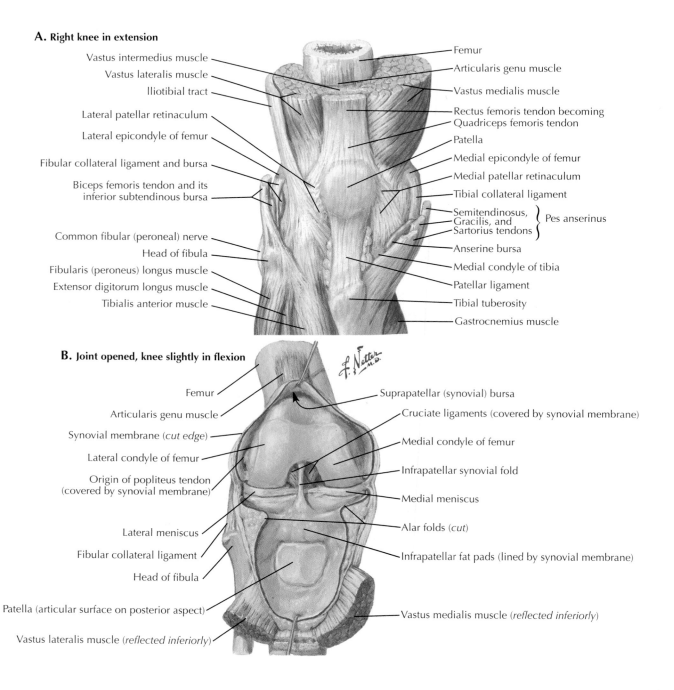

A. Right knee in extension

Vastus intermedius muscle
Vastus lateralis muscle
Iliotibial tract
Lateral patellar retinaculum
Lateral epicondyle of femur
Fibular collateral ligament and bursa
Biceps femoris tendon and its inferior subtendinous bursa
Common fibular (peroneal) nerve
Head of fibula
Fibularis (peroneus) longus muscle
Extensor digitorum longus muscle
Tibialis anterior muscle

Femur
Articularis genu muscle
Vastus medialis muscle
Rectus femoris tendon becoming Quadriceps femoris tendon
Patella
Medial epicondyle of femur
Medial patellar retinaculum
Tibial collateral ligament
Semitendinosus, Gracilis, and Sartorius tendons } Pes anserinus
Anserine bursa
Medial condyle of tibia
Patellar ligament
Tibial tuberosity
Gastrocnemius muscle

B. Joint opened, knee slightly in flexion

Femur
Articularis genu muscle
Synovial membrane (*cut edge*)
Lateral condyle of femur
Origin of popliteus tendon (covered by synovial membrane)
Lateral meniscus
Fibular collateral ligament
Head of fibula
Patella (articular surface on posterior aspect)
Vastus lateralis muscle (*reflected inferiorly*)

Suprapatellar (synovial) bursa
Cruciate ligaments (covered by synovial membrane)
Medial condyle of femur
Infrapatellar synovial fold
Medial meniscus
Alar folds (*cut*)
Infrapatellar fat pads (lined by synovial membrane)
Vastus medialis muscle (*reflected inferiorly*)

7.12 KNEE AND KNEE JOINT OVERVIEW

The femoral condyles articulate with tibial condyles to form the knee joint. The patella articulates with the femur and is embedded in the tendon of the quadriceps muscle group. From the patella to its insertion on the tibial tuberosity, it is called the *patellar ligament.*

Medial and lateral collateral ligaments prevent abduction and adduction of the joint, respectively. Inside the joint are medial and lateral fibrocartilage menisci, anterior and posterior cruciate ligaments, and fat pads. The ligaments and fat are covered by synovial membrane. The synovial joint cavity extends superiorly above the articular surface of the femur as the suprapatellar bursa.

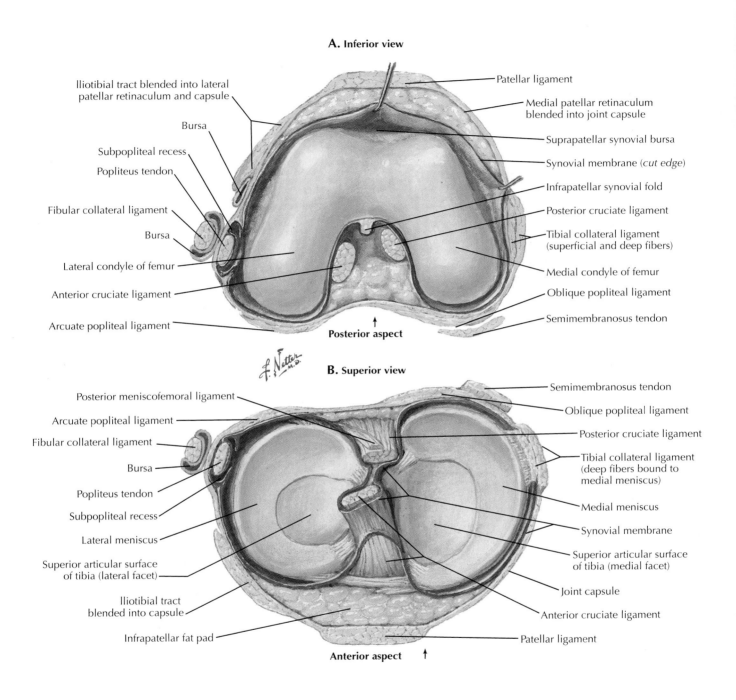

A. Inferior view

Iliotibial tract blended into lateral patellar retinaculum and capsule

Bursa

Subpopliteal recess

Popliteus tendon

Fibular collateral ligament

Bursa

Lateral condyle of femur

Anterior cruciate ligament

Arcuate popliteal ligament

Patellar ligament

Medial patellar retinaculum blended into joint capsule

Suprapatellar synovial bursa

Synovial membrane (*cut edge*)

Infrapatellar synovial fold

Posterior cruciate ligament

Tibial collateral ligament (superficial and deep fibers)

Medial condyle of femur

Oblique popliteal ligament

Semimembranosus tendon

Posterior aspect

B. Superior view

Posterior meniscofemoral ligament

Arcuate popliteal ligament

Fibular collateral ligament

Bursa

Popliteus tendon

Subpopliteal recess

Lateral meniscus

Superior articular surface of tibia (lateral facet)

Iliotibial tract blended into capsule

Infrapatellar fat pad

Semimembranosus tendon

Oblique popliteal ligament

Posterior cruciate ligament

Tibial collateral ligament (deep fibers bound to medial meniscus)

Medial meniscus

Synovial membrane

Superior articular surface of tibia (medial facet)

Joint capsule

Anterior cruciate ligament

Patellar ligament

Anterior aspect

7.13 KNEE JOINT INTERIOR

The medial (tibial) collateral ligament is a thickening of the fibrous joint capsule. The lateral (fibular) collateral ligament attaches to the head of the fibula and is separate from the joint capsule. The cruciate ligaments prevent anterior/posterior sliding of the femur and tibia on each other and are named according to their tibial attachments. The tibial collateral ligament attaches to the medial meniscus. The tendon of the popliteus muscle attaches to the femur and tibia but also enters the joint to attach to the lateral meniscus. Both menisci attach to the femur between the articular surfaces close to the cruciate ligaments. The C shape of the lateral meniscus is more closed than the medial meniscus.

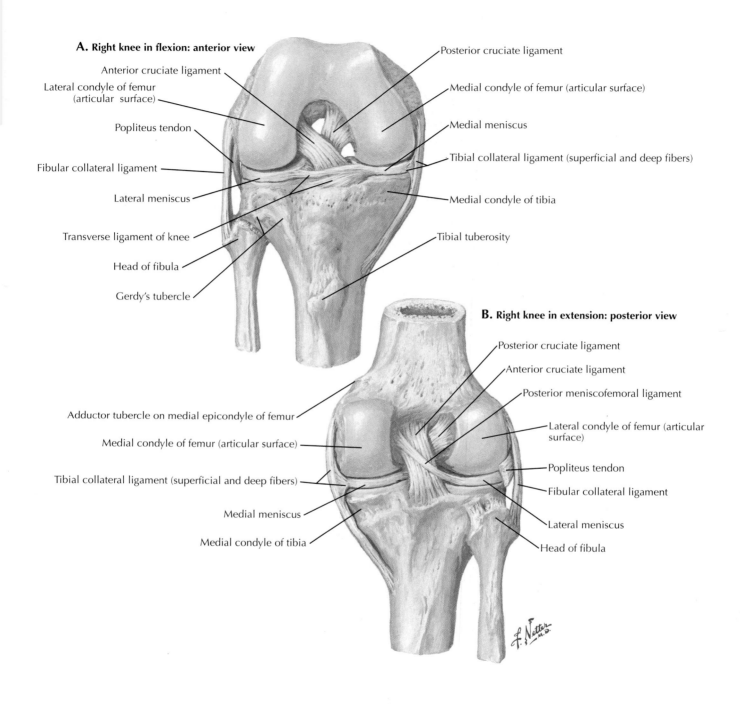

A. Right knee in flexion: anterior view

Anterior cruciate ligament

Lateral condyle of femur (articular surface)

Popliteus tendon

Fibular collateral ligament

Lateral meniscus

Transverse ligament of knee

Head of fibula

Gerdy's tubercle

Posterior cruciate ligament

Medial condyle of femur (articular surface)

Medial meniscus

Tibial collateral ligament (superficial and deep fibers)

Medial condyle of tibia

Tibial tuberosity

B. Right knee in extension: posterior view

Posterior cruciate ligament

Anterior cruciate ligament

Posterior meniscofemoral ligament

Lateral condyle of femur (articular surface)

Popliteus tendon

Fibular collateral ligament

Lateral meniscus

Head of fibula

Adductor tubercle on medial epicondyle of femur

Medial condyle of femur (articular surface)

Tibial collateral ligament (superficial and deep fibers)

Medial meniscus

Medial condyle of tibia

7.14 KNEE JOINT LIGAMENTS

These figures better illustrate the crossing nature and attachments of the cruciate ligaments and the relationship of the collateral ligaments to the fibrous joint capsule. The anterior cruciate ligament courses posteriorly and laterally from the tibia to its attachment to the lateral condyle of the femur. The posterior cruciate ligament attaches far back on the tibia and courses anteriorly and medially to the medial femoral condyle. Note the tendon of the popliteus muscle passing deep to the fibular (lateral) collateral ligament to its attachment to the femur and the lateral meniscus.

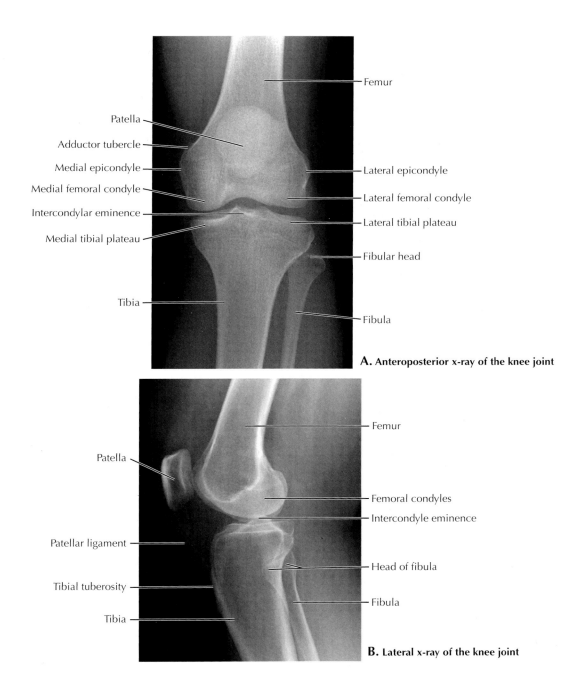

A. Anteroposterior x-ray of the knee joint

Labels (top image):
- Femur
- Patella
- Adductor tubercle
- Medial epicondyle
- Medial femoral condyle
- Intercondylar eminence
- Medial tibial plateau
- Tibia
- Lateral epicondyle
- Lateral femoral condyle
- Lateral tibial plateau
- Fibular head
- Fibula

B. Lateral x-ray of the knee joint

Labels (bottom image):
- Patella
- Patellar ligament
- Tibial tuberosity
- Tibia
- Femur
- Femoral condyles
- Intercondyle eminence
- Head of fibula
- Fibula

7.15 KNEE JOINT X-RAY

When evaluating an x-ray of the knee, look for signs of osteo-arthritis, which include joint space narrowing, osteophyte formation, and subchondral cysts. This can best be done on the anteroposterior (AP) view. Sometimes only one compartment (medial vs. lateral) is affected. The lateral view is good for evaluating the patella and to determine whether a joint effusion is present, which is often seen in the joint cavity superior to the patella (suprapatellar bursa) as a result of the fluid pushing the fat line anteriorly. When trauma has occurred, it is important not to miss a tibial plateau fracture, which might appear as a vertical line just lateral to the intercondylar eminence or as a depression of the tibial surface. The tibial plateau affects knee stability, motion, and alignment. In all positions the patella is in contact with the femur, and the femur in contact with the tibia. Early detection and treatment of tibial plateau fractures is important to minimize future patient disability that may result from post-traumatic arthritis.

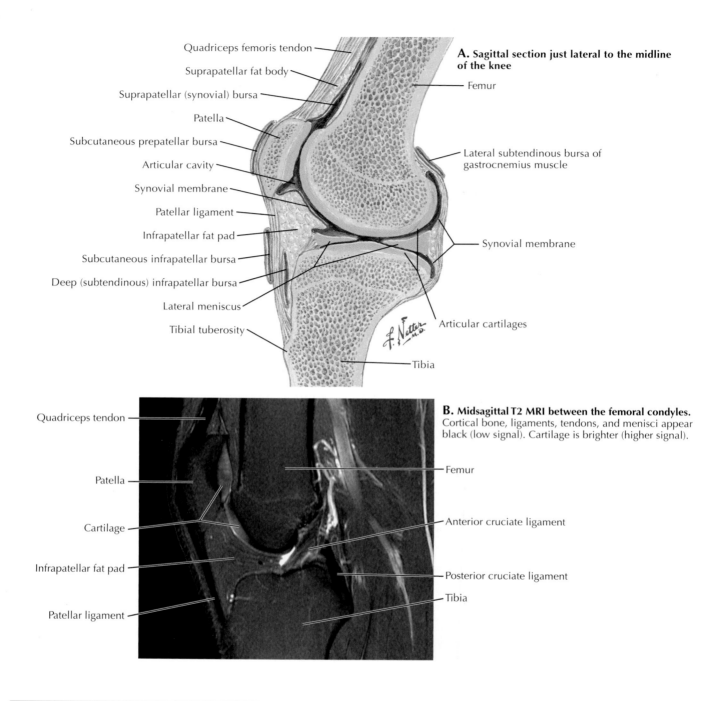

Quadriceps femoris tendon

Suprapatellar fat body

Suprapatellar (synovial) bursa

Patella

Subcutaneous prepatellar bursa

Articular cavity

Synovial membrane

Patellar ligament

Infrapatellar fat pad

Subcutaneous infrapatellar bursa

Deep (subtendinous) infrapatellar bursa

Lateral meniscus

Tibial tuberosity

A. Sagittal section just lateral to the midline of the knee

Femur

Lateral subtendinous bursa of gastrocnemius muscle

Synovial membrane

Articular cartilages

Tibia

Quadriceps tendon

Patella

Cartilage

Infrapatellar fat pad

Patellar ligament

B. Midsagittal T2 MRI between the femoral condyles. Cortical bone, ligaments, tendons, and menisci appear black (low signal). Cartilage is brighter (higher signal).

Femur

Anterior cruciate ligament

Posterior cruciate ligament

Tibia

7.16 SAGITTAL SECTION OF THE KNEE JOINT AND T2 MRI

MRI of the knee is the most frequently requested MRI joint study. It is the modality of choice for the evaluation of knee instability since the ligaments and the menisci involved in the stability of the knee are soft tissue structures and thus best seen on MRI. The two most common soft tissue injuries of the knee involve the cruciate ligaments and the menisci. Both cruciate ligaments are best evaluated using a sagittal T2-weighted image as shown in **B.** Whereas most normal ligaments appear black on MRI, the anterior cruciate ligament

(ACL) appears as a striated, intermediate-signal structure. When it is torn, it usually is simply not seen. Other injuries associated with an ACL tear include injury to the medial collateral ligament, a torn medial meniscus, or bone contusions to the tibia or femur, which appear as an area of increased signal on T2-weighted images. The posterior cruciate ligament appears as a gently curved, homogeneously low-signal structure. It is torn far less frequently than the ACL and is less often repaired when it is torn since it usually causes less instability in comparison to an ACL tear.

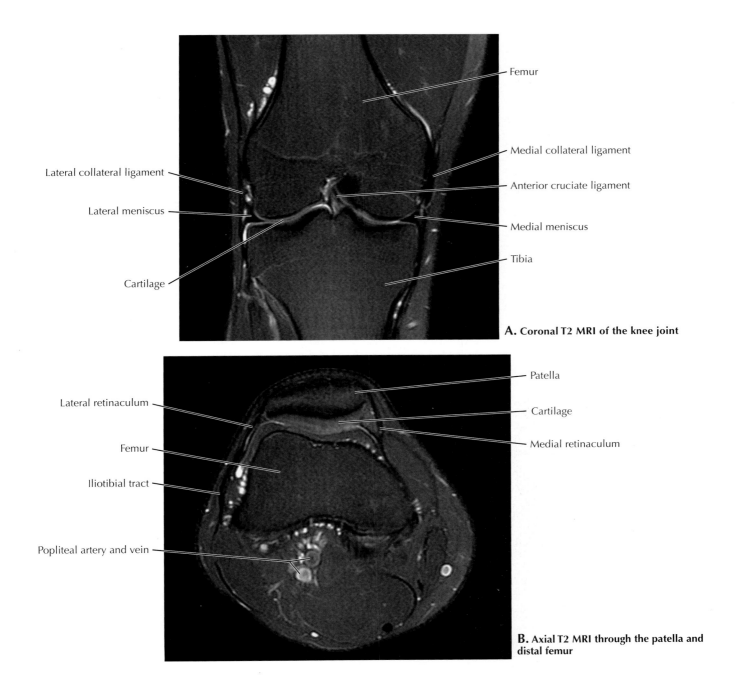

Femur

Medial collateral ligament

Lateral collateral ligament

Anterior cruciate ligament

Lateral meniscus

Medial meniscus

Tibia

Cartilage

A. Coronal T2 MRI of the knee joint

Patella

Lateral retinaculum

Cartilage

Femur

Medial retinaculum

Iliotibial tract

Popliteal artery and vein

B. Axial T2 MRI through the patella and distal femur

7.17 CORONAL AND AXIAL T2 MRI STUDIES OF THE KNEE

In **A,** a coronal image of the right knee, one can see the distal aspect of the ACL near its origin on the tibia. On either side of the knee joint are the hypointense medial and lateral collateral ligaments. The medial collateral ligament (MCL) is a thickening of the joint capsule and is more frequently injured than the lateral collateral ligament (LCL). The LCL is removed from the joint capsule and forms a complex with the biceps femoris tendon and the iliotibial tract. The menisci are C-shaped fibrocartilagenous structures that are thick peripherally and thin centrally. The menisci are visualized here as triangular structures with a typical low signal on the peripheral aspects of the knee joint. **B** is an axial image of the right knee through the distal femur and patella. The lateral and medial patellar retinacula can be seen on either side of the patella as low-signal structures. Just posterior to the lateral patellar retinaculum and lateral to the femur is another low-signal structure, the iliotibial tract (IT) or band. The IT is often the source of lateral knee pain at the level of the distal femur in runners. This is called *IT band syndrome,* and fluid may be seen on both sides of the IT when it is present.

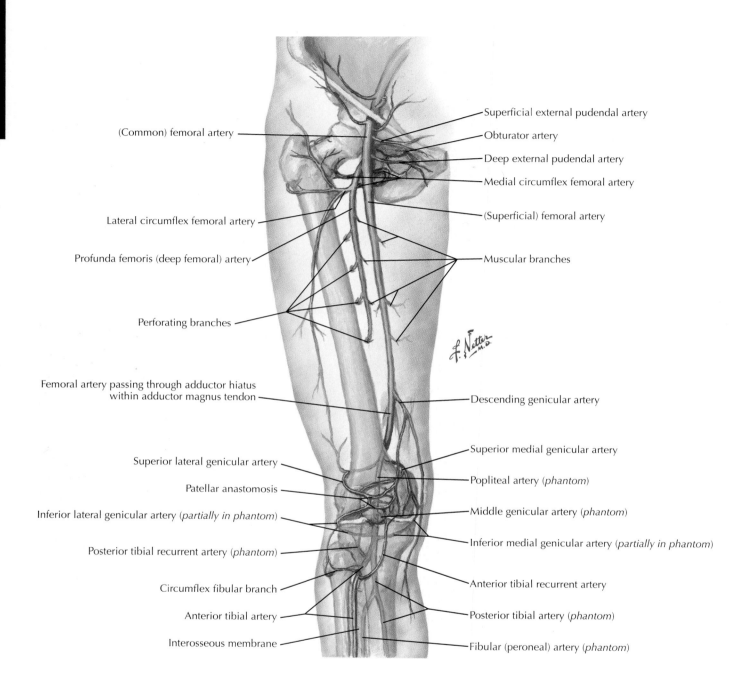

(Common) femoral artery

Lateral circumflex femoral artery

Profunda femoris (deep femoral) artery

Perforating branches

Femoral artery passing through adductor hiatus within adductor magnus tendon

Superior lateral genicular artery

Patellar anastomosis

Inferior lateral genicular artery (*partially in phantom*)

Posterior tibial recurrent artery (*phantom*)

Circumflex fibular branch

Anterior tibial artery

Interosseous membrane

Superficial external pudendal artery

Obturator artery

Deep external pudendal artery

Medial circumflex femoral artery

(Superficial) femoral artery

Muscular branches

Descending genicular artery

Superior medial genicular artery

Popliteal artery (*phantom*)

Middle genicular artery (*phantom*)

Inferior medial genicular artery (*partially in phantom*)

Anterior tibial recurrent artery

Posterior tibial artery (*phantom*)

Fibular (peroneal) artery (*phantom*)

7.18 ARTERIES OF THE THIGH AND KNEE

The entire blood supply to the lower extremity, with the exception of the adductor compartment, originates from the femoral artery, a continuation of the external iliac artery under the inguinal ligament. The deep femoral artery (profunda femoris artery) supplies the posterior flexor compartment of the thigh; no vessels accompany the sciatic nerve posteriorly. As a result of the embryonic medial rotation of the lower extremity, the femoral artery courses medially to the back of the knee through the hiatus in the adductor magnus tendon, where it becomes the popliteal artery. It gives rise to four genicular arteries (superior medial, superior lateral, inferior medial, inferior lateral) that anastomose extensively around the knee. Inferior to the knee the popliteal artery divides into the anterior and posterior tibial arteries, and the latter gives origin to the fibular (peroneal) artery.

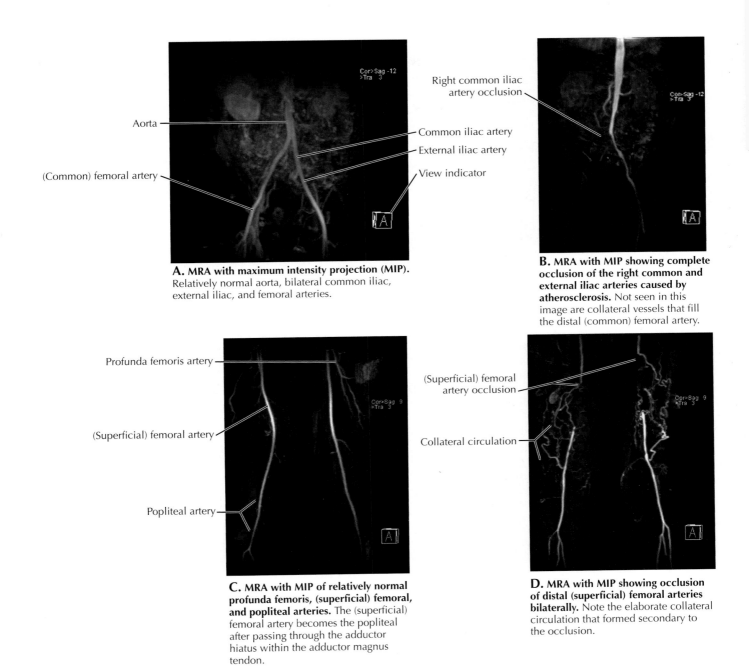

A. MRA with maximum intensity projection (MIP). Relatively normal aorta, bilateral common iliac, external iliac, and femoral arteries.

B. MRA with MIP showing complete occlusion of the right common and external iliac arteries caused by atherosclerosis. Not seen in this image are collateral vessels that fill the distal (common) femoral artery.

C. MRA with MIP of relatively normal profunda femoris, (superficial) femoral, and popliteal arteries. The (superficial) femoral artery becomes the popliteal after passing through the adductor hiatus within the adductor magnus tendon.

D. MRA with MIP showing occlusion of distal (superficial) femoral arteries bilaterally. Note the elaborate collateral circulation that formed secondary to the occlusion.

7.19 MAGNETIC RESONANCE ANGIOGRAPHY OF THE THIGH

As with the upper extremity, magnetic resonance angiography (MRA) is a useful imaging modality for detecting arterial stenoses, occlusions, and other pathology in the lower extremity vasculature. An intravenous (IV) catheter is inserted peripherally, typically in the arm, to inject a gadolinium-based contrast (**A**). As the contrast fills the vasculature, axial MRI images are obtained. Three-dimensional constructions of the arterial circulation are then visualized with maximum intensity projection (MIP) images. The MIP images are rotated on the monitor to improve the detection of pathology. A single two-dimensional image can often miss stenoses or make them appear less severe than they may actually be. Normal studies (**A** and **C**) are compared with filling defects from occlusions (**B** and **D**). When an artery occludes because of atherosclerosis, the process is gradual, thereby allowing for collateral artery formation (**D**).

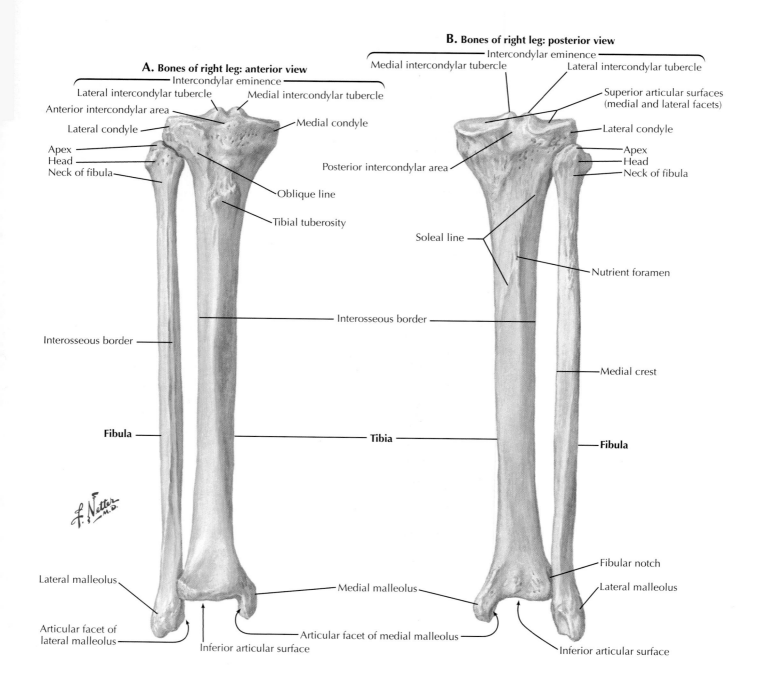

A. Bones of right leg: anterior view

Intercondylar eminence
Lateral intercondylar tubercle — Medial intercondylar tubercle
Anterior intercondylar area
Lateral condyle — Medial condyle
Apex
Head
Neck of fibula
Oblique line
Tibial tuberosity
Interosseous border
Interosseous border
Fibula — Tibia
Lateral malleolus
Articular facet of lateral malleolus
Inferior articular surface
Medial malleolus
Articular facet of medial malleolus

B. Bones of right leg: posterior view

Intercondylar eminence
Medial intercondylar tubercle — Lateral intercondylar tubercle
Superior articular surfaces (medial and lateral facets)
Lateral condyle
Apex
Head
Neck of fibula
Posterior intercondylar area
Soleal line
Nutrient foramen
Interosseous border
Medial crest
Fibula
Fibular notch
Lateral malleolus
Medial malleolus
Inferior articular surface

7.20 TIBIA AND FIBULA

The tibia articulates with the femur superiorly and the talus inferiorly. The tibial tuberosity is the attachment point of the quadriceps tendon. The head of the fibula articulates with the lateral condyle of the tibia, and the lateral malleolus ("little hammer") of the fibula articulates with the lateral surface of the trochlea of the talus. With the medial malleolus of the tibia on the medial surface of the trochlea, the tibia, fibula, and curving surface of the trochlea form a pure hinge joint for flexion/extension (plantar flexion/dorsiflexion, respectively) at the ankle.

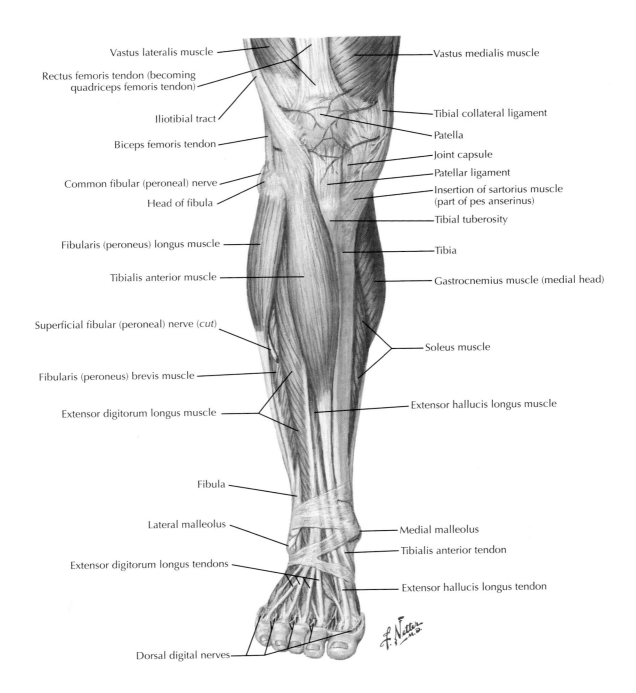

Vastus lateralis muscle

Rectus femoris tendon (becoming quadriceps femoris tendon)

Iliotibial tract

Biceps femoris tendon

Common fibular (peroneal) nerve

Head of fibula

Fibularis (peroneus) longus muscle

Tibialis anterior muscle

Superficial fibular (peroneal) nerve (*cut*)

Fibularis (peroneus) brevis muscle

Extensor digitorum longus muscle

Fibula

Lateral malleolus

Extensor digitorum longus tendons

Dorsal digital nerves

Vastus medialis muscle

Tibial collateral ligament

Patella

Joint capsule

Patellar ligament

Insertion of sartorius muscle (part of pes anserinus)

Tibial tuberosity

Tibia

Gastrocnemius muscle (medial head)

Soleus muscle

Extensor hallucis longus muscle

Medial malleolus

Tibialis anterior tendon

Extensor hallucis longus tendon

7.21 MUSCLES OF THE LEG: ANTERIOR VIEW

The anterior leg muscles are tibialis anterior, extensor digitorum, and extensor hallucis. The lateral compartment consists of fibularis (peroneus) longus and brevis muscles. All of these muscles are supplied by the common fibular nerve seen here coursing around the head of the fibula from the sciatic nerve at the back of the knee. The anterior muscles receive their blood from the anterior tibial artery, a terminal branch of the popliteal artery that passes above the interosseus membrane between the tibia and fibula.

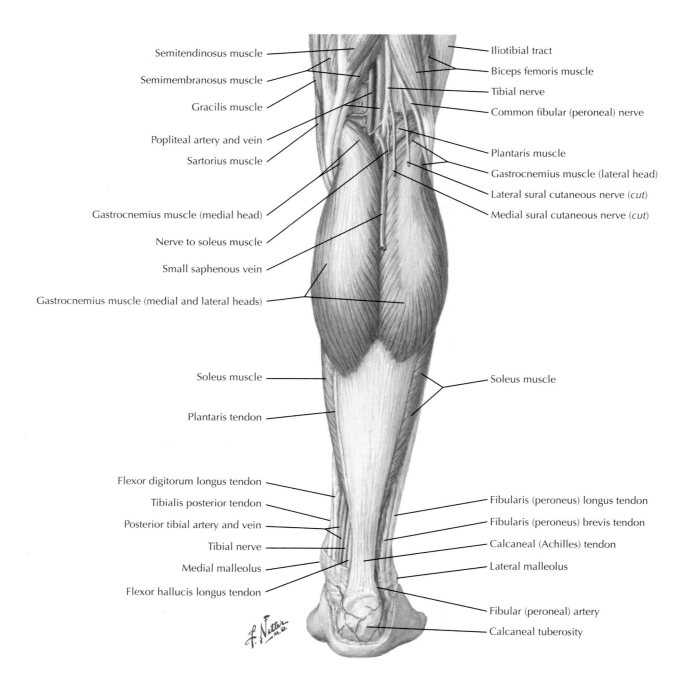

Semitendinosus muscle

Semimembranosus muscle

Gracilis muscle

Popliteal artery and vein

Sartorius muscle

Gastrocnemius muscle (medial head)

Nerve to soleus muscle

Small saphenous vein

Gastrocnemius muscle (medial and lateral heads)

Soleus muscle

Plantaris tendon

Flexor digitorum longus tendon

Tibialis posterior tendon

Posterior tibial artery and vein

Tibial nerve

Medial malleolus

Flexor hallucis longus tendon

Iliotibial tract

Biceps femoris muscle

Tibial nerve

Common fibular (peroneal) nerve

Plantaris muscle

Gastrocnemius muscle (lateral head)

Lateral sural cutaneous nerve (*cut*)

Medial sural cutaneous nerve (*cut*)

Soleus muscle

Fibularis (peroneus) longus tendon

Fibularis (peroneus) brevis tendon

Calcaneal (Achilles) tendon

Lateral malleolus

Fibular (peroneal) artery

Calcaneal tuberosity

7.22 MUSCLES OF THE LEG: POSTERIOR VIEW

The posterior leg muscles are flexor compartment muscles. The two large superficial muscles are the gastrocnemius and soleus muscles. Deep to them are the tibialis posterior, flexor digitorum longus, and flexor hallucis longus muscles. Their tendons pass to the medial side of the ankle. The flexor compartment is innervated by the tibial component of the sciatic nerve. Note the common fibular nerve coursing laterally to the fibularis and anterior compartment muscles. The blood supply to the posterior leg muscles is via the posterior tibial artery, a continuation of the popliteal artery, and its fibular (peroneal) branch.

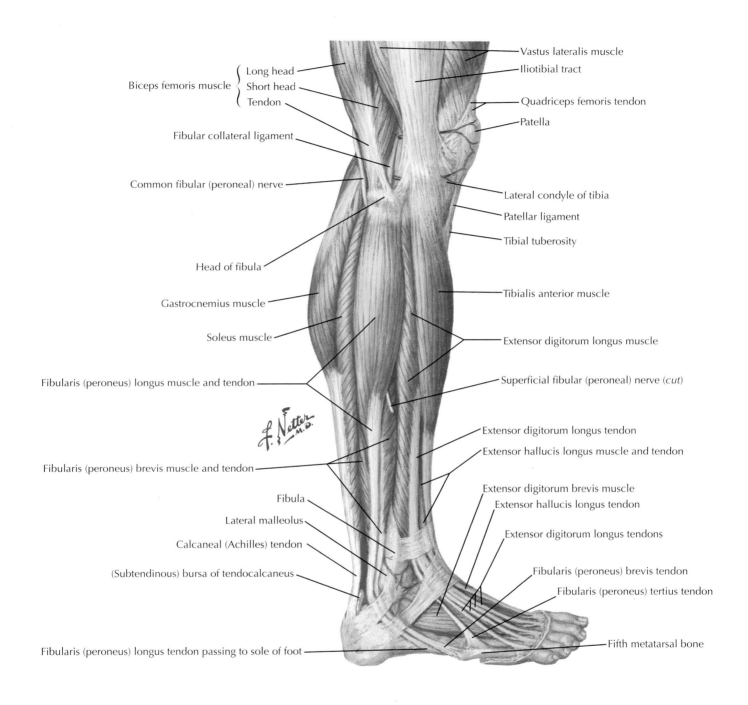

Biceps femoris muscle { Long head
Short head
Tendon

Vastus lateralis muscle

Iliotibial tract

Quadriceps femoris tendon

Patella

Fibular collateral ligament

Common fibular (peroneal) nerve

Lateral condyle of tibia

Patellar ligament

Tibial tuberosity

Head of fibula

Gastrocnemius muscle

Tibialis anterior muscle

Soleus muscle

Extensor digitorum longus muscle

Fibularis (peroneus) longus muscle and tendon

Superficial fibular (peroneal) nerve (*cut*)

Extensor digitorum longus tendon

Extensor hallucis longus muscle and tendon

Fibularis (peroneus) brevis muscle and tendon

Extensor digitorum brevis muscle

Extensor hallucis longus tendon

Fibula

Lateral malleolus

Extensor digitorum longus tendons

Calcaneal (Achilles) tendon

Fibularis (peroneus) brevis tendon

Fibularis (peroneus) tertius tendon

(Subtendinous) bursa of tendocalcaneus

Fifth metatarsal bone

Fibularis (peroneus) longus tendon passing to sole of foot

7.23 MUSCLES OF THE LEG: LATERAL VIEW

The lateral compartment of the leg contains the fibularis (peroneus) longus and brevis muscles that are everters and weak plantar flexors of the foot. They are supplied by the superficial branch of the common fibular nerve. The fibularis (peroneus) tertius muscle is the inferior part of extensor digitorum longus, but it has its own tendon that attaches to the fifth metatarsal close to the attachment of fibularis brevis. The tendon of fibularis longus extends under the foot to attach to the first metatarsal to form a "sling" with the tibialis anterior muscle.

A. Fascial compartments

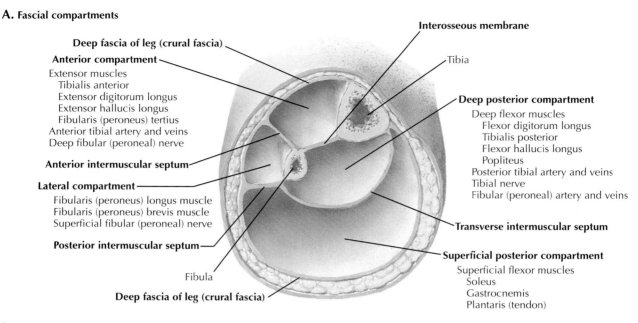

Deep fascia of leg (crural fascia)

Anterior compartment

Extensor muscles
  Tibialis anterior
  Extensor digitorum longus
  Extensor hallucis longus
  Fibularis (peroneus) tertius
Anterior tibial artery and veins
Deep fibular (peroneal) nerve

Anterior intermuscular septum

Lateral compartment

  Fibularis (peroneus) longus muscle
  Fibularis (peroneus) brevis muscle
  Superficial fibular (peroneal) nerve

Posterior intermuscular septum

Fibula

Deep fascia of leg (crural fascia)

Interosseous membrane

Tibia

Deep posterior compartment

Deep flexor muscles
  Flexor digitorum longus
  Tibialis posterior
  Flexor hallucis longus
  Popliteus
Posterior tibial artery and veins
Tibial nerve
Fibular (peroneal) artery and veins

Transverse intermuscular septum

Superficial posterior compartment

Superficial flexor muscles
  Soleus
  Gastrocnemis
  Plantaris (tendon)

B. Cross section just above middle of leg

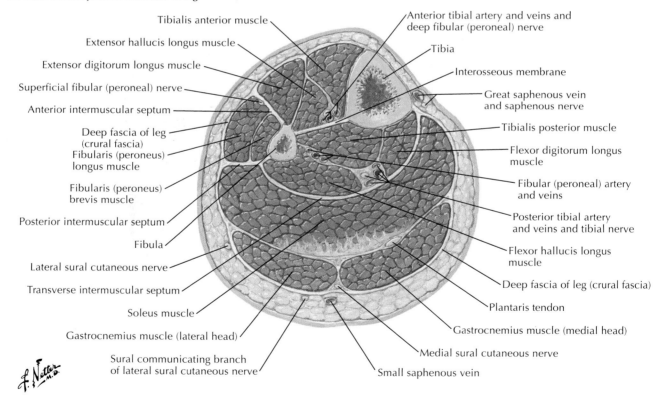

Tibialis anterior muscle

Extensor hallucis longus muscle

Extensor digitorum longus muscle

Superficial fibular (peroneal) nerve

Anterior intermuscular septum

Deep fascia of leg (crural fascia)
Fibularis (peroneus) longus muscle

Fibularis (peroneus) brevis muscle

Posterior intermuscular septum

Fibula

Lateral sural cutaneous nerve

Transverse intermuscular septum

Soleus muscle

Gastrocnemius muscle (lateral head)

Sural communicating branch of lateral sural cutaneous nerve

Anterior tibial artery and veins and deep fibular (peroneal) nerve

Tibia

Interosseous membrane

Great saphenous vein and saphenous nerve

Tibialis posterior muscle

Flexor digitorum longus muscle

Fibular (peroneal) artery and veins

Posterior tibial artery and veins and tibial nerve

Flexor hallucis longus muscle

Deep fascia of leg (crural fascia)

Plantaris tendon

Gastrocnemius muscle (medial head)

Medial sural cutaneous nerve

Small saphenous vein

7.24 LEG CROSS SECTION AND FASCIAL COMPARTMENTS

Although the leg muscle groups can be functionally divided into extensor (dorsiflexor), flexor (plantar-flexor), and lateral (everter) compartments, a more clinically useful grouping is by four fascial compartments where the flexors (plantar-flexors) are divided into superficial and deep groups. Swelling can occur in these compartments and can be relieved by cutting their fascia lengthwise.

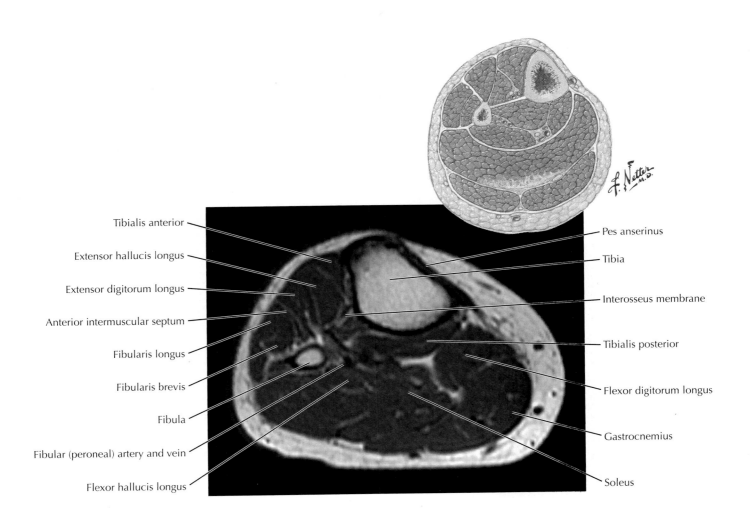

Tibialis anterior

Extensor hallucis longus

Extensor digitorum longus

Anterior intermuscular septum

Fibularis longus

Fibularis brevis

Fibula

Fibular (peroneal) artery and vein

Flexor hallucis longus

Pes anserinus

Tibia

Interosseus membrane

Tibialis posterior

Flexor digitorum longus

Gastrocnemius

Soleus

7.25   AXIAL T1 MRI THROUGH THE LEG

This is a T1-weighted axial image of the proximal right lower leg. The tibia and fibula are visualized here. On the anteromedial surface of the tibia is an area devoid of signal. This is the pes anserinus, which is the insertion point of the conjoined tendons (from anterior to posterior) of the sartorius, gracilis, and semitendinosus muscles. The clinical significance of the pes anserinus is that the bursa underlying the tendons can become irritated and inflamed from overuse and injury. This is often seen in athletes and is a cause of medial knee pain, swelling, and tenderness. Difficult to differentiate in this image are the lateral and medial heads of the gastrocnemius, soleus, flexor hallucis longus, and fibularis (peroneus) brevis muscles.

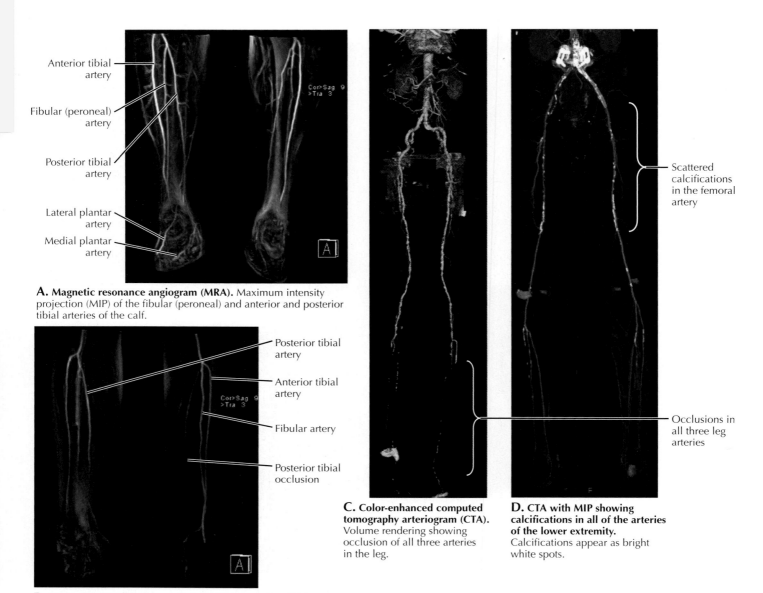

Anterior tibial artery

Fibular (peroneal) artery

Posterior tibial artery

Lateral plantar artery

Medial plantar artery

A. Magnetic resonance angiogram (MRA). Maximum intensity projection (MIP) of the fibular (peroneal) and anterior and posterior tibial arteries of the calf.

Posterior tibial artery

Anterior tibial artery

Fibular artery

Posterior tibial occlusion

B. MRA with MIP showing occlusion of left posterior tibial artery. Collateral artery forming from the distal fibular (peroneal) artery to the distal posterior tibial artery in the foot.

Scattered calcifications in the femoral artery

Occlusions in all three leg arteries

C. Color-enhanced computed tomography arteriogram (CTA). Volume rendering showing occlusion of all three arteries in the leg.

D. CTA with MIP showing calcifications in all of the arteries of the lower extremity. Calcifications appear as bright white spots.

7.26 VASCULAR STUDIES OF THE LOWER EXTREMITY: CTA/MRA OF THE LEG AND LOWER EXTREMITIES

A shows a normal, anterior view MRA of the arteries of the leg compared to an abnormal study (**B**) of a patient with occlusion of the posterior tibial artery. CT is also used to evaluate arteries (or veins) by computer reconstruction of the arteries from axial data as with MRA. CTA is excellent for showing calcifications (**D**). **C** is a color-enhanced, volume-rendering CT study of the arterial system from the heart to the feet that shows occlusions in the leg arteries. The choice of imaging modality is hospital dependent since some hospitals have superior MRI technology, whereas others have superior CT technology. The MIP images from MRA and the three-dimensional reconstructions from CTA provide adequate information to detect arterial stenoses and occlusions, along with other pathology.

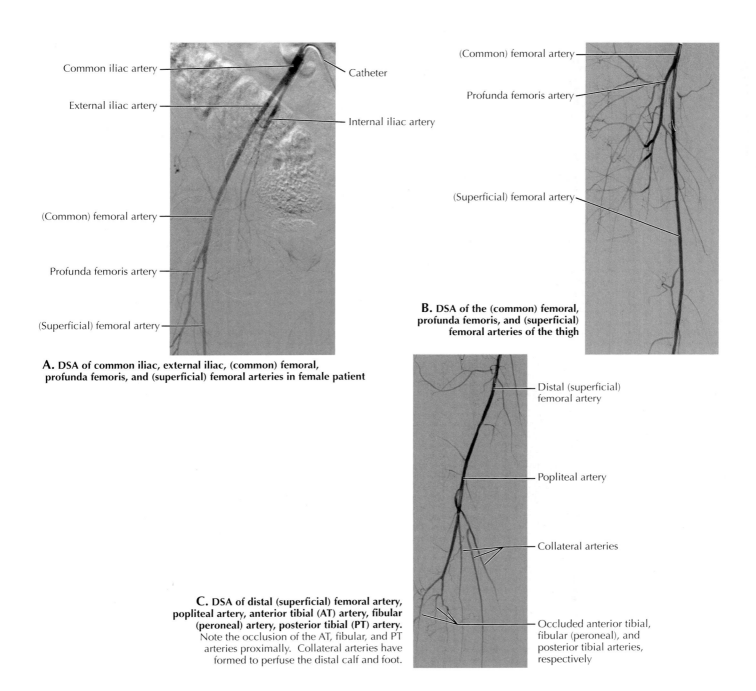

A. DSA of common iliac, external iliac, (common) femoral, profunda femoris, and (superficial) femoral arteries in female patient

Common iliac artery
External iliac artery
(Common) femoral artery
Profunda femoris artery
(Superficial) femoral artery
Catheter
Internal iliac artery

B. DSA of the (common) femoral, profunda femoris, and (superficial) femoral arteries of the thigh

(Common) femoral artery
Profunda femoris artery
(Superficial) femoral artery

C. DSA of distal (superficial) femoral artery, popliteal artery, anterior tibial (AT) artery, fibular (peroneal) artery, posterior tibial (PT) artery. Note the occlusion of the AT, fibular, and PT arteries proximally. Collateral arteries have formed to perfuse the distal calf and foot.

Distal (superficial) femoral artery
Popliteal artery
Collateral arteries
Occluded anterior tibial, fibular (peroneal), and posterior tibial arteries, respectively

7.27 DIGITAL SUBTRACTION ANGIOGRAPHY OF THE RIGHT LOWER EXTREMITY

Digital subtraction angiography (DSA) is another useful imaging tool to identify arterial pathology. To perform DSA, a catheter is typically inserted into the (common) femoral artery percutaneously (through the skin). For this patient, the left (common) femoral artery was accessed, and a catheter was passed retrograde through the external and common iliac arteries on the left to the aortic bifurcation, which then allowed for selection of the right common iliac artery (**A**). Iodinated contrast was injected, and fluoroscopic images were obtained using DSA. Multiple images of the same artery are usually obtained from different angles to most accurately detect arterial stenoses. The images in **C** reveal complete occlusion of all three vessels of the leg in this patient, with flow to the foot provided via collateral arteries that develop over time. This patient ultimately required a below-knee amputation because of the severe peripheral arterial disease in the distal right lower extremity.

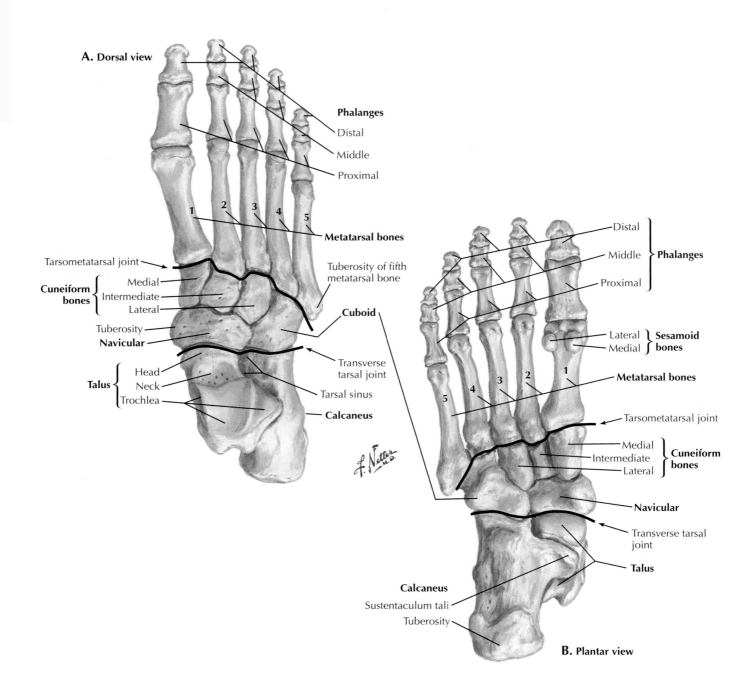

A. Dorsal view

Phalanges
- Distal
- Middle
- Proximal

1 2 3 4 5

Metatarsal bones

Tarsometatarsal joint

Cuneiform bones
- Medial
- Intermediate
- Lateral

Tuberosity

Navicular

Talus
- Head
- Neck
- Trochlea

Tuberosity of fifth metatarsal bone

Cuboid

Transverse tarsal joint

Tarsal sinus

Calcaneus

Distal

Middle — **Phalanges**

Proximal

Lateral — **Sesamoid bones**
Medial

Metatarsal bones

5 4 3 2 1

Tarsometatarsal joint

Medial
Intermediate — **Cuneiform bones**
Lateral

Navicular

Transverse tarsal joint

Talus

Calcaneus
Sustentaculum tali
Tuberosity

B. Plantar view

7.28 BONES OF THE FOOT: SUPERIOR AND INFERIOR VIEWS

The trochlea of the talus articulates with the tibia to form a hinge joint. The head of the talus pivots on the navicular bone in the transverse tarsal joint to produce much of the inversion and eversion movements of the foot. The sustentaculum tali of the calcaneus is a shelf of bone that supports ("sustains") the talus and has a groove for the tendon of the flexor hallucis longis muscle.

A. Lateral view

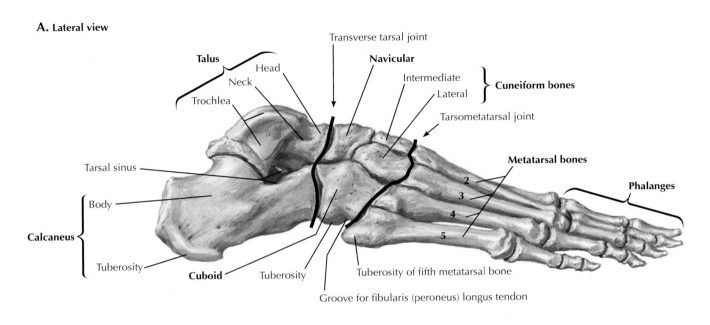

B. Medial view

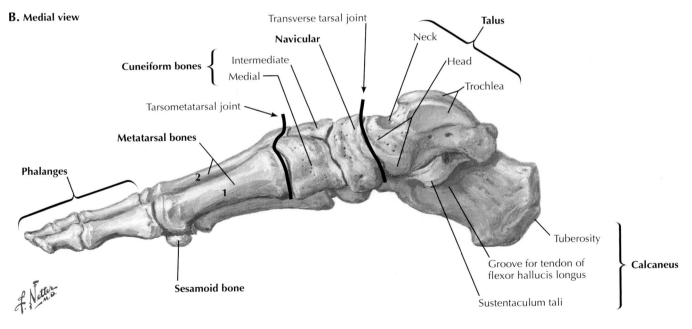

7.29 BONES OF THE FOOT: MEDIAL AND LATERAL VIEWS

A medial view of the foot illustrates the longitudinal arch of the foot and the convexity of the trochlea of the talus.

It also shows how the sesamoid bones elevate the tendon of flexor hallucis longus to give it more leverage in flexing the big toe.

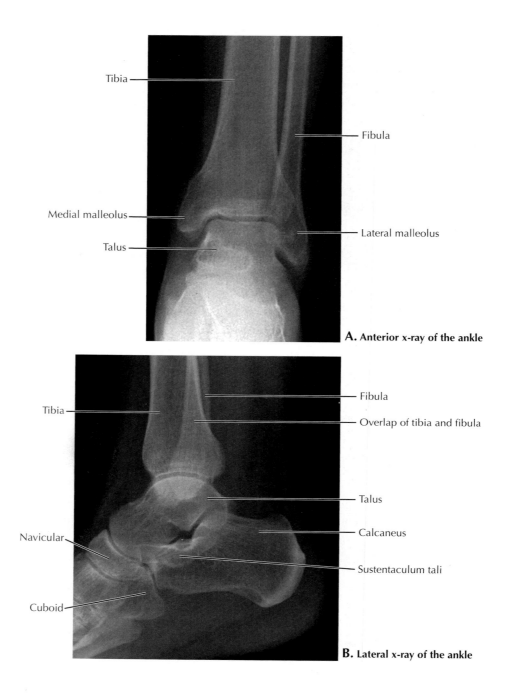

Tibia

Medial malleolus

Talus

Fibula

Lateral malleolus

A. Anterior x-ray of the ankle

Tibia

Navicular

Cuboid

Fibula

Overlap of tibia and fibula

Talus

Calcaneus

Sustentaculum tali

B. Lateral x-ray of the ankle

7.30 ANKLE X-RAYS

Normal imaging of the ankle involves the AP (**A**), lateral (**B**), and mortise (oblique) views. The vast majority of ankle x-rays are obtained to evaluate the effects of trauma. The most common fractures of the ankle involve either the medial or the lateral malleolus. **A** is a routine, non–weight-bearing AP view of the ankle. It is obtained with the patient supine, the heel on the cassette, and the toes pointed upward. On an AP view the talus and the tibia can be seen overlapping with the medial aspect of the distal fibula (lateral malleolus). The lateral view (**B**) shows the calcaneus and talus in profile. The base of the fifth metatarsal should be included. Fractures of the malleoli may be difficult to see on this view since they are all superimposed over one another and over the talus.

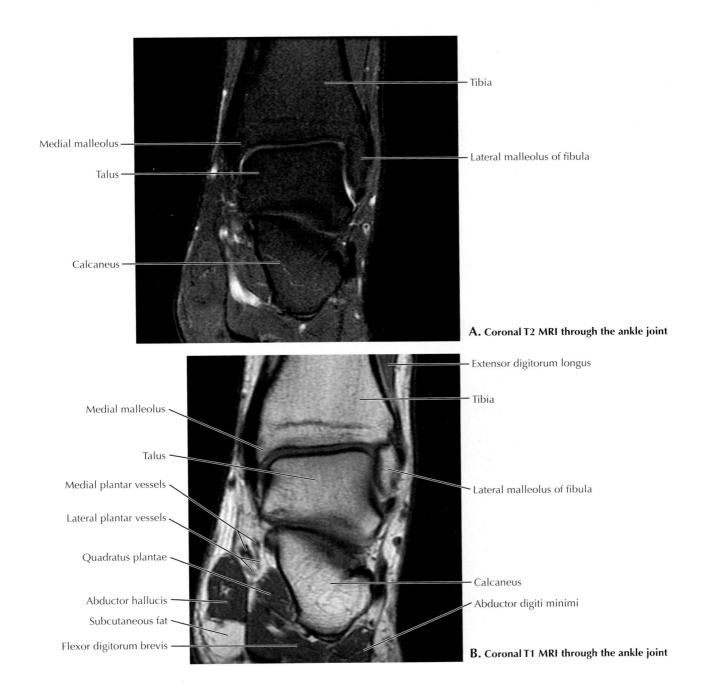

A. Coronal T2 MRI through the ankle joint

Labels (image A):
- Tibia
- Medial malleolus
- Lateral malleolus of fibula
- Talus
- Calcaneus

B. Coronal T1 MRI through the ankle joint

Labels (image B):
- Extensor digitorum longus
- Medial malleolus
- Tibia
- Talus
- Lateral malleolus of fibula
- Medial plantar vessels
- Lateral plantar vessels
- Quadratus plantae
- Calcaneus
- Abductor hallucis
- Abductor digiti minimi
- Subcutaneous fat
- Flexor digitorum brevis

7.31 CORONAL T1 AND T2 MRI OF THE ANKLE

The tibia, lateral malleolus, talus, and calcaneus bones are seen in these two coronal images of the left foot. The muscles are more clearly depicted in the T1-weighted image (**B**) as intermediate-signal structures. The extensor digitorum longus muscle is seen on the lateral aspect of the tibia. Distally in cross section from medial (left) to lateral are the abductor hallucis muscle, the flexor digitorum brevis muscle, the quadratus plantae muscle, and the abductor digiti minimi muscle. The high-signal structure seen in the T1-weighted image in the medial aspect of the foot between the abductor hallucis muscle and the flexor digitorum brevis muscle is normal subcutaneous fat.

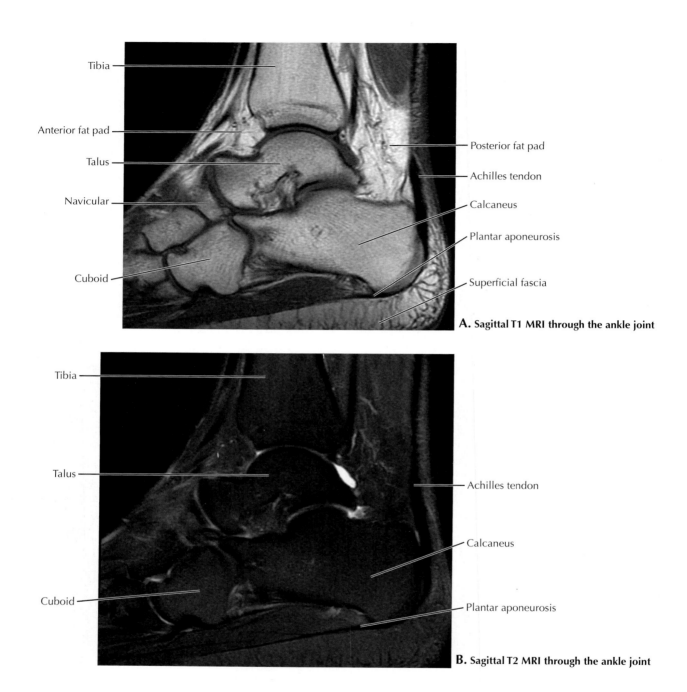

Tibia

Anterior fat pad

Talus

Navicular

Cuboid

Posterior fat pad

Achilles tendon

Calcaneus

Plantar aponeurosis

Superficial fascia

A. Sagittal T1 MRI through the ankle joint

Tibia

Talus

Cuboid

Achilles tendon

Calcaneus

Plantar aponeurosis

B. Sagittal T2 MRI through the ankle joint

7.32 SAGITTAL T1 AND T2 MRI OF THE ANKLE

MRI can be useful in the evaluation of ankle and foot tendons and ligaments. The Achilles tendon can be seen clearly on sagittal images of the ankle. In the sagittal T1-weighted (**A**) and T2-weighted (**B**) images, the distal aspect of the Achilles tendon is seen as a hypointense signal inserting on the calcaneus. A complete tear to the Achilles is most commonly seen in middle-age, unconditioned male athletes and is diagnosed by noting the absence of the tendon on one or more images. There is usually associated edema and hemorrhage (high signal on T2-weighted images). The plantar aponeurosis, which may the source of heel pain in a runner or middle-age obese women, is a fibrous connective tissue structure seen here as a thin hypointense area near its origin on the plantar aspect of the calcaneus. MRI can also be useful in evaluating stress fractures that are suspected but not clearly identified on conventional x-ray and the feet of persons with diabetes when determining the extent of spread of a wound seen superficially. MRI is also extremely sensitive in detecting and evaluating edema of bone marrow and surrounding bone (osteomyelitis).

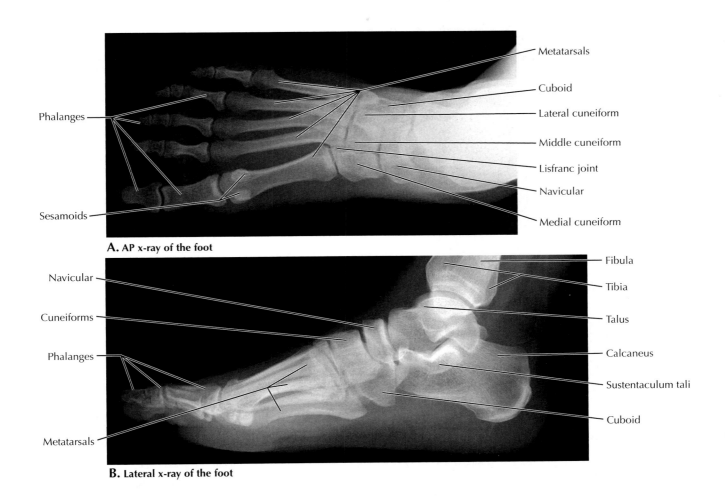

Phalanges

Sesamoids

Metatarsals

Cuboid

Lateral cuneiform

Middle cuneiform

Lisfranc joint

Navicular

Medial cuneiform

A. AP x-ray of the foot

Navicular

Cuneiforms

Phalanges

Metatarsals

Fibula

Tibia

Talus

Calcaneus

Sustentaculum tali

Cuboid

B. Lateral x-ray of the foot

7.33 X-RAYS OF THE FOOT

To evaluate the foot after trauma, AP (**A**), lateral (**B**), and oblique views should be ordered. A common fracture seen in the foot involves the fifth metatarsal and often occurs following overinversion of the foot. A Jones fracture is a fracture to the proximal portion of the fifth metatarsal. Other relatively common types of fractures seen in the foot are stress fractures involving the distal third of the second, third, or fourth metatarsals. These are typically seen in persons doing a lot of walking, marching (such as in army recruits), running, or dancing. Radiographic signs of stress fractures include a linear lucency with an adjacent periosteal reaction. When assessing a patient with arthritic complaints, AP and lateral views are usually sufficient. Gouty arthritis commonly affects the first metatarsophalangeal joint. Radiographic signs of gout include soft tissue swelling manifesting as a cloudy area of increased opacity around the joint, punched-out lesions in the bones near the joint, interosseous tophi (uric acid deposits), and joint-space narrowing.

8

HEAD AND NECK

HEAD AND NECK

8.1   SKULL: ANTERIOR VIEW

8.2   SKULL: ANTEROPOSTERIOR X-RAY

8.3   SKULL: ANTEROPOSTERIOR CALDWELL PROJECTION AND
       FACE/ORBIT DETAIL

8.4   SKULL: LATERAL VIEW

8.5   SKULL: MIDSAGITTAL SECTION

8.6   LATERAL X-RAY

8.7   CALVARIA

8.8   CRANIAL BASE: INFERIOR VIEW

8.9   CRANIAL BASE: SUPERIOR VIEW

8.10 SKULL OF THE NEWBORN

8.11 MANDIBLE

8.12 CERVICAL VERTEBRAE AND LATERAL X-RAY

8.13 ATLAS AND AXIS

8.14 IMAGING OF CERVICAL TRAUMA AND PATHOLOGY

8.15 SUPERFICIAL VESSELS, NERVES, AND MUSCLES OF THE NECK

8.16 ARTERIES OF ORAL AND PHARYNGEAL REGIONS

8.17 AXIAL CT AND CROSS SECTION OF THE NECK THROUGH C7 AND
       THE THYROID GLAND

8.18 AXIAL CT THROUGH C5 AND THE LARYNX

8.19 AXIAL CT THROUGH C3 AND THE HYOID BONE

8.20 SEARCH STRATEGY: NECK IMAGING OF LARYNGEAL TUMOR

8.21 CROSS AND CORONAL SECTIONS OF THE TONGUE AND SALIVARY GLANDS

8.22 AXIAL CT AT C2 AND C1

8.23 IMAGING PATHOLOGY OF THE ORAL CAVITY

8.24 LATERAL WALL OF THE NASAL CAVITY

8.25 THE NOSE, NASAL CAVITY, AND MAXILLARY SINUSES IN THE TRANSVERSE PLANE

8.26 PARANASAL AIR SINUSES

8.27 IMAGING OF THE PARANASAL SINUSES

8.28 CROSS AND CORONAL SECTIONS OF THE ORBIT

8.29 IMAGING OF THE ORBIT

8.30 IMAGING OF SINUS AND ORBIT PATHOLOGY

8.31 IMAGING OF SINUS AND ORBIT PATHOLOGY (CONT'D)

8.32 CORONAL SECTION OF THE HEAD THROUGH THE ORBIT, SINUSES, AND ORAL CAVITY: OVERVIEW

8.33 MIDSAGITTAL SECTION OF THE NASAL CAVITY, PHARYNX, ORAL CAVITY, AND NECK: OVERVIEW

8.34 T1 AND T2 MRI OF THE HEAD AND NECK IN MIDSAGITTAL SECTION

8.35 DURAL VENOUS SINUSES

8.36 DURAL VENOUS SINUSES (CONT'D)

8.37 THE CAVERNOUS SINUS

8.38 SUPERIOR SAGITTAL SINUS, MIDDLE MENINGEAL ARTERY, AND SUPERFICIAL CEREBRAL VEINS

8.39 IMAGING OF EPIDURAL AND SUBDURAL BLEEDING

8.40 ARTERIES FROM THE NECK TO THE BRAIN

8.41 VASCULAR STUDIES

8.42 EXTERNAL, MIDDLE, AND INNER EAR

8.43 CT OF THE TEMPORAL BONE AND EAR COMPARTMENTS

8.44 IMAGING OF TEMPORAL BONE/EAR PATHOLOGY

BRAIN

8.45 MIDSAGITTAL SECTION OF BRAIN; MEDIAL VIEW OF CEREBRUM

8.46 MIDSAGITTAL T1 MRI

8.47 VENTRICLES OF THE BRAIN

8.48 CIRCULATION OF CEREBROSPINAL FLUID AND HYDROCEPHALUS

8.49 FOURTH VENTRICLE AND SECTIONS OF THE CEREBELLUM

8.50 BRAINSTEM

8.51 CEREBELLUM

8.52 T1 SAGITTAL MRI NEAR THE MIDLINE

8.53 T1 SAGITTAL MRI THROUGH THE TEMPORAL LOBE

8.54 T1 SAGITTAL MRI THROUGH THE TEMPORAL LOBE (CONT'D)

8.55 T2 FLAIR CORONAL MRI THROUGH THE CEREBELLUM

8.56 T2 FLAIR CORONAL MRI THROUGH THE BRAINSTEM

8.57 T2 FLAIR CORONAL MRI THROUGH THE PONS AND THIRD VENTRICLE

8.58 T2 FLAIR CORONAL MRI THROUGH THE OPTIC CHIASM

8.59 T2 FLAIR CORONAL MRI THROUGH THE TEMPORAL LOBES

8.60 T2 FLAIR CORONAL MRI THROUGH THE FRONTAL LOBES

8.61 T1 AND T2 AXIAL MRI THROUGH THE MEDULLA

8.62 T1 AND T2 AXIAL MRI THROUGH THE CEREBELLUM, TEMPORAL LOBES, AND EYE

8.63 T1 AND T2 AXIAL MRI THROUGH THE UPPER CEREBELLUM

8.64 ARTERIES OF THE BRAIN: INFERIOR VIEW

8.65 CEREBRAL ARTERIAL CIRCLE (OF WILLIS)

8.66   T1 AND T2 AXIAL MRI THROUGH THE OPTIC CHIASM

8.67   T1 AND T2 AXIAL MRI THROUGH THE THALAMUS AND THIRD VENTRICLE

8.68   TRANSVERSE (AXIAL) SECTION OF THE BRAIN AT THE LEVEL OF
THE BASAL NUCLEI

8.69   T1 AND T2 AXIAL MRI THROUGH THE THALAMUS AND LATERAL VENTRICLES

8.70   THALAMUS

8.71   HIPPOCAMPUS AND FORNIX

8.72   T1 AND T2 AXIAL MRI THROUGH THE LATERAL VENTRICLES

8.73   T1 AND T2 AXIAL MRI THROUGH THE MIDDLE OF
THE CEREBRAL HEMISPHERES

8.74   T1 AND T2 AXIAL MRI THROUGH THE THALAMUS AND LATERAL VENTRICLES

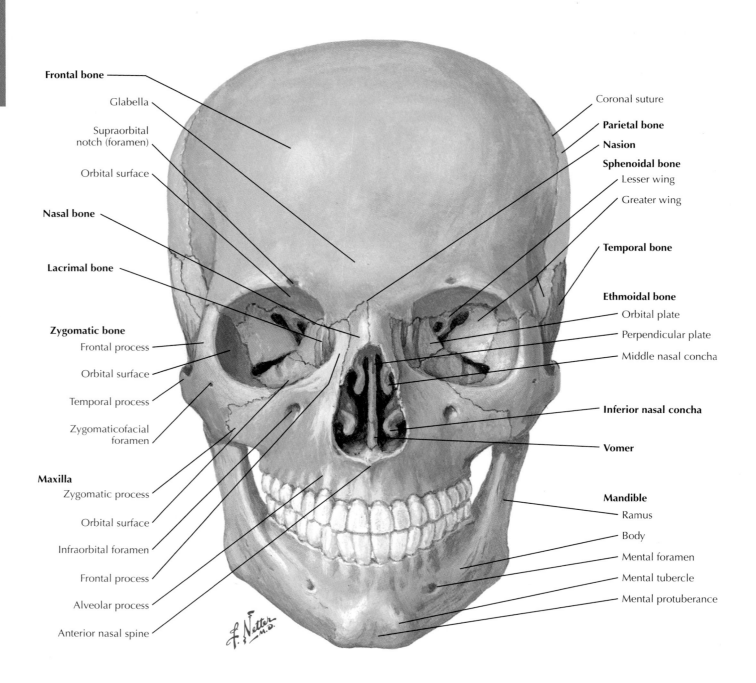

Frontal bone

Glabella

Supraorbital
notch (foramen)

Orbital surface

Nasal bone

Lacrimal bone

Zygomatic bone

Frontal process

Orbital surface

Temporal process

Zygomaticofacial
foramen

Maxilla

Zygomatic process

Orbital surface

Infraorbital foramen

Frontal process

Alveolar process

Anterior nasal spine

Coronal suture

Parietal bone

Nasion

Sphenoidal bone

Lesser wing

Greater wing

Temporal bone

Ethmoidal bone

Orbital plate

Perpendicular plate

Middle nasal concha

Inferior nasal concha

Vomer

Mandible

Ramus

Body

Mental foramen

Mental tubercle

Mental protuberance

8.1 SKULL: ANTERIOR VIEW

The prominent bones of the skull in an anterior view are the
frontal bone forming the anterior calvarium and roof of each
orbit, nasal bones, zygomatic bones of the cheek and lateral
wall of the orbit, maxilla, and mandible. The upper part of the
nasal septum and middle nasal conchae are parts of the
ethmoid bone; the lower part of the septum is the vomer.

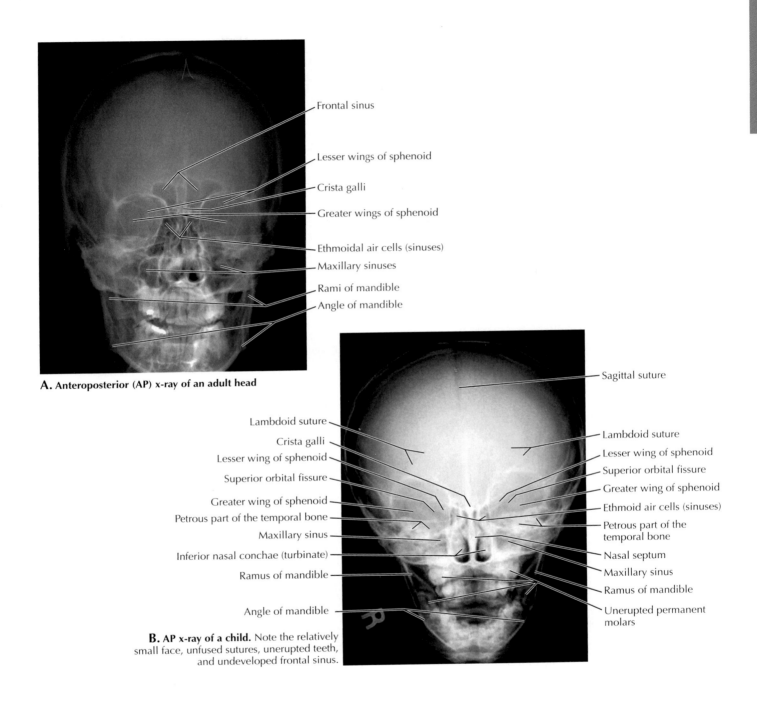

A. Anteroposterior (AP) x-ray of an adult head

Frontal sinus

Lesser wings of sphenoid

Crista galli

Greater wings of sphenoid

Ethmoidal air cells (sinuses)

Maxillary sinuses

Rami of mandible

Angle of mandible

Lambdoid suture

Crista galli

Lesser wing of sphenoid

Superior orbital fissure

Greater wing of sphenoid

Petrous part of the temporal bone

Maxillary sinus

Inferior nasal conchae (turbinate)

Ramus of mandible

Angle of mandible

Sagittal suture

Lambdoid suture

Lesser wing of sphenoid

Superior orbital fissure

Greater wing of sphenoid

Ethmoid air cells (sinuses)

Petrous part of the temporal bone

Nasal septum

Maxillary sinus

Ramus of mandible

Unerupted permanent molars

B. AP x-ray of a child. Note the relatively small face, unfused sutures, unerupted teeth, and undeveloped frontal sinus.

8.2 SKULL: ANTEROPOSTERIOR X-RAY

The most radiopaque (whitest) parts of the skull in an anterior x-ray are the petrous parts of the temporal bone and the overlap of the molar row of teeth in the maxilla and mandible. The head is positioned to superimpose the petrous temporal on the lower parts of the orbits to better view the inferior parts of the maxillary sinuses for fluid or blood (e.g., from trauma).

The most radiolucent (darkest) areas are from air in the mastoid air cells, nasal cavity, and paranasal sinuses (frontal, maxillary, and ethmoid). The ethmoid sinuses appear darker; they are superimposed on the sphenoid sinus behind it. Also note the increase in density where x-rays pass end-on through the flat bones at the periphery of the neurocranium and through the cribriform plate of the ethmoid bone.

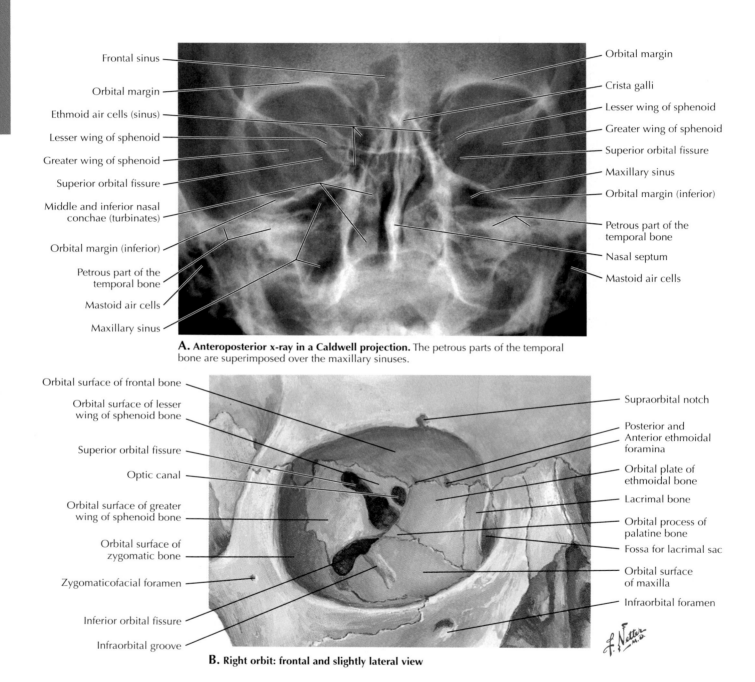

A. Anteroposterior x-ray in a Caldwell projection. The petrous parts of the temporal bone are superimposed over the maxillary sinuses.

Frontal sinus

Orbital margin

Ethmoid air cells (sinus)

Lesser wing of sphenoid

Greater wing of sphenoid

Superior orbital fissure

Middle and inferior nasal conchae (turbinates)

Orbital margin (inferior)

Petrous part of the temporal bone

Mastoid air cells

Maxillary sinus

Orbital margin

Crista galli

Lesser wing of sphenoid

Greater wing of sphenoid

Superior orbital fissure

Maxillary sinus

Orbital margin (inferior)

Petrous part of the temporal bone

Nasal septum

Mastoid air cells

Orbital surface of frontal bone

Orbital surface of lesser wing of sphenoid bone

Superior orbital fissure

Optic canal

Orbital surface of greater wing of sphenoid bone

Orbital surface of zygomatic bone

Zygomaticofacial foramen

Inferior orbital fissure

Infraorbital groove

Supraorbital notch

Posterior and Anterior ethmoidal foramina

Orbital plate of ethmoidal bone

Lacrimal bone

Orbital process of palatine bone

Fossa for lacrimal sac

Orbital surface of maxilla

Infraorbital foramen

B. Right orbit: frontal and slightly lateral view

8.3 SKULL: ANTEROPOSTERIOR CALDWELL PROJECTION AND FACE/ORBIT DETAIL

In an anteroposterior (AP) Caldwell view of the skull, the head is positioned so the petrous parts of the temporal bone are projected through the maxillary sinuses rather than the orbits. Orbital anatomy and pathology are better seen here; maxillary sinuses are better studied (e.g., for "blow-out" fractures) in a conventional film. A dominant feature of the orbit is the superior orbital fissure separating the greater and lesser wings of the sphenoid bone. The lateral surface of the greater wing of the sphenoid bone in the infratemporal fossa behind the orbit is also prominent.

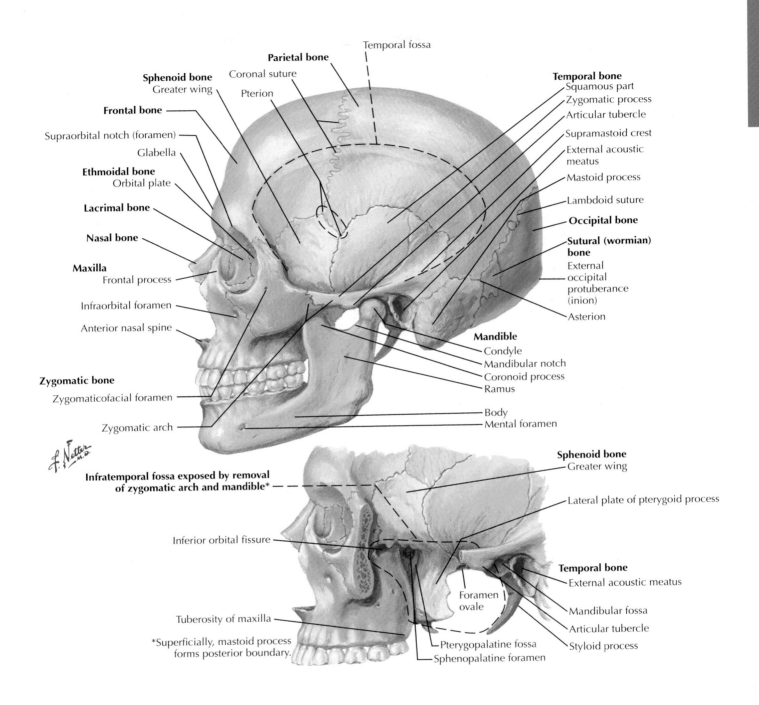

Temporal fossa

Parietal bone

Sphenoid bone Coronal suture
Greater wing

Pterion

Frontal bone

Supraorbital notch (foramen)

Glabella

Ethmoidal bone
Orbital plate

Lacrimal bone

Nasal bone

Maxilla
Frontal process

Infraorbital foramen

Anterior nasal spine

Zygomatic bone

Zygomaticofacial foramen

Zygomatic arch

Temporal bone
Squamous part
Zygomatic process
Articular tubercle
Supramastoid crest
External acoustic meatus
Mastoid process
Lambdoid suture
Occipital bone
Sutural (wormian) bone
External occipital protuberance (inion)
Asterion

Mandible
Condyle
Mandibular notch
Coronoid process
Ramus

Body
Mental foramen

Infratemporal fossa exposed by removal of zygomatic arch and mandible*

Inferior orbital fissure

Tuberosity of maxilla

*Superficially, mastoid process forms posterior boundary.

Sphenoid bone
Greater wing

Lateral plate of pterygoid process

Temporal bone
External acoustic meatus

Foramen ovale

Mandibular fossa
Articular tubercle
Styloid process

Pterygopalatine fossa
Sphenopalatine foramen

8.4 SKULL: LATERAL VIEW

The skull consists of a neurocranium surrounding the brain and a viscerocranium consisting of upper and lower jaws and the orbits. The coronal suture separates the frontal and parietal bones, the lambdoidal suture the parietal and occipital bones, and the squamous suture the parietal and temporal bones. Following the contour of the lateral surface of the neurocranium from superficial to deep are three fossae: the temporal fossa for the temporalis muscle; the infratemporal fossa for the pterygoid muscles, mandibular nerve, and maxillary artery; and the pterygopalatine fossa for the maxillary nerve and sphenopalatine artery.

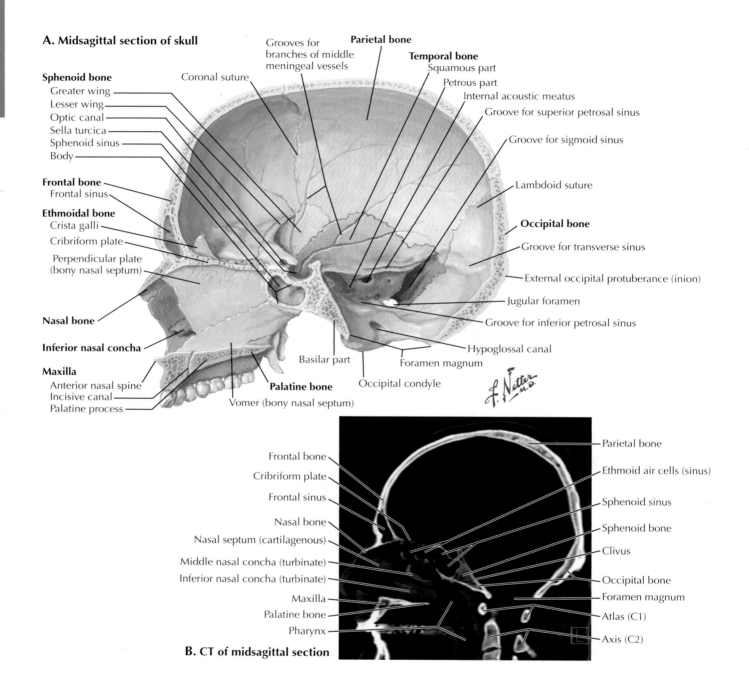

A. Midsagittal section of skull

Grooves for branches of middle meningeal vessels

Parietal bone

Temporal bone
Squamous part
Petrous part
Internal acoustic meatus

Coronal suture

Groove for superior petrosal sinus

Sphenoid bone
Greater wing
Lesser wing
Optic canal
Sella turcica
Sphenoid sinus
Body

Groove for sigmoid sinus

Lambdoid suture

Frontal bone
Frontal sinus

Occipital bone

Ethmoidal bone
Crista galli
Cribriform plate

Groove for transverse sinus

Perpendicular plate
(bony nasal septum)

External occipital protuberance (inion)

Jugular foramen

Nasal bone

Groove for inferior petrosal sinus

Inferior nasal concha

Hypoglossal canal

Basilar part

Maxilla
Anterior nasal spine
Incisive canal
Palatine process

Foramen magnum

Occipital condyle

Palatine bone

Vomer (bony nasal septum)

Frontal bone
Cribriform plate
Frontal sinus
Nasal bone
Nasal septum (cartilagenous)
Middle nasal concha (turbinate)
Inferior nasal concha (turbinate)
Maxilla
Palatine bone
Pharynx

Parietal bone
Ethmoid air cells (sinus)
Sphenoid sinus
Sphenoid bone
Clivus
Occipital bone
Foramen magnum
Atlas (C1)
Axis (C2)

B. CT of midsagittal section

8.5 SKULL: MIDSAGITTAL SECTION

The frontal sinus and sphenoidal sinus are cut in section. The sella turcica ("Turkish saddle") housing the hypophysis of the brain is an important landmark at the junction of the anterior and posterior cranial base between the viscerocranium and neurocranium. The petrous parts of the temporal bone separate the middle and posterior cranial fossae. Grooves on the neurocranial bones contain the middle meningeal vessel branches that supply these bones and the dura mater surrounding the brain.

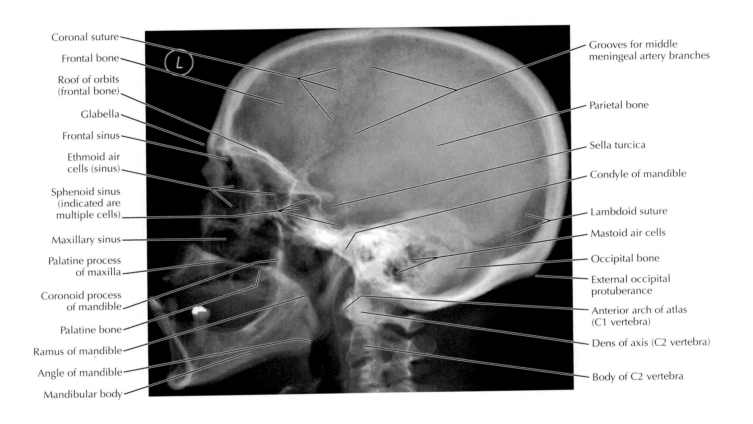

Coronal suture
Frontal bone
Roof of orbits (frontal bone)
Glabella
Frontal sinus
Ethmoid air cells (sinus)
Sphenoid sinus (indicated are multiple cells)
Maxillary sinus
Palatine process of maxilla
Coronoid process of mandible
Palatine bone
Ramus of mandible
Angle of mandible
Mandibular body

Grooves for middle meningeal artery branches
Parietal bone
Sella turcica
Condyle of mandible
Lambdoid suture
Mastoid air cells
Occipital bone
External occipital protuberance
Anterior arch of atlas (C1 vertebra)
Dens of axis (C2 vertebra)
Body of C2 vertebra

8.6 LATERAL X-RAY

Radiolucent air is apparent as dark areas in the mastoid air cells, paranasal air sinuses, and pharynx. The very dense opacity represents the petrous parts of the temporal bones superimposed on each other. Note the sella turcica, coronal and lambdoidal sutures, and atlas (C1) and axis (C2). The squamosal suture is not visible because the thin bones overlap at their articulation unlike the end-to-end articulations of thicker bone at the other sutures. Also note in the neurocranial bones the outer and inner tables of compact bone and the diploë (trabecular bone) in between.

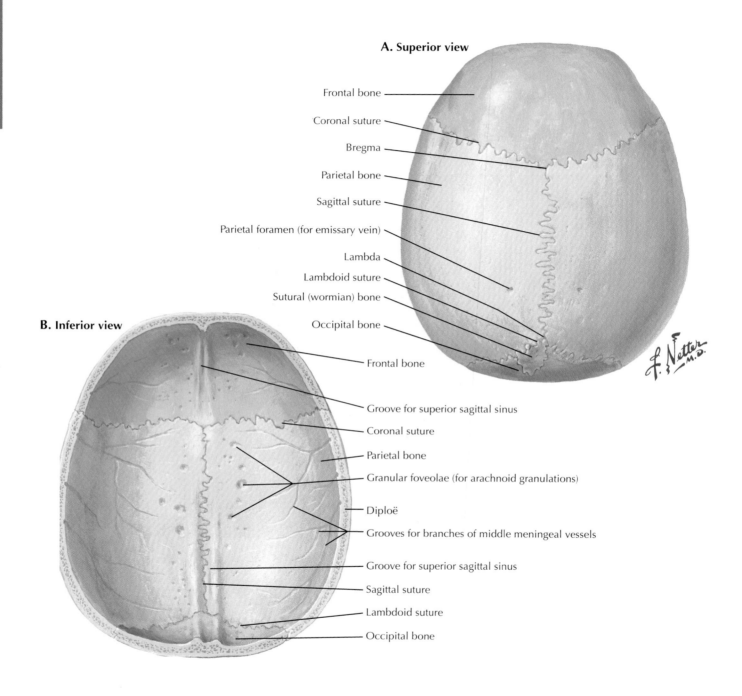

A. Superior view

Frontal bone

Coronal suture

Bregma

Parietal bone

Sagittal suture

Parietal foramen (for emissary vein)

Lambda

Lambdoid suture

Sutural (wormian) bone

Occipital bone

Frontal bone

B. Inferior view

Groove for superior sagittal sinus

Coronal suture

Parietal bone

Granular foveolae (for arachnoid granulations)

Diploë

Grooves for branches of middle meningeal vessels

Groove for superior sagittal sinus

Sagittal suture

Lambdoid suture

Occipital bone

8.7 CALVARIA

The sagittal suture separates the left and right parietal bones. From the frontal bone to the occipital bone is a groove for the superior sagittal sinus, a venous channel in the dura mater that receives blood from the brain. All dural sinuses converge on the internal jugular vein. Depressions on the parietal bone are for arachnoid granulations that penetrate lacunae, lateral extensions of the superior sagittal sinus. This is where cerebrospinal fluid (CSF) reenters the circulation. The parietal foramina and smaller foramina along the midline are for emissary veins that connect the scalp veins to the superior sagittal sinus.

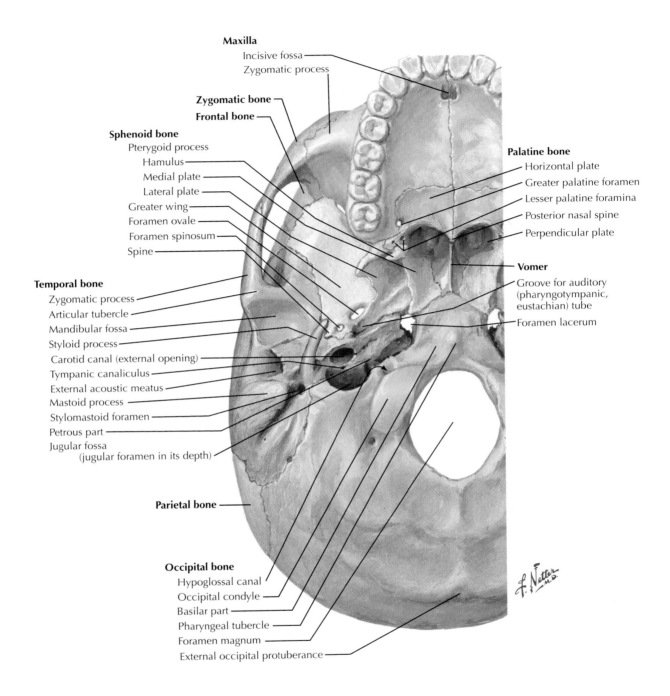

Maxilla
Incisive fossa
Zygomatic process

Zygomatic bone
Frontal bone

Sphenoid bone
Pterygoid process
Hamulus
Medial plate
Lateral plate
Greater wing
Foramen ovale
Foramen spinosum
Spine

Temporal bone
Zygomatic process
Articular tubercle
Mandibular fossa
Styloid process
Carotid canal (external opening)
Tympanic canaliculus
External acoustic meatus
Mastoid process
Stylomastoid foramen
Petrous part
Jugular fossa
(jugular foramen in its depth)

Parietal bone

Occipital bone
Hypoglossal canal
Occipital condyle
Basilar part
Pharyngeal tubercle
Foramen magnum
External occipital protuberance

Palatine bone
Horizontal plate
Greater palatine foramen
Lesser palatine foramina
Posterior nasal spine
Perpendicular plate

Vomer
Groove for auditory (pharyngotympanic, eustachian) tube
Foramen lacerum

8.8 CRANIAL BASE: INFERIOR VIEW

The cranial base is the inferior portion of the neurocranium that is the interface with the viscerocranium (facial skeleton) anteriorly. The petrous parts of the temporal bones extend medially between the occipital and sphenoid bones. The inferior extent of the upper jaw is the bony palate consisting of the maxilla and horizontal plate of the palatine bones. Behind the upper jaw are the medial and lateral pterygoid plates of the sphenoid bone. The nasal septum is the vomer posteriorly. Note the mandibular fossa of the temporal bone, the carotid and jugular canals, and the occipital condyles flanking the foramen magnum.

Bones

A. Superior view of cranial base

Foramina

Frontal bone
Sulcus of superior sagittal sinus
Frontal crest
Foramen cecum
Internal surface of orbital part

Ethmoid bone
Crista galli
Cribriform plate

Sphenoid bone
Lesser wing
Anterior clinoid process
Greater wing
Sulcus for middle meningeal
vessels (frontal branches)
Body
Sella turcica
Tuberculum sellae
Hypophyseal fossa
Posterior clinoid process
Dorsum sellae
Groove for internal carotid artery

Temporal bone
Squamous part
Petrous part
Sulcus of lesser petrosal nerve
Sulcus of greater petrosal nerve
Cartilage of auditory tube
Sulcus of superior petrosal sinus
Sulcus of sigmoid sinus

Parietal bone
Sulcus for middle meningeal
vessels (parietal branches)

Occipital bone
Basilar part
Sulcus of inferior petrosal sinus
Sulcus of transverse sinus
Sulcus of occipital sinus
Sulcus of superior sagittal sinus

Anterior cranial fossa
Middle cranial fossa
Posterior cranial fossa

Foramen cecum
Anterior ethmoidal foramen
Foramina of cribriform plate
Posterior ethmoidal foramen
Optic canal
Superior orbital fissure
Foramen rotundum
Foramen ovale
Foramen spinosum
Foramen lacerum
Hiatus of canal of lesser petrosal nerve
Hiatus of canal of greater petrosal nerve
Interior acoustic meatus
Vestibular aqueduct
Mastoid foramen (inconstant)
Jugular foramen
Condylar canal (inconstant)
Hypoglossal canal
Foramen magnum

Maxillary sinus
Sphenoid sinus
Clivus
Foramen lacerum
Mandibular condyle
Petrous part of temporal bone
External acoustic meatus
Foramen magnum (anterior half in the plane)
Mastoid air cells
Groove for
sigmoid sinus

Nasal septum
Foramen ovale
Foramen spinosum
Carotid canal
Petrous part of temporal bone
External acoustic meatus
Jugular foramen
Posterior cranial fossa
(with cerebellum)
Internal occipital protuberance
Occipital bone

**B. Axial CT through cranial base
and posterior cranial fossa.** The anterior
cranial base is above the plane of section.

8.9 CRANIAL BASE: SUPERIOR VIEW

The lesser wings of the sphenoid divide the anterior and middle cranial fossae, and the petrous parts of the temporal bone separate the middle and posterior cranial fossae. From anterior to posterior along the cranial base are the ethmoid bone (between the orbits), body of the sphenoid bone, and basilar part of the occipital bone. The anterior cranial fossa contains the cribriform plate of the ethmoid bone (for the olfactory nerve). The middle cranial fossa has the three openings for the three divisions of the trigeminal nerve: superior-orbital fissure, foramen rotundum, and foramen ovale. Next to the foramen ovale is the foramen spinosum for the middle meningeal artery.

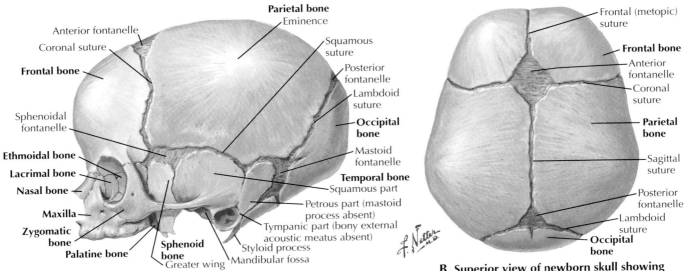

Anterior fontanelle
Coronal suture
Frontal bone
Sphenoidal fontanelle
Ethmoidal bone
Lacrimal bone
Nasal bone
Maxilla
Zygomatic bone
Palatine bone
Sphenoid bone
Greater wing

Parietal bone
Eminence
Squamous suture
Posterior fontanelle
Lambdoid suture
Occipital bone
Mastoid fontanelle
Temporal bone
Squamous part
Petrous part (mastoid process absent)
Tympanic part (bony external acoustic meatus absent)
Styloid process
Mandibular fossa

A. Lateral view of newborn skull

Frontal (metopic) suture
Frontal bone
Anterior fontanelle
Coronal suture
Parietal bone
Sagittal suture
Posterior fontanelle
Lambdoid suture
Occipital bone

B. Superior view of newborn skull showing fontanelles

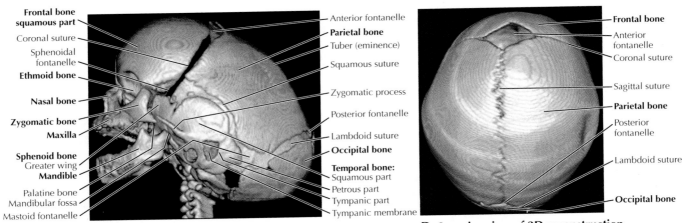

Frontal bone squamous part
Coronal suture
Sphenoidal fontanelle
Ethmoid bone
Nasal bone
Zygomatic bone
Maxilla
Sphenoid bone
Greater wing
Mandible
Palatine bone
Mandibular fossa
Mastoid fontanelle

Anterior fontanelle
Parietal bone
Tuber (eminence)
Squamous suture
Zygomatic process
Posterior fontanelle
Lambdoid suture
Occipital bone
Temporal bone:
Squamous part
Petrous part
Tympanic part
Tympanic membrane

C. Lateral view of 3D reconstruction from data derived from stacked CT axial slices. In infants, 3D reconstructions are used frequently for evaluating patients with craniosynostoses in which there is premature sutural closure that results in abnormal skull shape.

Frontal bone
Anterior fontanelle
Coronal suture
Sagittal suture
Parietal bone
Posterior fontanelle
Lambdoid suture
Occipital bone

D. Superior view of 3D reconstruction

8.10 SKULL OF THE NEWBORN

A newborn skull has a relatively large neurocranium and a relatively small viscerocranium. The bones of the cranial base develop via endochondral ossification. The flat bones of the neurocranium and the bones of the viscerocranium develop via intramembranous ossification. Unossified portions of the membranes called *fontanelles* are present anterior and posterior to the sagittal suture to facilitate deformation of the skull passing through the birth canal. The tympanic part of the temporal bone is a ring around the tympanic membrane at birth; there is no external acoustic meatus.

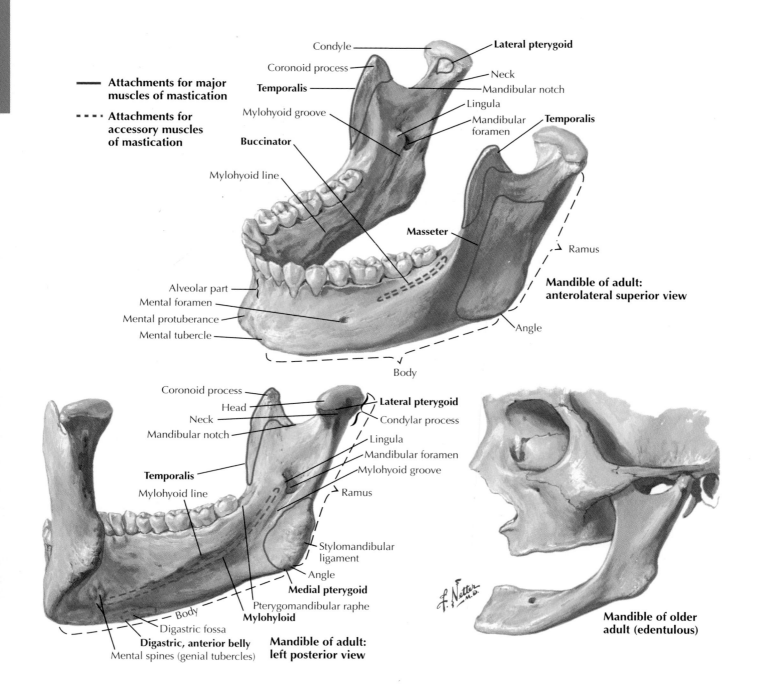

— Attachments for major muscles of mastication

- - - Attachments for accessory muscles of mastication

Condyle
Coronoid process
Temporalis
Mylohyoid groove
Buccinator
Mylohyoid line
Lateral pterygoid
Neck
Mandibular notch
Lingula
Mandibular foramen
Temporalis
Masseter
Ramus
Mandible of adult: anterolateral superior view
Alveolar part
Mental foramen
Mental protuberance
Mental tubercle
Angle
Body

Coronoid process
Head
Neck
Mandibular notch
Temporalis
Mylohyoid line
Lateral pterygoid
Condylar process
Lingula
Mandibular foramen
Mylohyoid groove
Ramus
Stylomandibular ligament
Angle
Medial pterygoid
Pterygomandibular raphe
Mylohyoid
Body
Digastric fossa
Digastric, anterior belly
Mental spines (genial tubercles)
Mandible of adult: left posterior view

Mandible of older adult (edentulous)

8.11 MANDIBLE

A mandible has a body with dense compact bone, an alveolar part containing the roots of the teeth, and a ramus. Parts of the latter include the angle, condyles for articulation with the temporal bones, and a coronoid process for attachment of the temporalis muscles. With the loss of teeth, the alveolar part of the mandible (and maxilla) is resorbed as a person grows older.

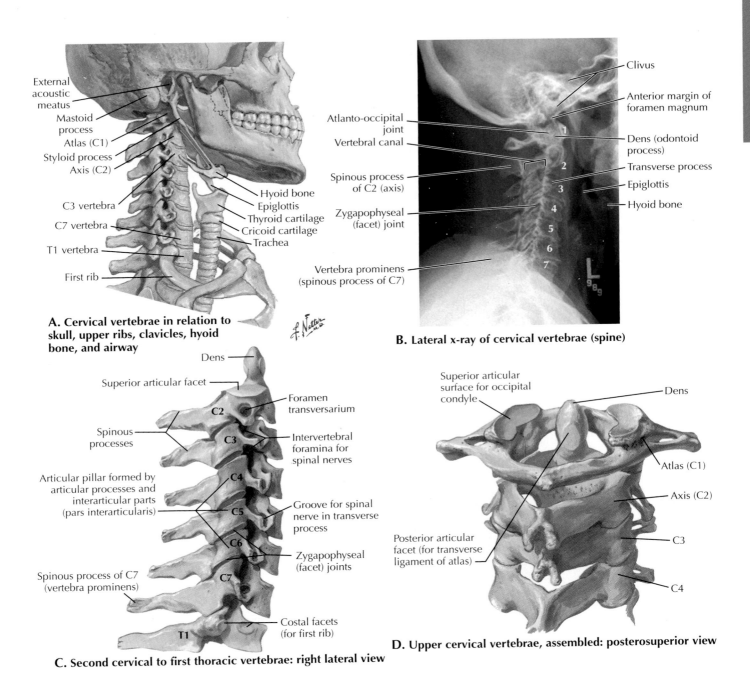

A. Cervical vertebrae in relation to skull, upper ribs, clavicles, hyoid bone, and airway

External acoustic meatus
Mastoid process
Atlas (C1)
Styloid process
Axis (C2)
C3 vertebra
C7 vertebra
T1 vertebra
First rib
Hyoid bone
Epiglottis
Thyroid cartilage
Cricoid cartilage
Trachea

B. Lateral x-ray of cervical vertebrae (spine)

Atlanto-occipital joint
Vertebral canal
Spinous process of C2 (axis)
Zygapophyseal (facet) joint
Vertebra prominens (spinous process of C7)
Clivus
Anterior margin of foramen magnum
Dens (odontoid process)
Transverse process
Epiglottis
Hyoid bone

C. Second cervical to first thoracic vertebrae: right lateral view

Dens
Superior articular facet
Spinous processes
Articular pillar formed by articular processes and interarticular parts (pars interarticularis)
Spinous process of C7 (vertebra prominens)
Foramen transversarium
Intervertebral foramina for spinal nerves
Groove for spinal nerve in transverse process
Zygapophyseal (facet) joints
Costal facets (for first rib)

D. Upper cervical vertebrae, assembled: posterosuperior view

Superior articular surface for occipital condyle
Posterior articular facet (for transverse ligament of atlas)
Dens
Atlas (C1)
Axis (C2)
C3
C4

8.12 CERVICAL VERTEBRAE AND LATERAL X-RAY

The seven cervical vertebrae are characterized by transverse foramina in the transverse processes. The first six are for passage of the vertebral arteries; the seventh is vestigial. The articulations between superior and inferior articular processes of adjacent vertebrae (facet joints) are flat and relatively horizontal. In the x-ray note the vertebral canal posterior to the vertebral bodies and the overlap of the dens (odontoid process) of C2 with the occipital condyles of the atlanto-occipital joint. The foramen magnum in this x-ray is obscured by the temporal bones. Its anterior margin can be located by extrapolating the lines of the clivus and the anterior wall of the vertebral canal. The projections of these lines converge on the anterior lip of the foramen magnum.

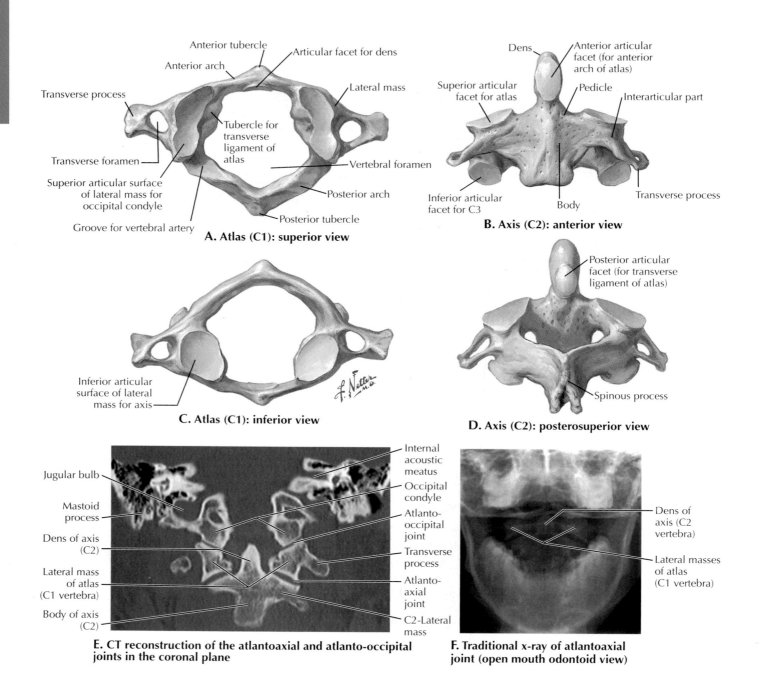

A. Atlas (C1): superior view

B. Axis (C2): anterior view

C. Atlas (C1): inferior view

D. Axis (C2): posterosuperior view

E. CT reconstruction of the atlantoaxial and atlanto-occipital joints in the coronal plane

F. Traditional x-ray of atlantoaxial joint (open mouth odontoid view)

8.13 ATLAS AND AXIS

With the ability to reconstruct different planes, computed tomography (CT) has largely replaced the open mouth C1/C2 x-rays. The atlas is the widest cervical vertebra, and it lacks a body (centrum). It articulates superiorly with the occipital condyles in a hinge joint for flexion and extension. Together with the skull, it pivots on the dens (odontoid process) of the axis (C2). The dens is the body of C1 that fuses to the axis during development.

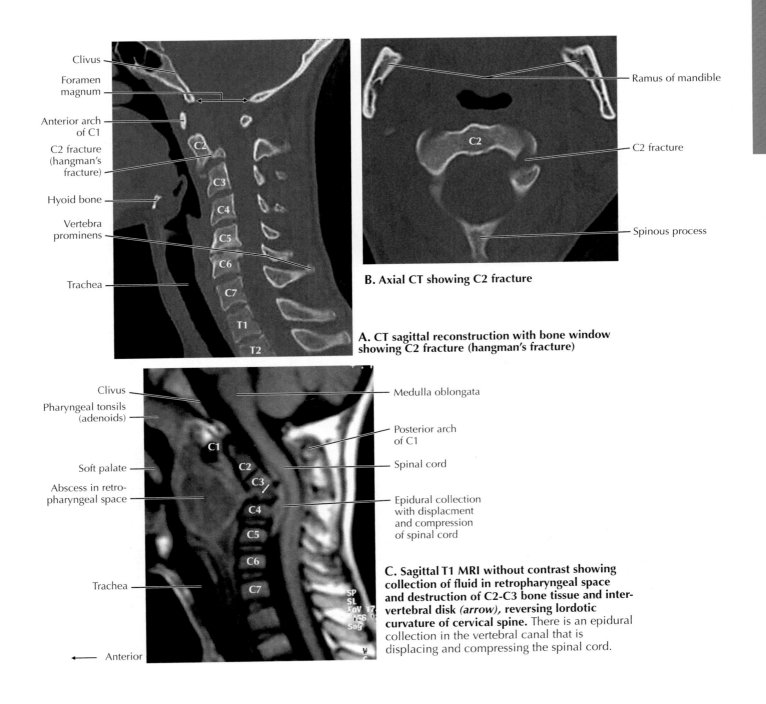

Clivus
Foramen magnum
Anterior arch of C1
C2 fracture (hangman's fracture)
Hyoid bone
Vertebra prominens
Trachea

C2, C3, C4, C5, C6, C7, T1, T2

Ramus of mandible
C2 fracture
Spinous process

B. Axial CT showing C2 fracture

A. CT sagittal reconstruction with bone window showing C2 fracture (hangman's fracture)

Clivus
Pharyngeal tonsils (adenoids)
Soft palate
Abscess in retro-pharyngeal space
Trachea
Anterior

Medulla oblongata
Posterior arch of C1
Spinal cord
Epidural collection with displacment and compression of spinal cord

C. Sagittal T1 MRI without contrast showing collection of fluid in retropharyngeal space and destruction of C2-C3 bone tissue and inter-vertebral disk *(arrow)*, reversing lordotic curvature of cervical spine. There is an epidural collection in the vertebral canal that is displacing and compressing the spinal cord.

8.14 IMAGING OF CERVICAL TRAUMA AND PATHOLOGY

Part of the systematic search strategy for the study of any image of the spine includes a close inspection of the size, shape, and alignment of the vertebral bodies. The anterior and posterior walls of the vertebral bodies and the posterior wall vertebral canal are known as the anterior spinal line, posterior spinal line, and spinolaminar line, respectively. The patient in **A** and **B** was in an automobile accident and has a fracture of the C2 body (hangman's fracture) and dislocation of the atlantoaxial joint (C1/C2). The dens is below the arch of the atlas, and the vertebral canal and spinal cord are displaced posteriorly below C1. There are also compression fractures of the C5 and C6 vertebral bodies. Note the increased density of bone, the narrow intervertebral space, and the posterior protrusion of bone into the vertebral canal. Other components of a search strategy include the evaluation of vertebral bodies for metastases and lesions (see Chapter 2, p. 27), other components of the vertebrae, plus the soft tissues anterior to the vertebral column (**C** [a different patient than in **A** and **B**]).

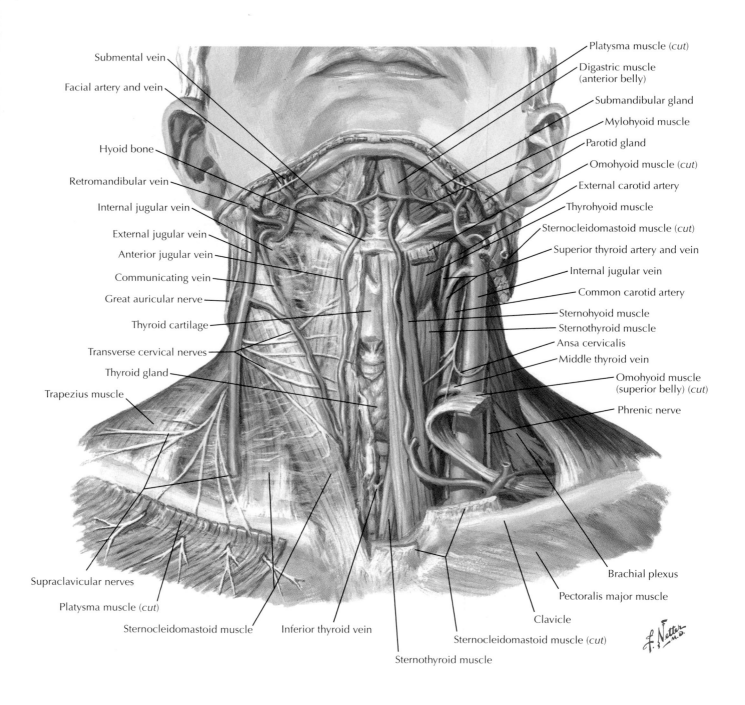

Submental vein

Facial artery and vein

Hyoid bone

Retromandibular vein

Internal jugular vein

External jugular vein

Anterior jugular vein

Communicating vein

Great auricular nerve

Thyroid cartilage

Transverse cervical nerves

Thyroid gland

Trapezius muscle

Supraclavicular nerves

Platysma muscle (cut)

Sternocleidomastoid muscle

Inferior thyroid vein

Sternothyroid muscle

Platysma muscle (cut)

Digastric muscle (anterior belly)

Submandibular gland

Mylohyoid muscle

Parotid gland

Omohyoid muscle (cut)

External carotid artery

Thyrohyoid muscle

Sternocleidomastoid muscle (cut)

Superior thyroid artery and vein

Internal jugular vein

Common carotid artery

Sternohyoid muscle

Sternothyroid muscle

Ansa cervicalis

Middle thyroid vein

Omohyoid muscle (superior belly) (cut)

Phrenic nerve

Brachial plexus

Pectoralis major muscle

Clavicle

Sternocleidomastoid muscle (cut)

8.15 SUPERFICIAL VESSELS, NERVES, AND MUSCLES OF THE NECK

The large, superficial sternocleidomastoid and trapezius muscles define the contours of the neck. Deep and anterior to the sternocleidomastoid muscle are the thin, infrahyoid "strap" muscles that are named by their attachments: omohyoid (reflected on one side); sternohyoid; and deep to these, the sternothyroid and thyrohyoid muscles. The hyoid bone is at vertebral level C3. At C5 is the thyroid cartilage of the larynx, and at C7 is the thyroid gland anterior to the trachea. The external jugular vein courses superficial to the sternocleidomastoid muscle. Deep to the muscle is the carotid sheath containing the internal jugular vein, common carotid artery, and vagus nerve.

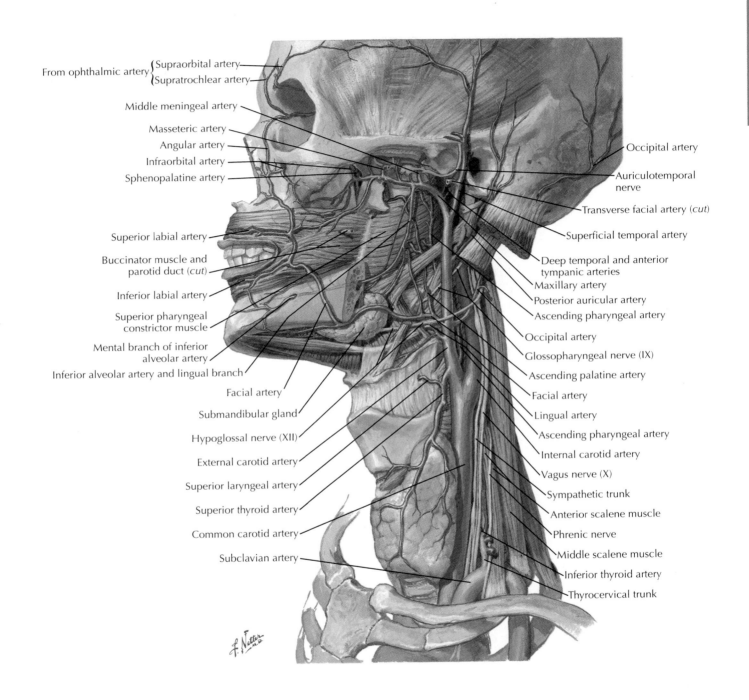

From ophthalmic artery {Supraorbital artery
Supratrochlear artery

Middle meningeal artery

Masseteric artery

Angular artery

Infraorbital artery

Sphenopalatine artery

Superior labial artery

Buccinator muscle and parotid duct (cut)

Inferior labial artery

Superior pharyngeal constrictor muscle

Mental branch of inferior alveolar artery

Inferior alveolar artery and lingual branch

Facial artery

Submandibular gland

Hypoglossal nerve (XII)

External carotid artery

Superior laryngeal artery

Superior thyroid artery

Common carotid artery

Subclavian artery

Occipital artery

Auriculotemporal nerve

Transverse facial artery (cut)

Superficial temporal artery

Deep temporal and anterior tympanic arteries

Maxillary artery

Posterior auricular artery

Ascending pharyngeal artery

Occipital artery

Glossopharyngeal nerve (IX)

Ascending palatine artery

Facial artery

Lingual artery

Ascending pharyngeal artery

Internal carotid artery

Vagus nerve (X)

Sympathetic trunk

Anterior scalene muscle

Phrenic nerve

Middle scalene muscle

Inferior thyroid artery

Thyrocervical trunk

8.16 ARTERIES OF ORAL AND PHARYNGEAL REGIONS

The deeper muscles of the neck are the three scalene muscles (anterior, middle, and posterior) that attach to the first and second ribs and the constrictors of the pharynx. The inferior constrictor muscle attaches anteriorly to the thyroid cartilage of the larynx, the middle constrictor muscle to the hyoid bone (not seen clearly here), and the superior constrictor muscle to the buccinator muscle. The common carotid artery bifurcates in the carotid sheath into the external and internal carotid arteries around the level of C4.

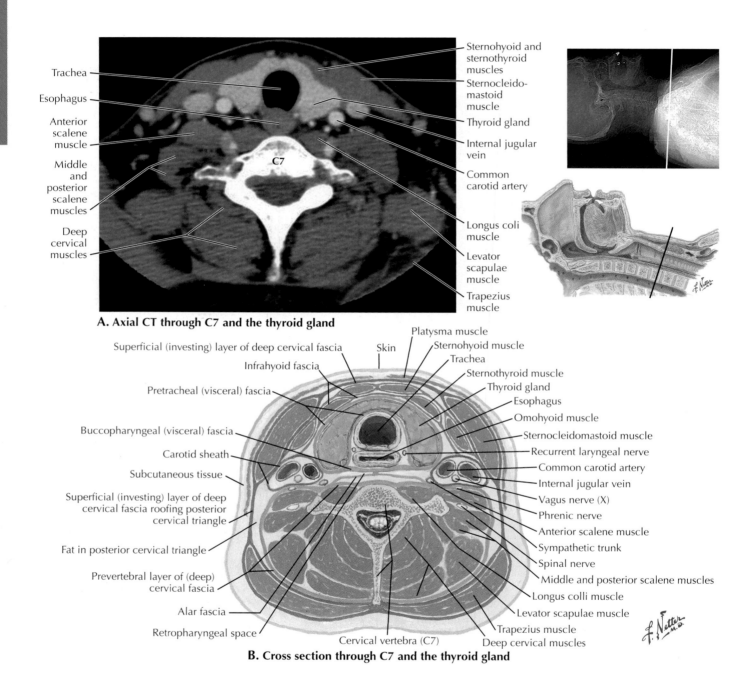

A. Axial CT through C7 and the thyroid gland

Trachea

Esophagus

Anterior scalene muscle

Middle and posterior scalene muscles

Deep cervical muscles

C7

Sternohyoid and sternothyroid muscles

Sternocleido-mastoid muscle

Thyroid gland

Internal jugular vein

Common carotid artery

Longus coli muscle

Levator scapulae muscle

Trapezius muscle

Superficial (investing) layer of deep cervical fascia

Infrahyoid fascia

Pretracheal (visceral) fascia

Buccopharyngeal (visceral) fascia

Carotid sheath

Subcutaneous tissue

Superficial (investing) layer of deep cervical fascia roofing posterior cervical triangle

Fat in posterior cervical triangle

Prevertebral layer of (deep) cervical fascia

Alar fascia

Retropharyngeal space

Skin

Platysma muscle

Sternohyoid muscle

Trachea

Sternothyroid muscle

Thyroid gland

Esophagus

Omohyoid muscle

Sternocleidomastoid muscle

Recurrent laryngeal nerve

Common carotid artery

Internal jugular vein

Vagus nerve (X)

Phrenic nerve

Anterior scalene muscle

Sympathetic trunk

Spinal nerve

Middle and posterior scalene muscles

Longus colli muscle

Levator scapulae muscle

Trapezius muscle

Deep cervical muscles

Cervical vertebra (C7)

B. Cross section through C7 and the thyroid gland

8.17 AXIAL CT AND CROSS SECTION OF THE NECK THROUGH C7 AND THE THYROID GLAND

The fascias of the neck envelop a visceral unit that includes the trachea/larynx, esophagus, and thyroid gland and a vertebral unit consisting of the vertebral column and surrounding muscles. The carotid sheath contains the common carotid artery, internal jugular vein, and vagus nerve. An axial (transverse) section of the neck at the level of the seventh cervical vertebra (C7) is through the thyroid gland (**A** and **B**). CT (**A**) is used for evaluation of the neck because of rapid scanning that can be obtained during a breath hold. Magnetic resonance imaging (MRI) can be used as well but is often less well tolerated by patients with significant pathologies. In addition, artifact from motion such as breathing and swallowing can degrade images.

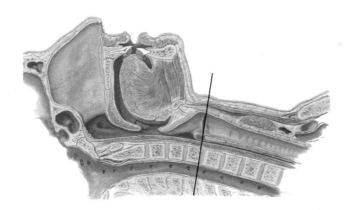

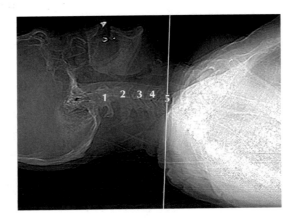

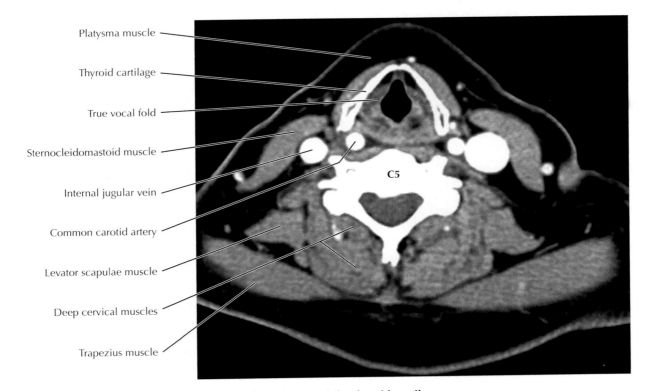

Platysma muscle

Thyroid cartilage

True vocal fold

Sternocleidomastoid muscle

Internal jugular vein

Common carotid artery

Levator scapulae muscle

Deep cervical muscles

Trapezius muscle

C5

Axial CT through C5 and the thyroid cartilage

8.18 AXIAL CT THROUGH C5 AND THE LARYNX

The larynx is the most prominent structure at the level of C5. In this axial CT, the section is through the true vocal folds and thyroid cartilage of the larynx. It is above the level of the cricoid cartilage. Between the larynx and C5 vertebra is the carotid sheath containing the internal jugular vein and common carotid artery. Note that the left internal jugular vein is much larger than the right. The sternocleidomastoid and trapezius muscles define the contour of the neck at all levels.

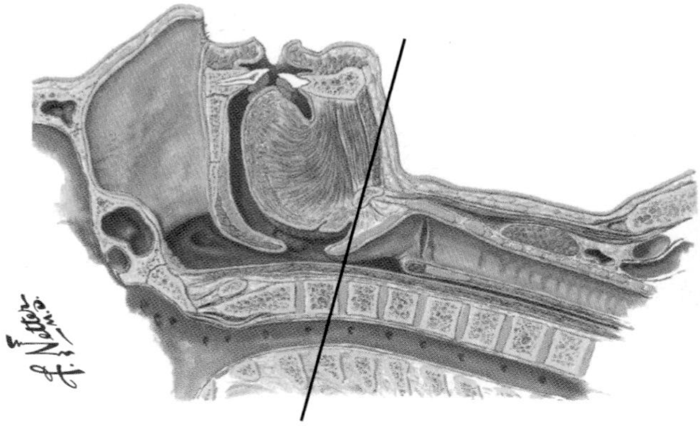

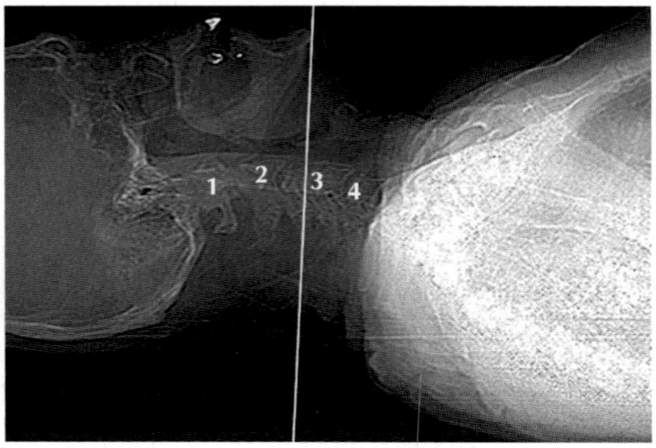
1
2
3
4

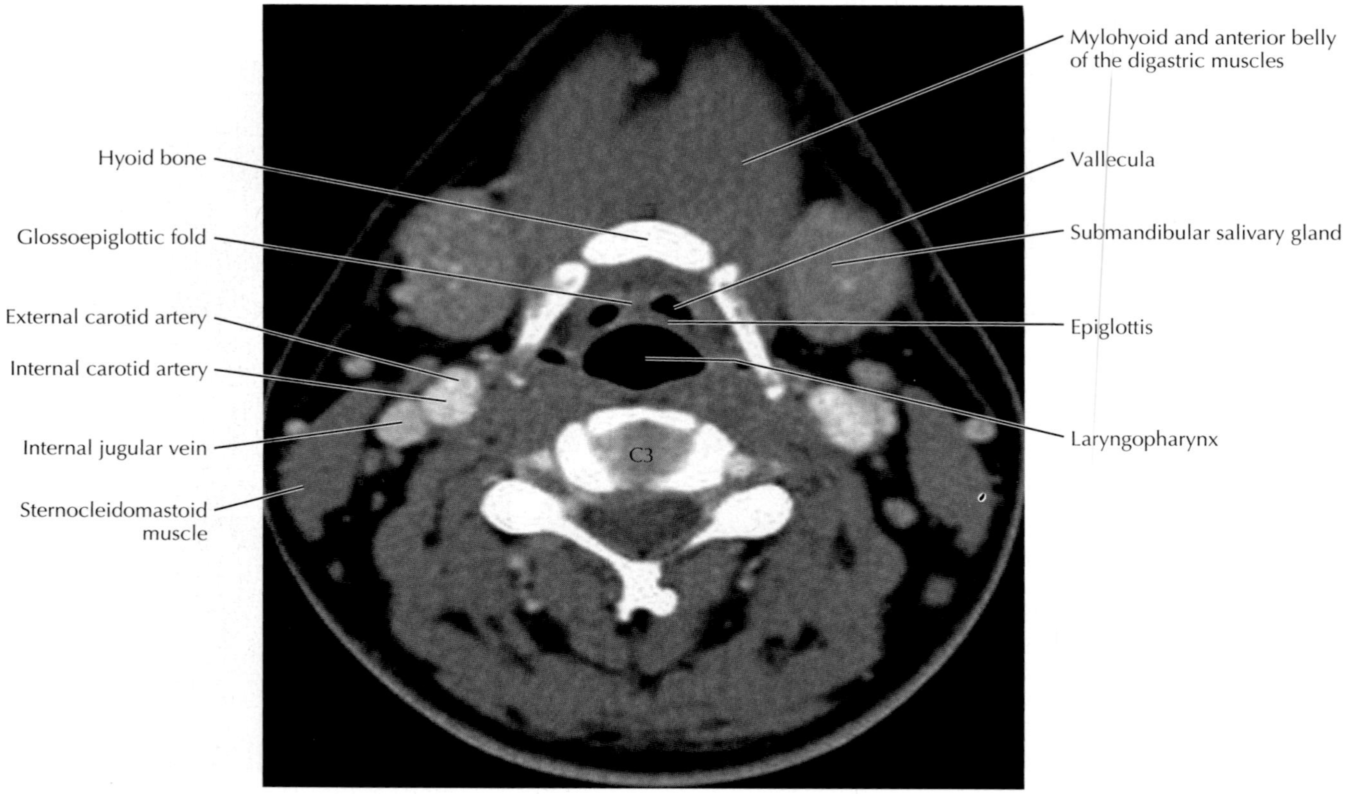
Hyoid bone
Glossoepiglottic fold
External carotid artery
Internal carotid artery
Internal jugular vein
Sternocleidomastoid muscle
C3
Mylohyoid and anterior belly of the digastric muscles
Vallecula
Submandibular salivary gland
Epiglottis
Laryngopharynx

Axial CT through C3 and the hyoid bone

8.19 AXIAL CT THROUGH C3 AND THE HYOID BONE

A section at C3 passes through the hyoid bone and epiglottis, just below the mandible in this individual. The projecting contour anteriorly indicates that the plane is close to the mandible, and the mylohyoid and anterior belly of the digastric muscles and the submandibular glands are visible. This is also at the level of the division of the common carotid artery into its internal and external branches.

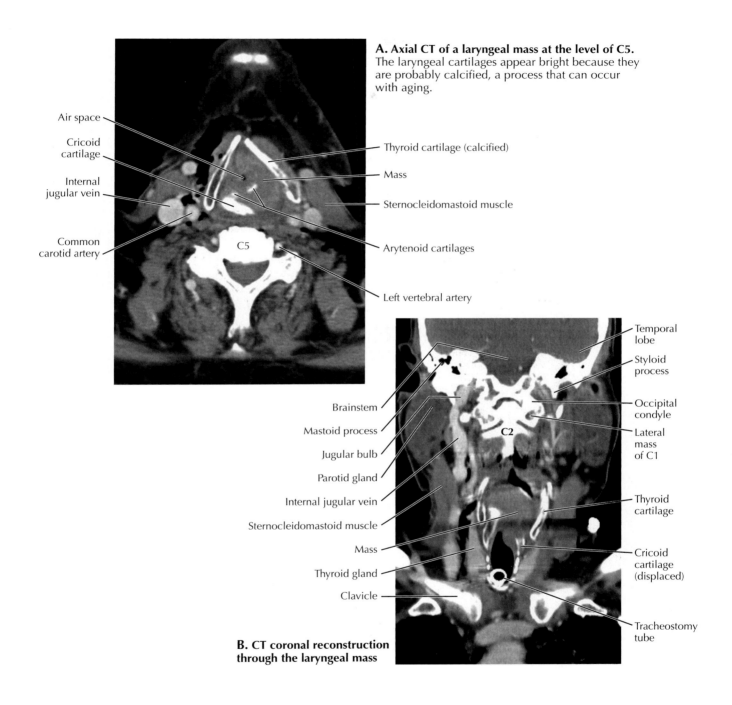

A. Axial CT of a laryngeal mass at the level of C5.
The laryngeal cartilages appear bright because they are probably calcified, a process that can occur with aging.

Air space

Cricoid cartilage

Internal jugular vein

Common carotid artery

Thyroid cartilage (calcified)

Mass

Sternocleidomastoid muscle

Arytenoid cartilages

C5

Left vertebral artery

Temporal lobe

Styloid process

Occipital condyle

Lateral mass of C1

Brainstem

Mastoid process

Jugular bulb

Parotid gland

Internal jugular vein

Sternocleidomastoid muscle

Mass

Thyroid gland

Clavicle

C2

Thyroid cartilage

Cricoid cartilage (displaced)

Tracheostomy tube

B. CT coronal reconstruction through the laryngeal mass

8.20 SEARCH STRATEGY: NECK IMAGING OF LARYNGEAL TUMOR

In addition to an analysis of the vertebral compartment (p. 199), a search strategy for the interpretation of neck images includes careful, systematic study of spaces, blood vessels, lymph nodes, organs of the visceral compartment, and other structures and layers visible in the image. **A** and **B** are views of a mass in the larynx on the left. In the axial image (**A**), the thyroid cartilage of the larynx is pushed laterally on the left. The mass is eroding and displacing inferiorly the cricoid cartilage on the left and compromising the air space in the larynx. The coronal view (**B**) shows an airway tube in the trachea and the mass filling much of the interior of the larynx.

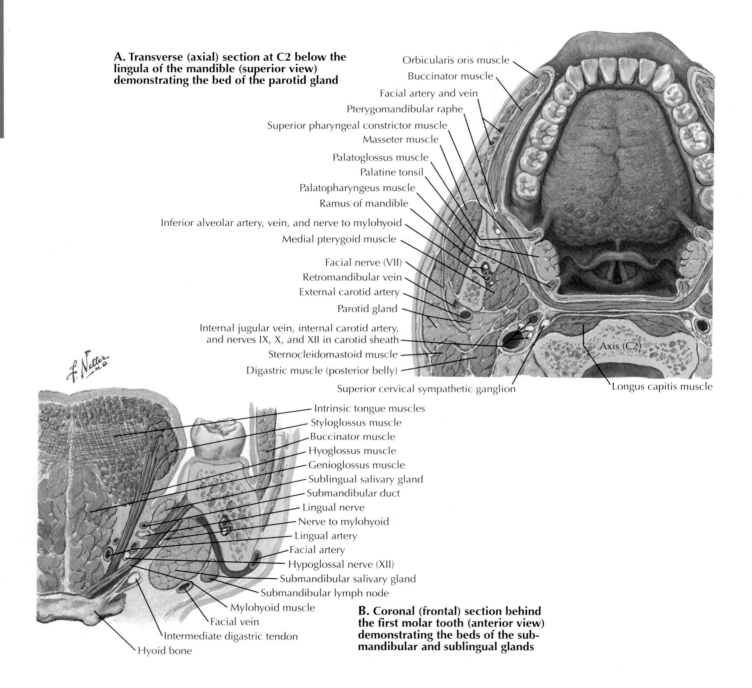

A. Transverse (axial) section at C2 below the lingula of the mandible (superior view) demonstrating the bed of the parotid gland

Orbicularis oris muscle
Buccinator muscle
Facial artery and vein
Pterygomandibular raphe
Superior pharyngeal constrictor muscle
Masseter muscle
Palatoglossus muscle
Palatine tonsil
Palatopharyngeus muscle
Ramus of mandible
Inferior alveolar artery, vein, and nerve to mylohyoid
Medial pterygoid muscle
Facial nerve (VII)
Retromandibular vein
External carotid artery
Parotid gland
Internal jugular vein, internal carotid artery, and nerves IX, X, and XII in carotid sheath
Sternocleidomastoid muscle
Digastric muscle (posterior belly)
Superior cervical sympathetic ganglion
Axis (C2)
Longus capitis muscle

Intrinsic tongue muscles
Styloglossus muscle
Buccinator muscle
Hyoglossus muscle
Genioglossus muscle
Sublingual salivary gland
Submandibular duct
Lingual nerve
Nerve to mylohyoid
Lingual artery
Facial artery
Hypoglossal nerve (XII)
Submandibular salivary gland
Submandibular lymph node
Mylohyoid muscle
Facial vein
Intermediate digastric tendon
Hyoid bone

B. Coronal (frontal) section behind the first molar tooth (anterior view) demonstrating the beds of the sub-mandibular and sublingual glands

8.21 CROSS AND CORONAL SECTIONS OF THE TONGUE AND SALIVARY GLANDS

A is a horizontal (axial) section. The buccinator muscle lining the oral cavity is continuous with the superior constrictor muscle of the pharynx. The masseter muscle is superficial to the ramus of the mandible; the medial pterygoid muscle is deep to it. The parotid gland extends deep to the mandibular ramus, and it is traversed in part by the external carotid artery and the facial nerve. **B** is a coronal section. The mylohyoid muscle is the floor of the oral cavity. The sublingual gland on each side is superior to it, and the submandibular gland is inferior to it, although it hooks around the muscle posteriorly to extend into the oral cavity, where its duct passes anteriorly to the lingual frenulum. The inferior half of the tongue is the genioglossus muscle, the fibers of which blend with the intrinsic tongue muscles in the superior half of the tongue.

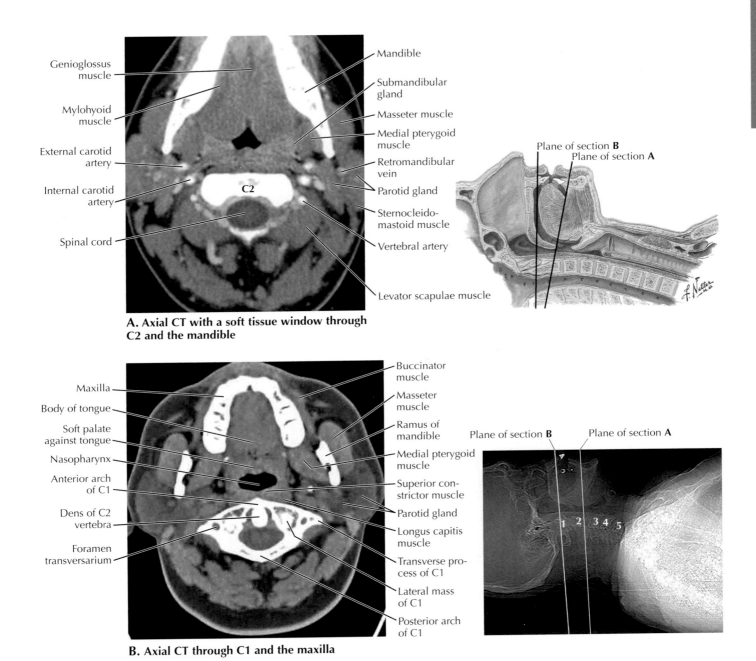

Genioglossus muscle

Mylohyoid muscle

External carotid artery

Internal carotid artery

Spinal cord

Mandible

Submandibular gland

Masseter muscle

Medial pterygoid muscle

Retromandibular vein

Parotid gland

Sternocleido-mastoid muscle

Vertebral artery

Levator scapulae muscle

Plane of section **B**

Plane of section **A**

A. Axial CT with a soft tissue window through C2 and the mandible

Maxilla

Body of tongue

Soft palate against tongue

Nasopharynx

Anterior arch of C1

Dens of C2 vertebra

Foramen transversarium

Buccinator muscle

Masseter muscle

Ramus of mandible

Medial pterygoid muscle

Superior con-strictor muscle

Parotid gland

Longus capitis muscle

Transverse pro-cess of C1

Lateral mass of C1

Posterior arch of C1

Plane of section **B**

Plane of section **A**

B. Axial CT through C1 and the maxilla

8.22 AXIAL CT AT C2 AND C1

A plane at the level of C2 (**A**) includes the mandible and genioglossus and mylohyoid muscles. The plane in this patient is low on the mandibular ramus at the most inferior attachment of the medial pterygoid muscle, and the submandibular gland is visible. The masseter muscle is superficial to the ramus, and the parotid gland wraps around the posterior margin of the ramus. The common carotid artery has just divided into its external and internal branches. At C1 (**B**), the plane is through the maxilla, intrinsic tongue muscles, and nasopharynx. The patient is breathing through the nose, and the soft palate compresses the oropharynx against the tongue. The medial pterygoid and masseter muscles are prominent in their attachments to the mandibular ramus.

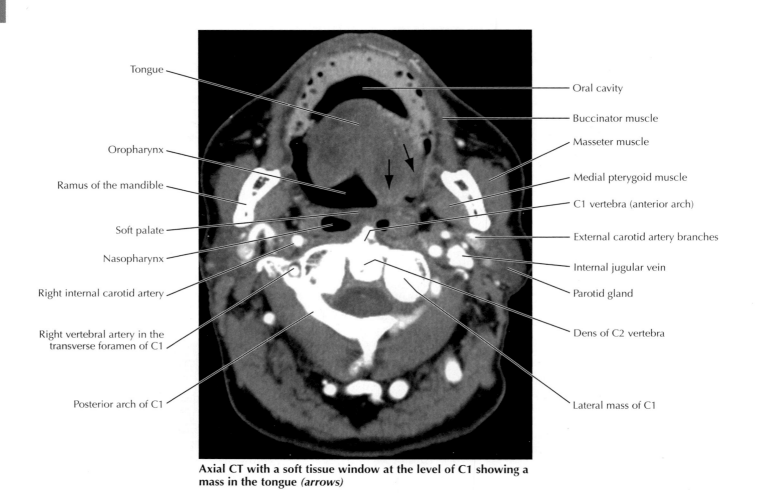

Tongue

Oropharynx

Ramus of the mandible

Soft palate

Nasopharynx

Right internal carotid artery

Right vertebral artery in the transverse foramen of C1

Posterior arch of C1

Oral cavity

Buccinator muscle

Masseter muscle

Medial pterygoid muscle

C1 vertebra (anterior arch)

External carotid artery branches

Internal jugular vein

Parotid gland

Dens of C2 vertebra

Lateral mass of C1

Axial CT with a soft tissue window at the level of C1 showing a mass in the tongue *(arrows)*

8.23 IMAGING PATHOLOGY OF THE ORAL CAVITY

A mass in the tongue projecting into the oropharynx on the left is visible in this image. The patient is breathing through the mouth, with the soft palate elevated against the posterior wall of the pharynx.

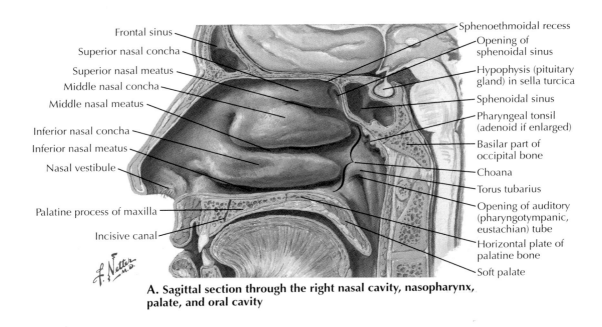

Frontal sinus
Superior nasal concha
Superior nasal meatus
Middle nasal concha
Middle nasal meatus
Inferior nasal concha
Inferior nasal meatus
Nasal vestibule
Palatine process of maxilla
Incisive canal

Sphenoethmoidal recess
Opening of sphenoidal sinus
Hypophysis (pituitary gland) in sella turcica
Sphenoidal sinus
Pharyngeal tonsil (adenoid if enlarged)
Basilar part of occipital bone
Choana
Torus tubarius
Opening of auditory (pharyngotympanic, eustachian) tube
Horizontal plate of palatine bone
Soft palate

A. Sagittal section through the right nasal cavity, nasopharynx, palate, and oral cavity

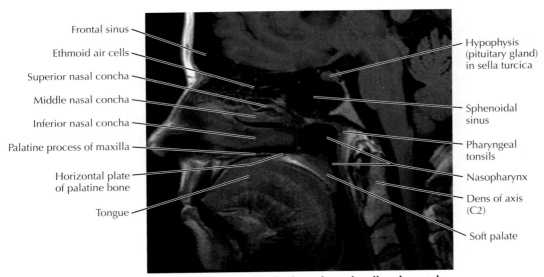

Frontal sinus
Ethmoid air cells
Superior nasal concha
Middle nasal concha
Inferior nasal concha
Palatine process of maxilla
Horizontal plate of palatine bone
Tongue

Hypophysis (pituitary gland) in sella turcica
Sphenoidal sinus
Pharyngeal tonsils
Nasopharynx
Dens of axis (C2)
Soft palate

B. Sagittal T1 MRI through the lateral nasal wall and nasopharynx

8.24 LATERAL WALL OF THE NASAL CAVITY

Scroll-like superior, middle, and inferior nasal conchae occupy the lateral wall of each nasal cavity (**A**). The spaces below conchae are called meati. The bony palate consisting of the maxilla and palatine bones separates the nasal and oral cavities. The soft palate separates the nasopharynx from the oropharynx. The nasolacrimal duct drains tears into the inferior meatus. Mucus from the frontal sinus, maxillary sinus, and anterior ethmoid air cells drains into the hiatus semilunaris of the middle meatus. Posterior ethmoid air cells drain into the superior meatus. The sphenoid sinus drains into the highest space in the nasal cavity above the superior concha, the sphenoethmoidal recess. The auditory tube from the middle ear cavity opens in the nasopharynx to balance pressure on both sides of the tympanic membrane (eardrum).

A. Cross section of the nose and maxillary sinuses

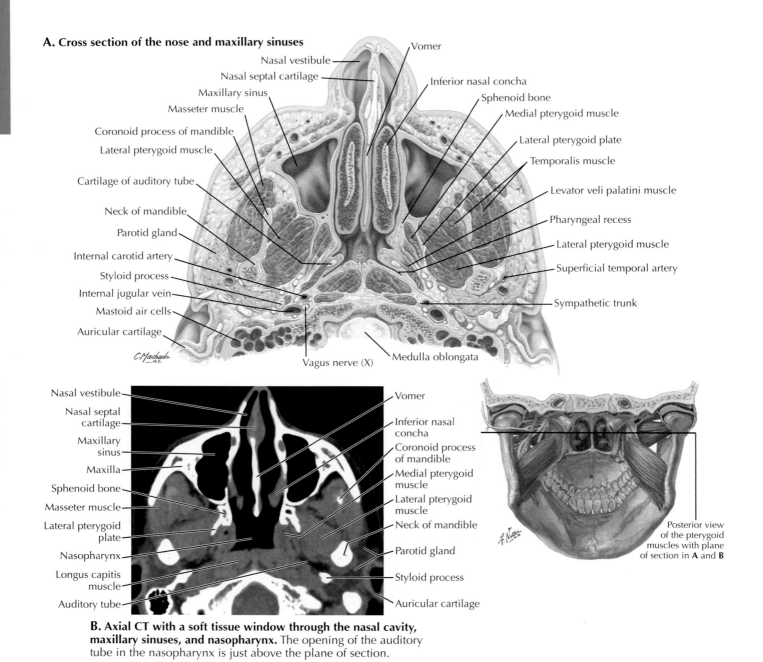

Vomer

Nasal vestibule

Nasal septal cartilage

Inferior nasal concha

Maxillary sinus

Sphenoid bone

Masseter muscle

Medial pterygoid muscle

Coronoid process of mandible

Lateral pterygoid plate

Lateral pterygoid muscle

Temporalis muscle

Cartilage of auditory tube

Levator veli palatini muscle

Neck of mandible

Pharyngeal recess

Parotid gland

Lateral pterygoid muscle

Internal carotid artery

Superficial temporal artery

Styloid process

Internal jugular vein

Sympathetic trunk

Mastoid air cells

Auricular cartilage

Vagus nerve (X)

Medulla oblongata

Nasal vestibule

Vomer

Nasal septal cartilage

Inferior nasal concha

Maxillary sinus

Coronoid process of mandible

Maxilla

Medial pterygoid muscle

Sphenoid bone

Lateral pterygoid muscle

Masseter muscle

Neck of mandible

Lateral pterygoid plate

Parotid gland

Nasopharynx

Longus capitis muscle

Styloid process

Auditory tube

Auricular cartilage

Posterior view of the pterygoid muscles with plane of section in **A** and **B**

B. Axial CT with a soft tissue window through the nasal cavity, maxillary sinuses, and nasopharynx. The opening of the auditory tube in the nasopharynx is just above the plane of section.

8.25 THE NOSE, NASAL CAVITY, AND MAXILLARY SINUSES IN THE TRANSVERSE PLANE

The section is through the maxillary sinuses, inferior nasal conchae, nasopharynx, and mastoid air cells. Note the opening of the auditory tube (which is just above the level of section in the CT). The plane is near the top of the mandible through the coronoid process and neck above most of the medial pterygoid muscle. At this level the lateral pterygoid muscle extends from the lateral pterygoid plate to the neck of the condyle and articular disk. The soft tissue window in the axial CT (**B**) is useful for the identification of masses and other soft tissue pathology that might extend into the air spaces of nose, nasal cavity, nasopharynx, and maxillary sinuses.

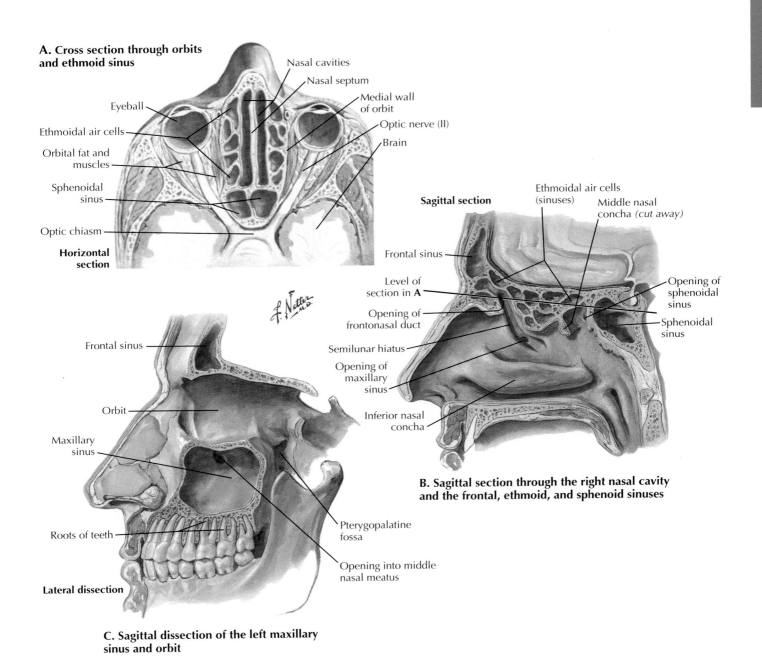

A. Cross section through orbits and ethmoid sinus

Nasal cavities

Nasal septum

Eyeball

Medial wall of orbit

Ethmoidal air cells

Optic nerve (II)

Orbital fat and muscles

Brain

Sphenoidal sinus

Optic chiasm

Horizontal section

Sagittal section

Ethmoidal air cells (sinuses)

Middle nasal concha *(cut away)*

Frontal sinus

Opening of sphenoidal sinus

Level of section in **A**

Sphenoidal sinus

Opening of frontonasal duct

Semilunar hiatus

Opening of maxillary sinus

Frontal sinus

Inferior nasal concha

Orbit

B. Sagittal section through the right nasal cavity and the frontal, ethmoid, and sphenoid sinuses

Maxillary sinus

Roots of teeth

Pterygopalatine fossa

Opening into middle nasal meatus

Lateral dissection

C. Sagittal dissection of the left maxillary sinus and orbit

8.26 PARANASAL AIR SINUSES

The orbits are bounded by paranasal air sinuses. Between the orbits is the ethmoid bone with its ethmoid air cells (ethmoid sinus); the large chamber of each maxillary sinus is below the orbit. Continuous with the ethmoid air cells anteriorly and superiorly is the frontal sinus, and posterior to the ethmoid air cells is the sphenoid sinus in the body of the sphenoid bone.

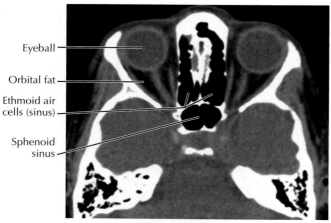

Eyeball

Orbital fat

Ethmoid air
cells (sinus)

Sphenoid
sinus

**A. Axial CT through the ethmoid and sphenoid
sinuses and orbits**

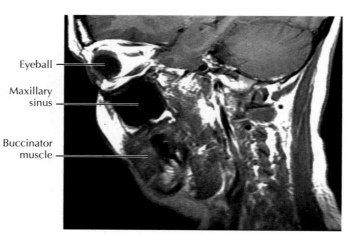

Eyeball

Maxillary
sinus

Buccinator
muscle

**B. Parasagittal T1 MRI through an orbit and
maxillary sinus**

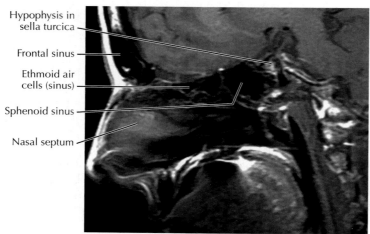

Hypophysis in
sella turcica

Frontal sinus

Ethmoid air
cells (sinus)

Sphenoid sinus

Nasal septum

**C. Midsagittal T1 MRI through the frontal, ethmoid,
and sphenoid sinuses**

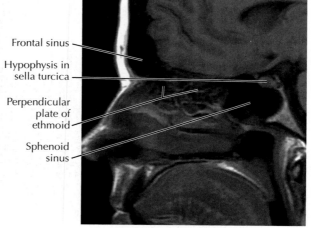

Frontal sinus

Hypophysis in
sella turcica

Perpendicular
plate of
ethmoid

Sphenoid
sinus

**D. Midsagittal T1 MRI through the upper
bony nasal septum**

8.27 IMAGING OF
THE PARANASAL SINUSES

A through **D** are axial and sagittal sections that show the paranasal sinuses. The sections in **A** and **B** also capture the orbit. The air in the sinuses appears black in both CT and MRI, which makes them prominent features in any image. The section in **D** is close to the perpendicular plate of the ethmoid

bone, the upper part of the nasal septum. Large ethmoid air cells are not seen. CT is excellent for evaluating bones of the orbits and paranasal sinuses and aeration status of the paranasal sinuses. MRI is better at evaluating the nature of soft tissues, especially if masses are present. MRI is also excellent for evaluating intraorbital pathology.

A. Horizontal section

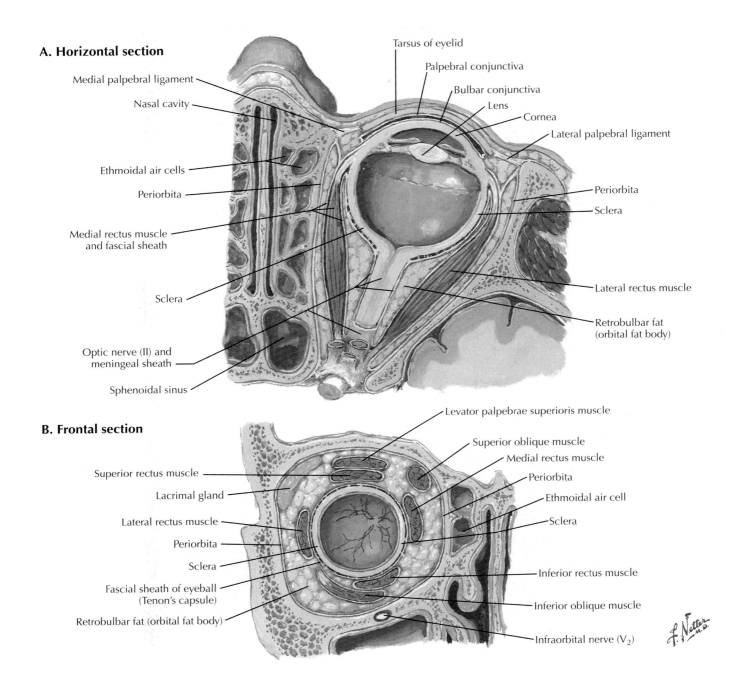

Medial palpebral ligament

Nasal cavity

Ethmoidal air cells

Periorbita

Medial rectus muscle
and fascial sheath

Sclera

Optic nerve (II) and
meningeal sheath

Sphenoidal sinus

Tarsus of eyelid

Palpebral conjunctiva

Bulbar conjunctiva

Lens

Cornea

Lateral palpebral ligament

Periorbita

Sclera

Lateral rectus muscle

Retrobulbar fat
(orbital fat body)

B. Frontal section

Levator palpebrae superioris muscle

Superior oblique muscle

Medial rectus muscle

Periorbita

Ethmoidal air cell

Sclera

Inferior rectus muscle

Inferior oblique muscle

Infraorbital nerve (V₂)

Superior rectus muscle

Lacrimal gland

Lateral rectus muscle

Periorbita

Sclera

Fascial sheath of eyeball
(Tenon's capsule)

Retrobulbar fat (orbital fat body)

8.28 CROSS AND CORONAL SECTIONS OF THE ORBIT

Six extraocular eye muscles attach to each eyeball (oculus) in the orbit: four rectus muscles (superior, inferior, medial, and lateral) and two oblique muscles (superior and inferior). The levator palpebrae superiorus runs above superior rectus into the upper eyelid. The lacrimal gland produces tears in the upper lateral aspect of the orbit. The optic nerve is surrounded by meninges, and the dura mater is continuous anteriorly with the sclera, the thick, connective tissue framework of the eye. The visual axes of the eyes are AP, but the axes of the orbits and optic nerves diverge laterally.

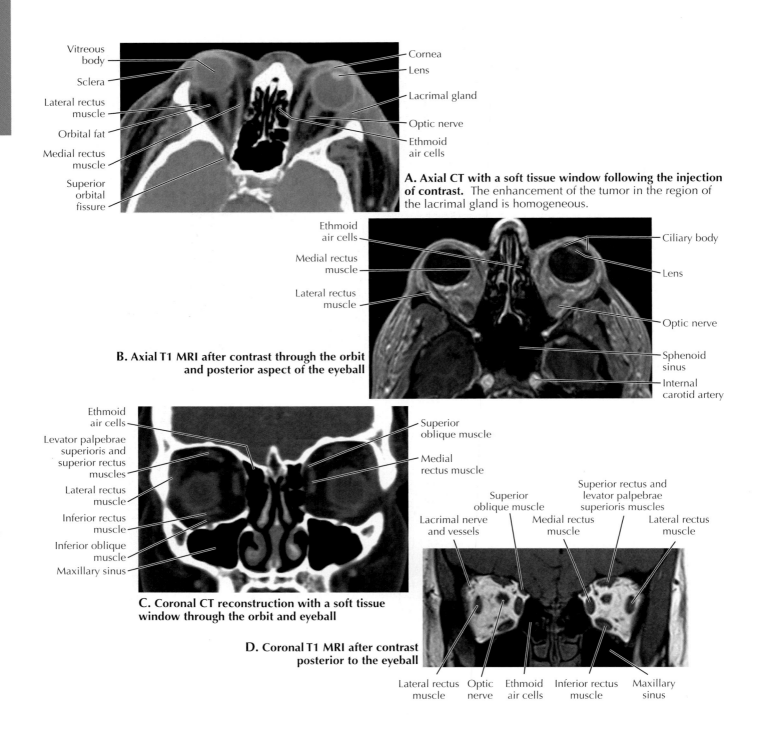

Vitreous body
Sclera
Lateral rectus muscle
Orbital fat
Medial rectus muscle
Superior orbital fissure

Cornea
Lens
Lacrimal gland
Optic nerve
Ethmoid air cells

A. Axial CT with a soft tissue window following the injection of contrast. The enhancement of the tumor in the region of the lacrimal gland is homogeneous.

Ethmoid air cells
Medial rectus muscle
Lateral rectus muscle

Ciliary body
Lens
Optic nerve
Sphenoid sinus
Internal carotid artery

B. Axial T1 MRI after contrast through the orbit and posterior aspect of the eyeball

Ethmoid air cells
Levator palpebrae superioris and superior rectus muscles
Lateral rectus muscle
Inferior rectus muscle
Inferior oblique muscle
Maxillary sinus

Superior oblique muscle
Medial rectus muscle

C. Coronal CT reconstruction with a soft tissue window through the orbit and eyeball

Superior oblique muscle
Lacrimal nerve and vessels
Medial rectus muscle
Superior rectus and levator palpebrae superioris muscles
Lateral rectus muscle

D. Coronal T1 MRI after contrast posterior to the eyeball

Lateral rectus muscle   Optic nerve   Ethmoid air cells   Inferior rectus muscle   Maxillary sinus

8.29 IMAGING OF THE ORBIT

The coronal section in **C** is posterior to the midline of the eyeball, and there is space between the extraocular muscles and the sclera. The inferior oblique muscle is not seen in **D** because the section is at the back of the orbit posterior to the eye; the muscle originates near the anterior margin of maxilla. CT is useful for evaluating the bony orbit, for hematomas as a result of trauma, and for foreign bodies. MRI is more sensitive for the detection of masses and inflammatory lesions.

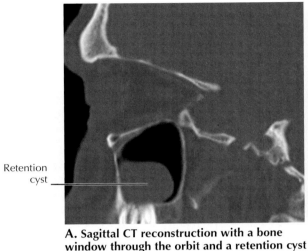

Retention cyst

A. Sagittal CT reconstruction with a bone window through the orbit and a retention cyst in the maxillary sinus

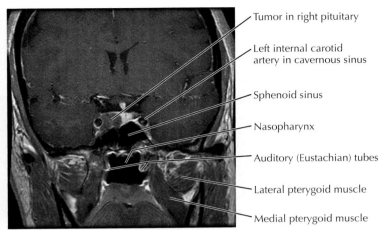

Tumor in right pituitary

Left internal carotid artery in cavernous sinus

Sphenoid sinus

Nasopharynx

Auditory (Eustachian) tubes

Lateral pterygoid muscle

Medial pterygoid muscle

B. MRI in the coronal plane through the sphenoid sinus, nasopharynx, and a tumor in the right half of the pituitary gland

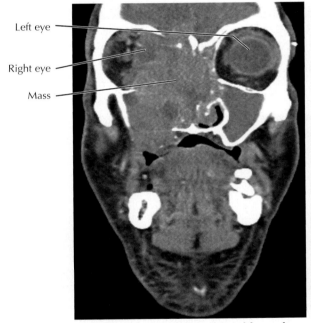

Left eye

Right eye

Mass

C. Coronal CT reconstruction with a soft tissue window showing a large mass in the right side of the face

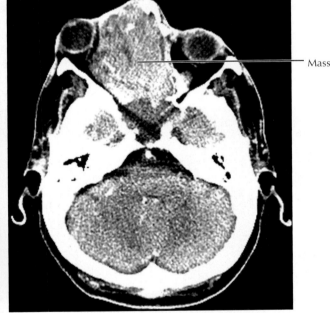

Mass

D. Axial contrast-enhanced CT showing the extent of the mass in the transverse plane

8.30 IMAGING OF SINUS AND ORBIT PATHOLOGY

The paranasal sinuses are air-filled, mucus-lined spaces in the bones that appear black in imaging studies. It is easy to see if they contain blood, mucus, fluid, masses, or other pathology. Compare one side with the other. **A** shows a mucus retention cyst in the maxillary sinus. **B** shows asymmetry of the sphenoid sinus in the coronal plane from a small tumor (microadenoma) of the pituitary gland that is projecting into the sphenoid sinus on the right side. **C** and **D** are coronal and axial CTs showing the extent of a large mass in the right side of the face. It has filled the ethmoid sinus, right maxillary sinus, and most of the nasal cavity. It has invaded the oral cavity and right orbit, obliterating the medial orbital wall and protruding the right eyeball. Note how the left maxillary sinus is filled with mucus or fluid from obstruction of its outflow into the nasal cavity.

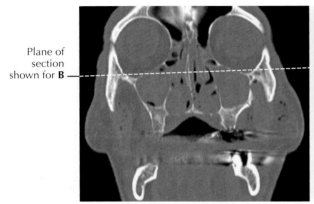

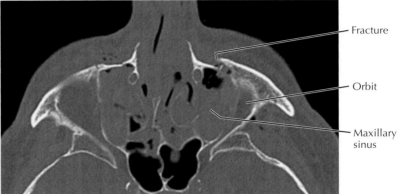

Plane of
section
shown for **B**

Fracture

Orbit

Maxillary
sinus

A. Coronal CT reconstruction showing soft tissue density, most likely blood, in the maxillary and ethmoid sinuses and nasal cavity

B. Axial CT of the same patient as in A (plane of section indicated in A) showing fracture of the roof of the left maxillary sinus (floor of the orbit) and multiple fractures of the ethmoid bone. The sphenoid sinus is mostly clear.

Mass

Mass

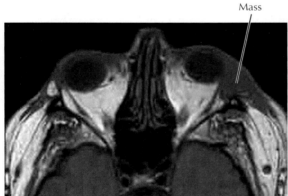

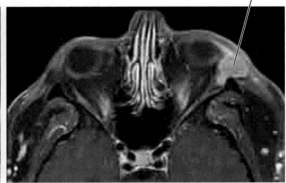

C. Axial T1 MRI through the orbits before vascular contrast showing a mass in the lacrimal region of the left orbit

D. Axial T1 MRI with a fat saturation sequence of the same patient in C after the administration of contrast

8.31 IMAGING OF SINUS AND ORBIT PATHOLOGY (CONT'D)

The CT images in **A** and **B** show fractures of the relatively thin bone of the floor and medial walls of the orbits with filling of the ethmoid and maxillary sinuses and nasal cavity with blood. The mass in the lacrimal region of the orbit in **C** and **D** is visualized with MRI before vascular contrast (**C**) and after vascular contrast (**D**). Its homogeneous appearance after contrast indicates that it is not a fluid-filled cyst or other nonvascular mass.

Coronal section

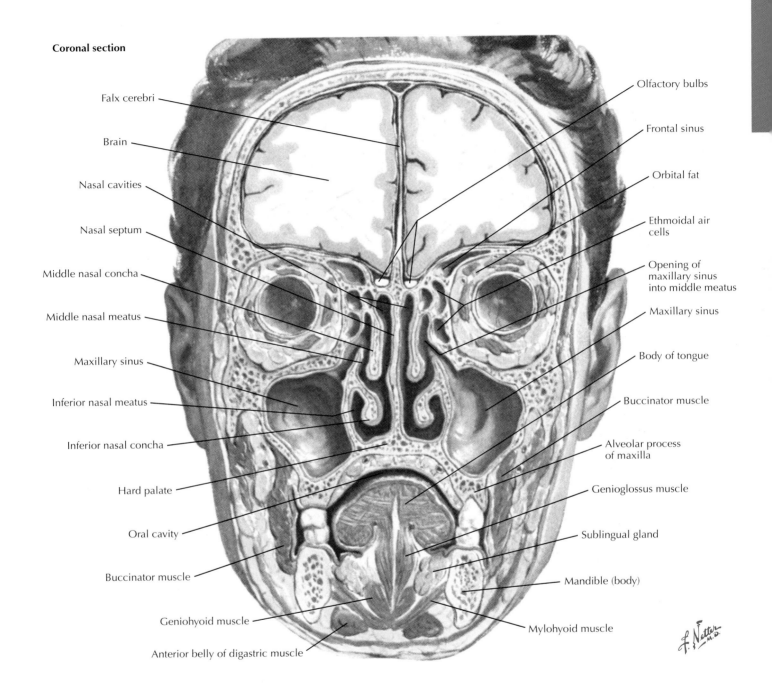

Falx cerebri

Brain

Nasal cavities

Nasal septum

Middle nasal concha

Middle nasal meatus

Maxillary sinus

Inferior nasal meatus

Inferior nasal concha

Hard palate

Oral cavity

Buccinator muscle

Geniohyoid muscle

Anterior belly of digastric muscle

Olfactory bulbs

Frontal sinus

Orbital fat

Ethmoidal air cells

Opening of maxillary sinus into middle meatus

Maxillary sinus

Body of tongue

Buccinator muscle

Alveolar process of maxilla

Genioglossus muscle

Sublingual gland

Mandible (body)

Mylohyoid muscle

8.32 CORONAL SECTION OF THE HEAD THROUGH THE ORBIT, SINUSES, AND ORAL CAVITY: OVERVIEW

Review in this coronal section of the head the relationships of the orbit, nasal cavity, oral cavity, maxillary sinus, frontal and ethmoid sinuses, and frontal lobes of the brain. Captured in this plane are the openings of the maxillary sinuses in the middle meati. Bounding the oral cavity are the bony (hard) palate above, the buccinator muscles laterally, and the mylohyoid muscle comprising the floor. In the anterior cranial fossa of the skull with the brain are sections through the superior sagittal sinus, the falx cerebri (originating from the crista galli of the ethmoid bone), and olfactory bulbs on the cribriform plate of the ethmoid bone.

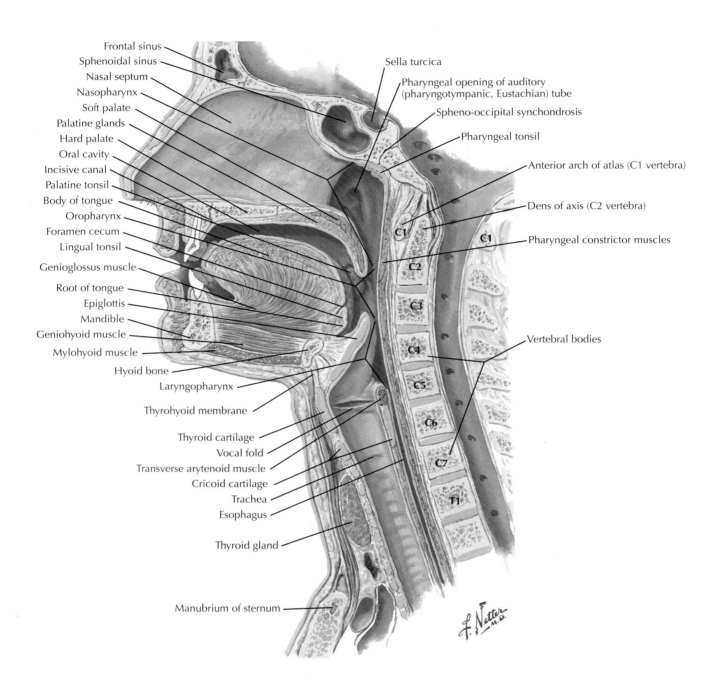

Frontal sinus
Sphenoidal sinus
Nasal septum
Nasopharynx
Soft palate
Palatine glands
Hard palate
Oral cavity
Incisive canal
Palatine tonsil
Body of tongue
Oropharynx
Foramen cecum
Lingual tonsil
Genioglossus muscle
Root of tongue
Epiglottis
Mandible
Geniohyoid muscle
Mylohyoid muscle
Hyoid bone
Laryngopharynx
Thyrohyoid membrane
Thyroid cartilage
Vocal fold
Transverse arytenoid muscle
Cricoid cartilage
Trachea
Esophagus
Thyroid gland
Manubrium of sternum

Sella turcica
Pharyngeal opening of auditory (pharyngotympanic, Eustachian) tube
Spheno-occipital synchondrosis
Pharyngeal tonsil
Anterior arch of atlas (C1 vertebra)
Dens of axis (C2 vertebra)
Pharyngeal constrictor muscles
Vertebral bodies

C1
C2
C3
C4
C5
C6
C7
T1

8.33 MIDSAGITTAL SECTION OF THE NASAL CAVITY, PHARYNX, ORAL CAVITY, AND NECK: OVERVIEW

Review in this median (midsagittal) section the anatomical relationships between structures in the face and neck. Included are the frontal and sphenoid sinuses; nasal cavity; oral cavity; and subdivisions of the pharynx, larynx, trachea, esophagus, cranial base, and cervical vertebrae. Also note the sella turcica, auditory tube, tonsils (pharyngeal, palatine, and lingual), genioglossus muscle, hyoid bone, vocal fold, and thyroid gland anterior to tracheal rings. Compare these structures with their appearance in MRI on the following page.

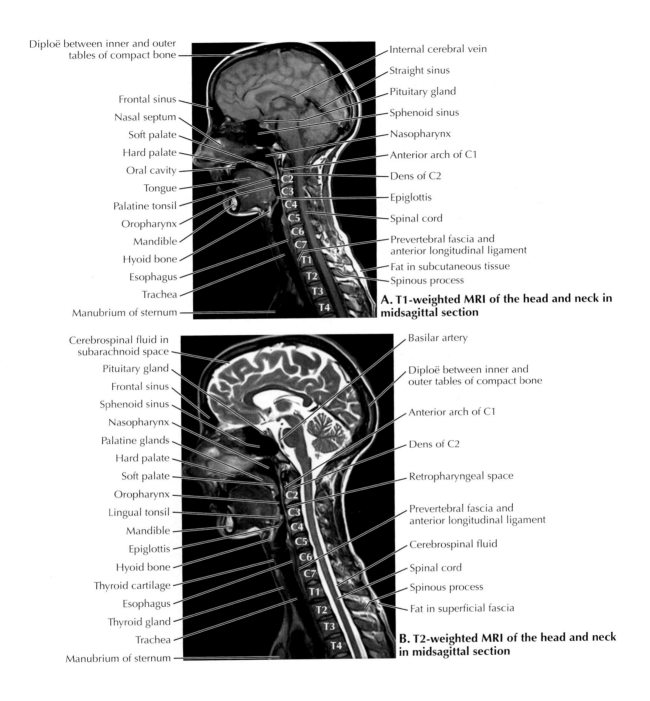

Diploë between inner and outer tables of compact bone

Frontal sinus
Nasal septum
Soft palate
Hard palate
Oral cavity
Tongue
Palatine tonsil
Oropharynx
Mandible
Hyoid bone
Esophagus
Trachea
Manubrium of sternum

Internal cerebral vein
Straight sinus
Pituitary gland
Sphenoid sinus
Nasopharynx
Anterior arch of C1
Dens of C2
Epiglottis
Spinal cord
Prevertebral fascia and anterior longitudinal ligament
Fat in subcutaneous tissue
Spinous process

C2
C3
C4
C5
C6
C7
T1
T2
T3
T4

A. T1-weighted MRI of the head and neck in midsagittal section

Cerebrospinal fluid in subarachnoid space
Pituitary gland
Frontal sinus
Sphenoid sinus
Nasopharynx
Palatine glands
Hard palate
Soft palate
Oropharynx
Lingual tonsil
Mandible
Epiglottis
Hyoid bone
Thyroid cartilage
Esophagus
Thyroid gland
Trachea
Manubrium of sternum

Basilar artery
Diploë between inner and outer tables of compact bone
Anterior arch of C1
Dens of C2
Retropharyngeal space
Prevertebral fascia and anterior longitudinal ligament
Cerebrospinal fluid
Spinal cord
Spinous process
Fat in superficial fascia

C2
C3
C4
C5
C6
C7
T1
T2
T3
T4

B. T2-weighted MRI of the head and neck in midsagittal section

8.34 T1 AND T2 MRI OF THE HEAD AND NECK IN MIDSAGITTAL SECTION

A review of the entire head and neck provides a good overview of the differences in tissue densities seen in T1-weighted compared to T2-weighted MRI. In a T1 MRI (**A**), air and compact bone appear black, and fat white. Fluid and blood are also dark, whereas spongy bone and most soft tissues have an intermediate density. The most prominent difference in a T2 MRI (**B**) is that fluid appears bright white in addition to fat.

Note the bright CSF around the brain and spinal cord. The signals for fat, bone, and soft tissues are similar in T1 and T2. Note how compact bone appears as a black rim around vertebral bodies, manubrium, and mandible in both figures. As we proceed to the study of meninges and dural sinuses, note the relationship between the appearance of CSF in the subarachnoid space and the inner and outer tables of compact bone in the neurocranium.

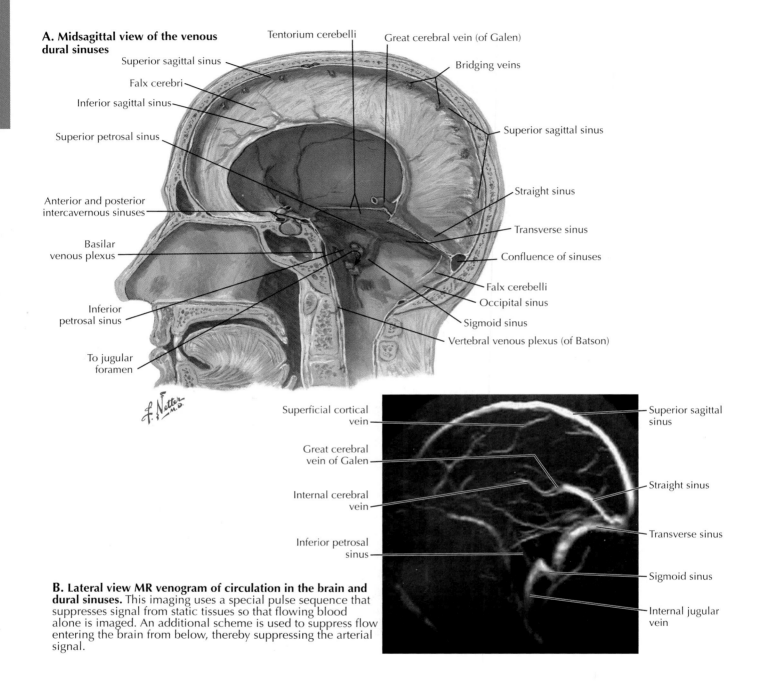

A. Midsagittal view of the venous dural sinuses

Tentorium cerebelli

Great cerebral vein (of Galen)

Superior sagittal sinus

Bridging veins

Falx cerebri

Inferior sagittal sinus

Superior sagittal sinus

Superior petrosal sinus

Straight sinus

Anterior and posterior intercavernous sinuses

Transverse sinus

Basilar venous plexus

Confluence of sinuses

Falx cerebelli

Occipital sinus

Inferior petrosal sinus

Sigmoid sinus

Vertebral venous plexus (of Batson)

To jugular foramen

Superficial cortical vein

Superior sagittal sinus

Great cerebral vein of Galen

Internal cerebral vein

Straight sinus

Transverse sinus

Inferior petrosal sinus

Sigmoid sinus

Internal jugular vein

B. Lateral view MR venogram of circulation in the brain and dural sinuses. This imaging uses a special pulse sequence that suppresses signal from static tissues so that flowing blood alone is imaged. An additional scheme is used to suppress flow entering the brain from below, thereby suppressing the arterial signal.

8.35 DURAL VENOUS SINUSES

Dural sinuses are venous channels in the dura mater that receive blood from the orbits, brain, and neurocranial bones and carry it to the internal jugular veins. The superior sagittal sinus and straight sinus in the falx cerebri converge on the transverse sinuses that course in the back edge of the tentorium cerebelli. Internal cerebral veins converge on the great cerebral vein of Galen, which joins the inferior sagittal sinus to form the straight sinus. The transverse sinuses continue as the sigmoid sinuses, which in turn exit the skull as the internal jugular veins. Blood from the orbits and deep brain enter the cavernous sinus that surrounds the body of the sphenoid bone. From there, blood passes into the sigmoid sinuses via the superior and inferior petrosal sinuses.

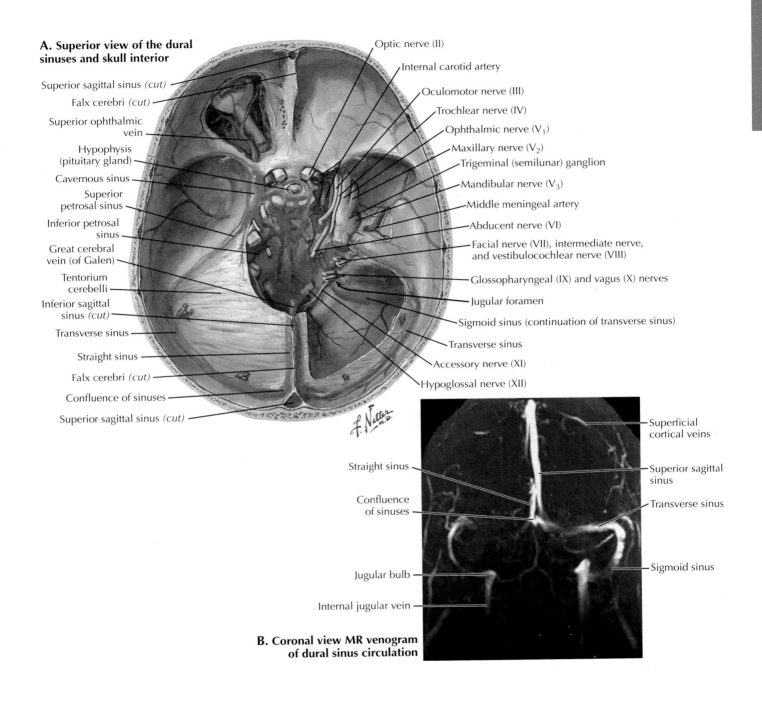

A. Superior view of the dural sinuses and skull interior

Superior sagittal sinus *(cut)*

Falx cerebri *(cut)*

Superior ophthalmic vein

Hypophysis (pituitary gland)

Cavernous sinus

Superior petrosal sinus

Inferior petrosal sinus

Great cerebral vein (of Galen)

Tentorium cerebelli

Inferior sagittal sinus *(cut)*

Transverse sinus

Straight sinus

Falx cerebri *(cut)*

Confluence of sinuses

Superior sagittal sinus *(cut)*

Optic nerve (II)

Internal carotid artery

Oculomotor nerve (III)

Trochlear nerve (IV)

Ophthalmic nerve (V₁)

Maxillary nerve (V₂)

Trigeminal (semilunar) ganglion

Mandibular nerve (V₃)

Middle meningeal artery

Abducent nerve (VI)

Facial nerve (VII), intermediate nerve, and vestibulocochlear nerve (VIII)

Glossopharyngeal (IX) and vagus (X) nerves

Jugular foramen

Sigmoid sinus (continuation of transverse sinus)

Transverse sinus

Accessory nerve (XI)

Hypoglossal nerve (XII)

Straight sinus

Confluence of sinuses

Jugular bulb

Internal jugular vein

Superficial cortical veins

Superior sagittal sinus

Transverse sinus

Sigmoid sinus

B. Coronal view MR venogram of dural sinus circulation

8.36 DURAL VENOUS SINUSES (CONT'D)

In superior and coronal views it is easier to appreciate the junction of the superior sagittal and straight sinuses at the confluence of sinuses and the left and right transverse sinuses continuing as the sigmoid sinuses. Most of the blood in the superior sagittal sinus typically flows into the left transverse sinus, and most of the blood in the straight sinus usually goes to the right transverse sinus. The patient in **B** has aplasia (congenital underdevelopment) of the right transverse sinus. The blood from both the superior sagittal sinus and straight sinus flows to the left side, where the transverse sinus, sigmoid sinus, and internal jugular vein are enlarged to accommodate the increased volume of flow.

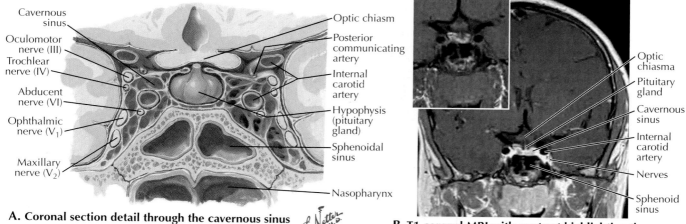

Cavernous sinus
Oculomotor nerve (III)
Trochlear nerve (IV)
Abducent nerve (VI)
Ophthalmic nerve (V₁)
Maxillary nerve (V₂)

Optic chiasm
Posterior communicating artery
Internal carotid artery
Hypophysis (pituitary gland)
Sphenoidal sinus
Nasopharynx

A. Coronal section detail through the cavernous sinus

Optic chiasma
Pituitary gland
Cavernous sinus
Internal carotid artery
Nerves
Sphenoid sinus

B. T1 coronal MRI with contrast highlighting the cavernous sinus. The insert shows the precontrast image. The image is captured several minutes after the introduction of contrast; slow-moving blood in the cavernous sinus is bright, and fast-moving blood in the internal carotid artery and superior sagittal sinus is black.

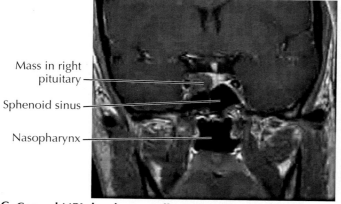

Mass in right pituitary
Sphenoid sinus
Nasopharynx

C. Coronal MRI showing a small tumor (microadenoma) in the right half of the pituitary gland filling the cavernous sinus on that side

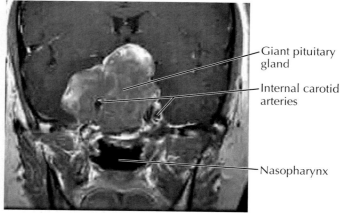

Giant pituitary gland
Internal carotid arteries
Nasopharynx

D. Coronal MRI showing a greatly enlarged pituitary gland obliterating the cavernous sinus and sphenoid sinus. The internal carotid arteries are still visible.

8.37 THE CAVERNOUS SINUS

The cavernous sinus flanks the body of the sphenoid bone and has anatomical relationships that are clinically significant. Passing through the sinus are the internal carotid artery, the three motor nerves to the orbit, and the ophthalmic and maxillary divisions of the trigeminal nerve. In the middle of the cavernous sinus is the pituitary gland. The cavernous sinus receives blood from the orbits and deeper parts of the brain.

Its outflow is to the sigmoid sinus via the petrosal sinuses. Contrast in the cavernous sinus (**B**) makes it easier to see masses that might arise from the pituitary gland (**C** and **D**), meninges, nerves, or other sources and impair the functions of the nerves in the sinus. The internal carotid artery may rupture in the sinus, causing a large arteriovenous shunt that reverses the flow of blood through the ophthalmic veins and deep cerebral veins.

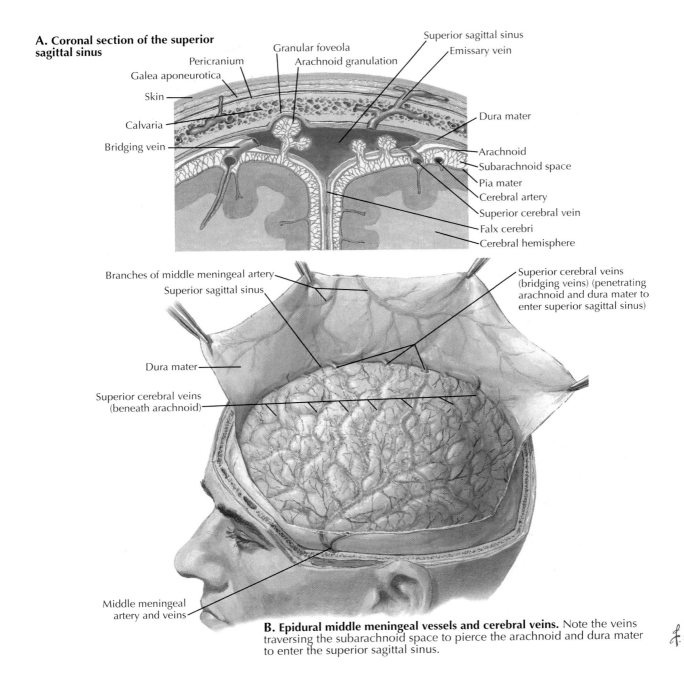

A. Coronal section of the superior sagittal sinus

Galea aponeurotica
Pericranium
Skin
Calvaria
Bridging vein

Granular foveola
Arachnoid granulation

Superior sagittal sinus
Emissary vein

Dura mater
Arachnoid
Subarachnoid space
Pia mater
Cerebral artery
Superior cerebral vein
Falx cerebri
Cerebral hemisphere

Branches of middle meningeal artery
Superior sagittal sinus

Dura mater

Superior cerebral veins (beneath arachnoid)

Middle meningeal artery and veins

Superior cerebral veins (bridging veins) (penetrating arachnoid and dura mater to enter superior sagittal sinus)

B. Epidural middle meningeal vessels and cerebral veins. Note the veins traversing the subarachnoid space to pierce the arachnoid and dura mater to enter the superior sagittal sinus.

8.38 SUPERIOR SAGITTAL SINUS, MIDDLE MENINGEAL ARTERY, AND SUPERFICIAL CEREBRAL VEINS

The superior sagittal sinus, like other dural sinuses, receives venous blood from the brain and neurocranial bones and is connected to veins of the scalp via emissary veins. It is also the only location where CSF enters the venous circulation. Tufts of arachnoid called *arachnoid granulations* pierce the superior sagittal sinus and its lateral extensions (lacunae) to act as simple valves for the diffusion of CSF into the blood. The blood supply to the neurocranial bones and dura is by the middle meningeal branch of the maxillary artery. Rupture of this artery from a blow to the thin bones on the side of the skull results in serious bleeding in an epidural location. Venous bleeding from head trauma is usually subdural. The cerebral veins often tear where they enter the dural sinuses, and blood accumulates between the arachnoid and the dura mater.

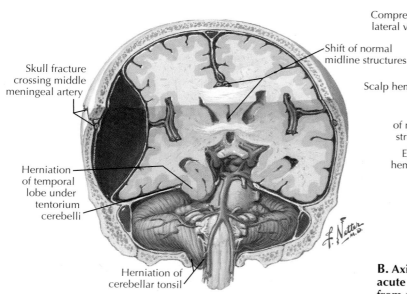

A. Coronal section showing an epidural hematoma from a skull fracture tearing the middle meningeal artery

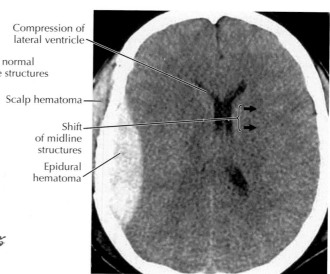

B. Axial CT with a soft tissue (brain) window showing an acute epidural hematoma and scalp hematoma in a patient from a motor vehicle accident. Note the depression of the bony contour on the right.

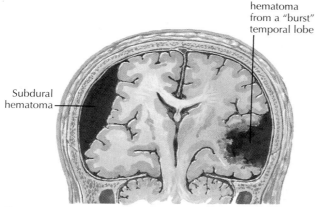

C. Coronal section showing an acute, venous, subdural hematoma on the left and a subarachnoid, arterial hematoma on the right originating from a temporal lobe intracerebral hematoma ("burst" temporal lobe) (e.g., from trauma or a ruptured aneurysm)

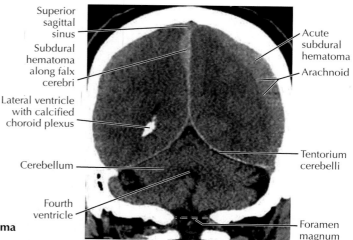

D. Coronal CT reconstruction showing an acute subdural hematoma on the left and along the right side of the falx cerebi. This patient was also in an automobile accident.

8.39 IMAGING OF EPIDURAL AND SUBDURAL BLEEDING

If the middle meningeal artery ruptures, high-pressure arterial blood separates the dura from the bone, producing an epidural accumulation of blood that is convex toward the brain (**A** and **B**). The increased pressure on cranial nerves, vessels, and brain tissue in general is a medical emergency. Subdural bleeding (**C** and **D**) is usually venous blood. A blow to the head puts tension on the cerebral veins, and they typically tear at their attachment to the dural sinuses. The blood extends between the dura and arachnoid, which are only held together by the pressure of the CSF in the subarachnoid space. The profile of the venous accumulation of blood is more irregular and less convex toward the brain compared with epidural bleeding. Subarachnoid bleeding into the CSF (**C**) follows the contours of the surface of the brain and is arterial if it is from an intracerebral hematoma.

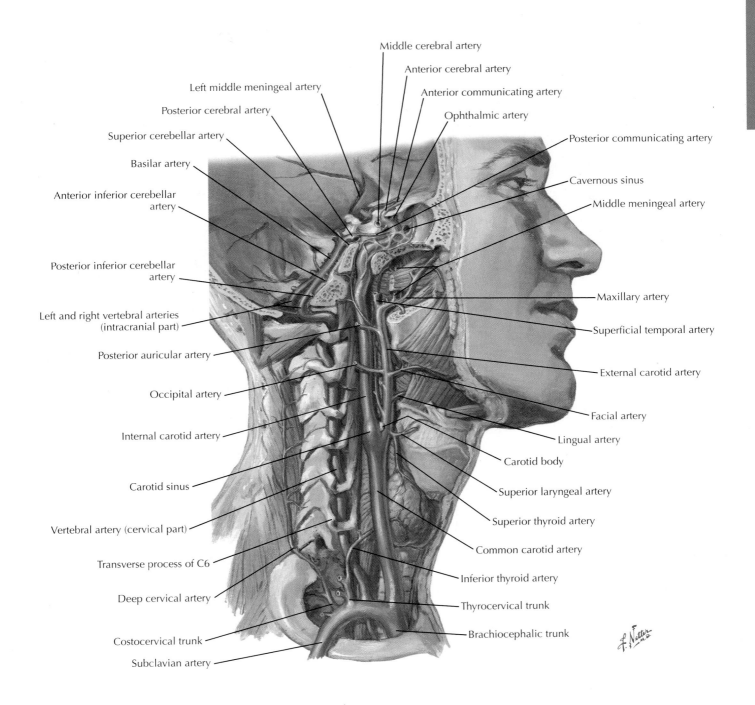

Middle cerebral artery

Anterior cerebral artery

Anterior communicating artery

Ophthalmic artery

Posterior communicating artery

Cavernous sinus

Middle meningeal artery

Left middle meningeal artery

Posterior cerebral artery

Superior cerebellar artery

Basilar artery

Anterior inferior cerebellar artery

Posterior inferior cerebellar artery

Left and right vertebral arteries (intracranial part)

Posterior auricular artery

Occipital artery

Internal carotid artery

Carotid sinus

Vertebral artery (cervical part)

Transverse process of C6

Deep cervical artery

Costocervical trunk

Subclavian artery

Maxillary artery

Superficial temporal artery

External carotid artery

Facial artery

Lingual artery

Carotid body

Superior laryngeal artery

Superior thyroid artery

Common carotid artery

Inferior thyroid artery

Thyrocervical trunk

Brachiocephalic trunk

8.40 ARTERIES FROM THE NECK TO THE BRAIN

The brain receives its blood supply from the vertebral and internal carotid arteries. The vertebral arteries form the basilar artery, which divides into the posterior cerebral arteries. The internal carotid arteries continue as the middle cerebral arteries and give off the anterior cerebral arteries. The orbits are also supplied by the internal carotid arteries via their ophthalmic branches. The external carotid arteries supply the nasal cavities, oral cavity, muscles of mastication, structures of the face, and most of the anterior neck down through the upper half of the thyroid gland.

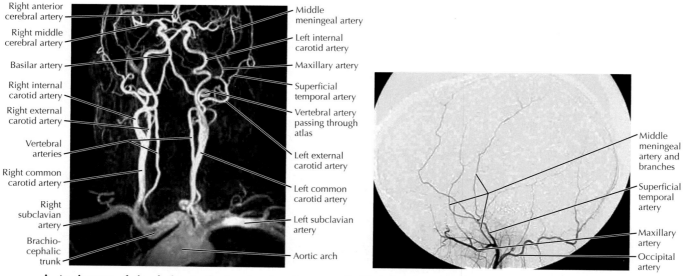

Right anterior cerebral artery

Right middle cerebral artery

Basilar artery

Right internal carotid artery

Right external carotid artery

Vertebral arteries

Right common carotid artery

Right subclavian artery

Brachio-cephalic trunk

Middle meningeal artery

Left internal carotid artery

Maxillary artery

Superficial temporal artery

Vertebral artery passing through atlas

Left external carotid artery

Left common carotid artery

Left subclavian artery

Aortic arch

A. Angiogram of circulation to the head and neck

Middle meningeal artery and branches

Superficial temporal artery

Maxillary artery

Occipital artery

B. Digital catheter angiogram of the left external carotid artery

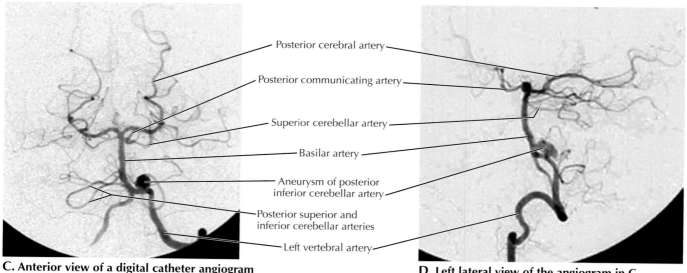

Posterior cerebral artery

Posterior communicating artery

Superior cerebellar artery

Basilar artery

Aneurysm of posterior inferior cerebellar artery

Posterior superior and inferior cerebellar arteries

Left vertebral artery

C. Anterior view of a digital catheter angiogram of the left vertebral artery with retrograde flow into the right vertebral artery

D. Left lateral view of the angiogram in C

8.41 VASCULAR STUDIES

Vascular imaging studies of the head and neck detect aneurysms (dilations) (**C** and **D**), arteriovenous malformations, vessels leaking from trauma, and the reduction in blood flow from compression of arteries (e.g., from tumors) or narrowing of the lumen from plaque formation, which occurs often in the common carotid arteries. **A** is an angiogram in which contrast is introduced into the arch of the aorta, filling the common carotid and vertebral arteries and their branches on both sides. **B, C,** and **D** are digital subtraction angiograms. In digital angiography a "mask" image is obtained before administration of contrast. Following injection of the contrast agent into a specific vessel, the mask image is subtracted electronically. This leaves only the image of the contrast in the blood vessels, which can be rotated to view from any angle. Interventions can also be performed through the catheter at the time of the study, such as the placement of stents, balloon dilation of narrow vessels, stripping of the arterial intima, or injection of clot-dissolving agents.

Frontal section

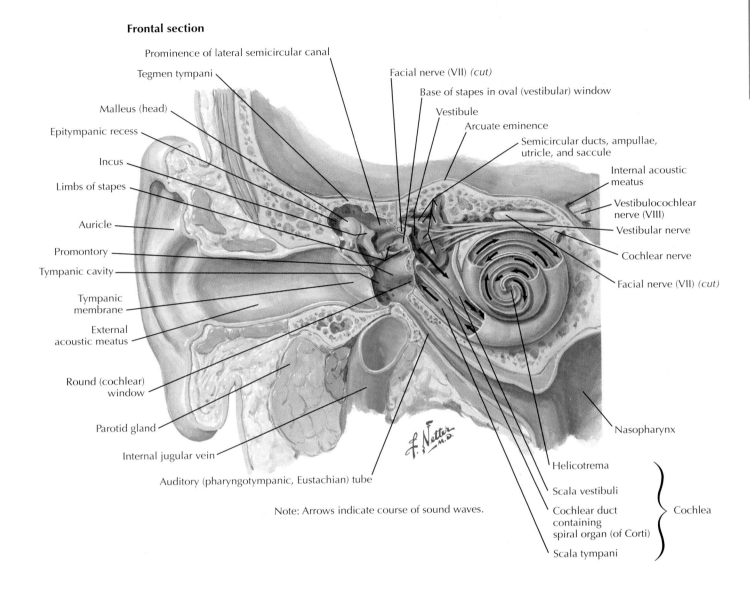

Prominence of lateral semicircular canal

Tegmen tympani

Malleus (head)

Epitympanic recess

Incus

Limbs of stapes

Auricle

Promontory

Tympanic cavity

Tympanic membrane

External acoustic meatus

Round (cochlear) window

Parotid gland

Internal jugular vein

Auditory (pharyngotympanic, Eustachian) tube

Note: Arrows indicate course of sound waves.

Facial nerve (VII) *(cut)*

Base of stapes in oval (vestibular) window

Vestibule

Arcuate eminence

Semicircular ducts, ampullae, utricle, and saccule

Internal acoustic meatus

Vestibulocochlear nerve (VIII)

Vestibular nerve

Cochlear nerve

Facial nerve (VII) *(cut)*

Nasopharynx

Helicotrema

Scala vestibuli

Cochlear duct containing spiral organ (of Corti)

Scala tympani

Cochlea

8.42 EXTERNAL, MIDDLE, AND INNER EAR

The three compartments of the ear are contained within the temporal bone. The external ear consists of the auricle and the external acoustic meatus, which transmit sound waves to the tympanic membrane (eardrum). The air-filled tympanic cavity (middle ear) has three ear ossicles that carry the sound vibrations from the tympanic membrane to the cochlea of the inner ear, where sound vibrations are converted into electrical impulses in the auditory branch of the vestibulocochlear nerve (cranial nerve VIII). The tympanic cavity is connected to the nasopharynx anteriorly by the auditory (Eustachian) tube to balance pressure on both sides of the eardrum and posteriorly to the mastoid air cells. The inner ear also contains the vestibular apparatus containing the three semicircular canals, utricle, and saccule that register positional sense, balance, rotations, and linear acceleration. This information is conveyed via the vestibular branch of nerve VIII. Inferior to the middle ear cavity is the jugular bulb. The facial nerve (VII) is superior to the tympanic cavity and then passes inferiorly along its posterior wall.

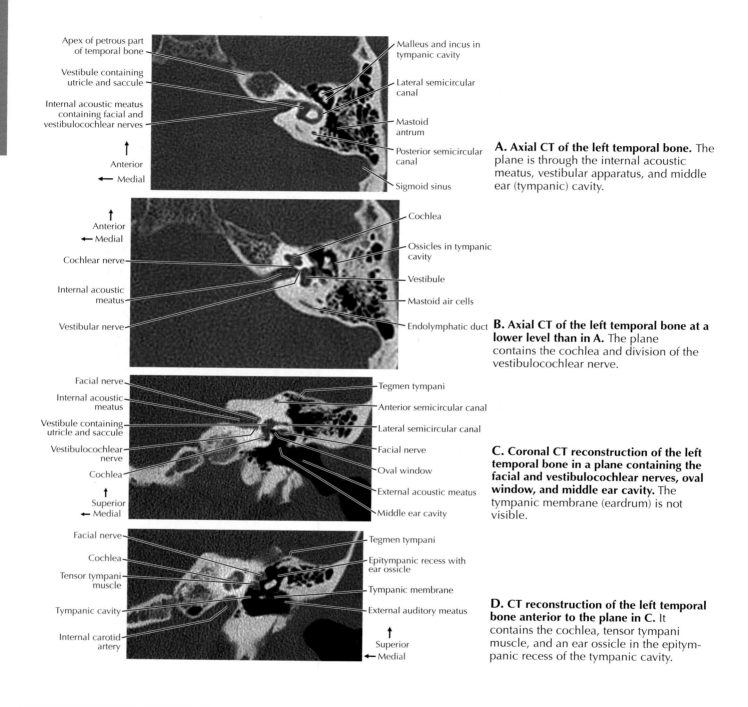

Apex of petrous part of temporal bone

Vestibule containing utricle and saccule

Internal acoustic meatus containing facial and vestibulocochlear nerves

Anterior
← Medial

Malleus and incus in tympanic cavity

Lateral semicircular canal

Mastoid antrum

Posterior semicircular canal

Sigmoid sinus

A. Axial CT of the left temporal bone. The plane is through the internal acoustic meatus, vestibular apparatus, and middle ear (tympanic) cavity.

Anterior
← Medial

Cochlear nerve

Internal acoustic meatus

Vestibular nerve

Cochlea

Ossicles in tympanic cavity

Vestibule

Mastoid air cells

Endolymphatic duct

B. Axial CT of the left temporal bone at a lower level than in A. The plane contains the cochlea and division of the vestibulocochlear nerve.

Facial nerve

Internal acoustic meatus

Vestibule containing utricle and saccule

Vestibulocochlear nerve

Cochlea

Superior
← Medial

Tegmen tympani

Anterior semicircular canal

Lateral semicircular canal

Facial nerve

Oval window

External acoustic meatus

Middle ear cavity

C. Coronal CT reconstruction of the left temporal bone in a plane containing the facial and vestibulocochlear nerves, oval window, and middle ear cavity. The tympanic membrane (eardrum) is not visible.

Facial nerve

Cochlea

Tensor tympani muscle

Tympanic cavity

Internal carotid artery

Superior
← Medial

Tegmen tympani

Epitympanic recess with ear ossicle

Tympanic membrane

External auditory meatus

D. CT reconstruction of the left temporal bone anterior to the plane in C. It contains the cochlea, tensor tympani muscle, and an ear ossicle in the epitympanic recess of the tympanic cavity.

8.43 CT OF THE TEMPORAL BONE AND EAR COMPARTMENTS

Study of the tiny structures and compartments in the temporal bone with CT bone windows requires thin slice acquisition—0.6 or 1.25 mm rather than the more typical 5 mm—and the slices are overlapped in plane reconstructions to provide greater detail. The inner ear organs are enclosed in dense cortical bone, the bright white signal in the illustrations. The cochlea is anterior and a bit inferior to the vestibular apparatus, and each plane of section predominantly captures one or the other. The facial and vestibulocochlear nerves enter the internal acoustic meatus of the petrous part of the temporal bone (**B**). The vestibulocochlear nerve (**C**) divides into anterior cochlear and posterior vestibular branches (**B**). The cochlear branch then passes inferiorly to the cochlea. Note the continuity of the tympanic cavity (middle ear) with the mastoid air cells (**A**). The tensor tympani muscle (**D**) is in the roof of the auditory tube (not shown). The epitympanic recess is the extension of the middle ear cavity above the level of the tympanic membrane (**D**).

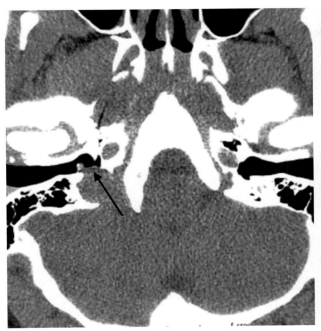

A. Axial CT showing the jugular bulb extending into the middle ear cavity *(arrow)*

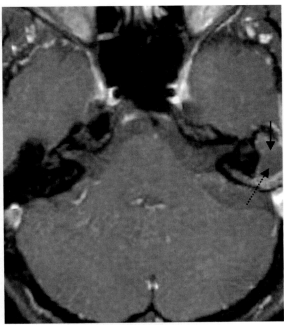

B. MRI showing a mass (cholesteatoma) in the epitympanic recess *(solid arrow)* **and mastoid antrum** *(dashed arrow)*

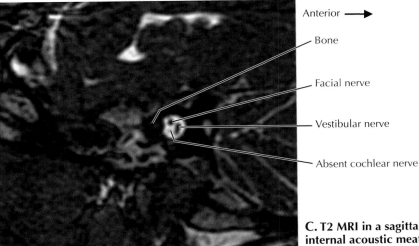

Anterior ⟶

Bone

Facial nerve

Vestibular nerve

Absent cochlear nerve

C. T2 MRI in a sagittal plane through the internal acoustic meatus of a deaf patient with congenital absence of the cochlear nerve

8.44 IMAGING OF TEMPORAL BONE/EAR PATHOLOGY

Imaging studies of the temporal bone require careful evaluation of the spaces and the selection of modalities that best highlight soft tissue structures. **A** shows an anatomical variation that impacts function of the middle ear. The sigmoid sinus curves upward under the middle ear cavity as the jugular bulb, the beginning of the internal jugular vein. Here the jugular bulb projects through the bony floor of the tympanic cavity. The MRI in **B** shows a mass in the tympanic cavity extending into the mastoid antrum. It is a congenital cholesteatoma, a cyst with keratinized epithelial debris and cholesterol. It shows the typical lack of enhancement when T1 with vascular contrast is used. In **C**, landmarks are hard to discern; but the T2 MRI clearly shows the congenital lack of the cochlear nerve in the internal acoustic meatus within dense, cortical bone *(black)*.

Sagittal section of brain in situ

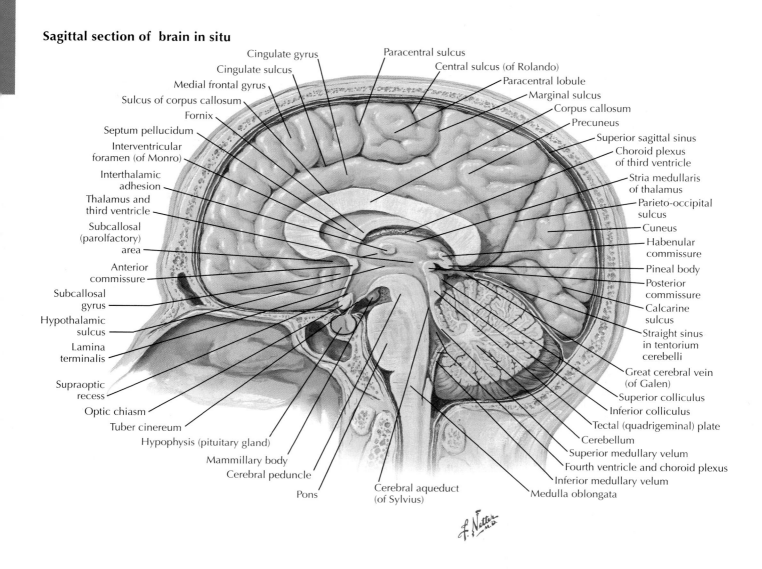

Cingulate gyrus
Cingulate sulcus
Medial frontal gyrus
Sulcus of corpus callosum
Fornix
Septum pellucidum
Interventricular foramen (of Monro)
Interthalamic adhesion
Thalamus and third ventricle
Subcallosal (parolfactory) area
Anterior commissure
Subcallosal gyrus
Hypothalamic sulcus
Lamina terminalis
Supraoptic recess
Optic chiasm
Tuber cinereum
Hypophysis (pituitary gland)
Mammillary body
Cerebral peduncle
Pons

Paracentral sulcus
Central sulcus (of Rolando)
Paracentral lobule
Marginal sulcus
Corpus callosum
Precuneus
Superior sagittal sinus
Choroid plexus of third ventricle
Stria medullaris of thalamus
Parieto-occipital sulcus
Cuneus
Habenular commissure
Pineal body
Posterior commissure
Calcarine sulcus
Straight sinus in tentorium cerebelli
Great cerebral vein (of Galen)
Superior colliculus
Inferior colliculus
Tectal (quadrigeminal) plate
Cerebellum
Superior medullary velum
Fourth ventricle and choroid plexus
Inferior medullary velum
Medulla oblongata
Cerebral aqueduct (of Sylvius)

8.45 MIDSAGITTAL SECTION OF BRAIN; MEDIAL VIEW OF CEREBRUM

The subdivisions of the brain are, from superior to inferior, the large cerebral hemispheres (telencephalon) and the smaller diencephalon (thalamus and related structures) that together make up the cerebrum (prosencephalon), the narrow midbrain (mesencephalon) seen here as the tectal plate and cerebral peduncle, the pons anteriorly and the cerebellum posteriorly (metencephalon), and the tapering medulla oblongata (myelencephalon) that is continuous with the spinal cord at the foramen magnum. Each cerebral hemisphere is divided into four lobes from anterior to posterior: the frontal lobe, the parietal lobe, the occipital lobe and, inferiorly, the temporal lobe (out of the plane of section). The corpus callosum is a large bundle of commissural fibers connecting functionally related areas in the two hemispheres. Inferior to the corpus callosum is the C-shaped fornix, a smaller bundle of fibers that project from the hippocampal formation in the temporal lobe to primarily the mammillary body of the hypothalamus.

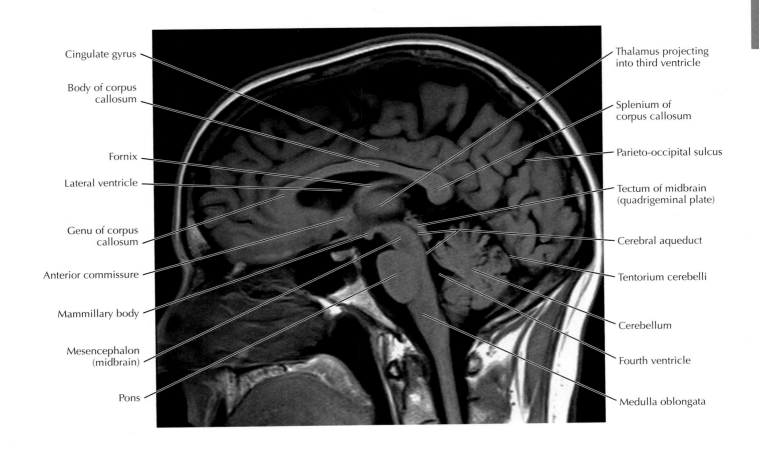

Cingulate gyrus

Body of corpus callosum

Fornix

Lateral ventricle

Genu of corpus callosum

Anterior commissure

Mammillary body

Mesencephalon (midbrain)

Pons

Thalamus projecting into third ventricle

Splenium of corpus callosum

Parieto-occipital sulcus

Tectum of midbrain (quadrigeminal plate)

Cerebral aqueduct

Tentorium cerebelli

Cerebellum

Fourth ventricle

Medulla oblongata

8.46 MIDSAGITTAL T1 MRI

In general, when the neuroradiologist reviews a series of MR images, the anatomy is scrutinized for normalcy rather than searching for specific abnormal findings first. For example, the junction of the gray and white matter is evaluated; if it is normal, the next structure is evaluated. If it is abnormal, a differential diagnosis of pathologies that could blur that interface is constructed within the context of the patient's history. This search strategy is more comprehensive than a search for particular pathologies, most of which are unlikely to be found. This midsagittal MRI is T1-weighted, in which fluid, compact bone, and air have dark signal and subcutaneous fat and bone marrow have bright signal. Brain tissue is gray, with white matter being a bit lighter than gray matter. Very evident in the section is CSF in the ventricles and surrounding the brain and spinal cord. Although close to the midline, the falx cerebri is out of the plane, and a mammillary body and part of a lateral ventricle are seen. The midsagittal T1-weighted MR image of the brain is where many neuroradiologists begin when evaluating a series of images for pathology. Abnormalities that are usually first recognized sagittally include pituitary tumors, abnormally sized CSF spaces (ventricles, cisterns, and subarachnoid space), and pathology within the corpus callosum.

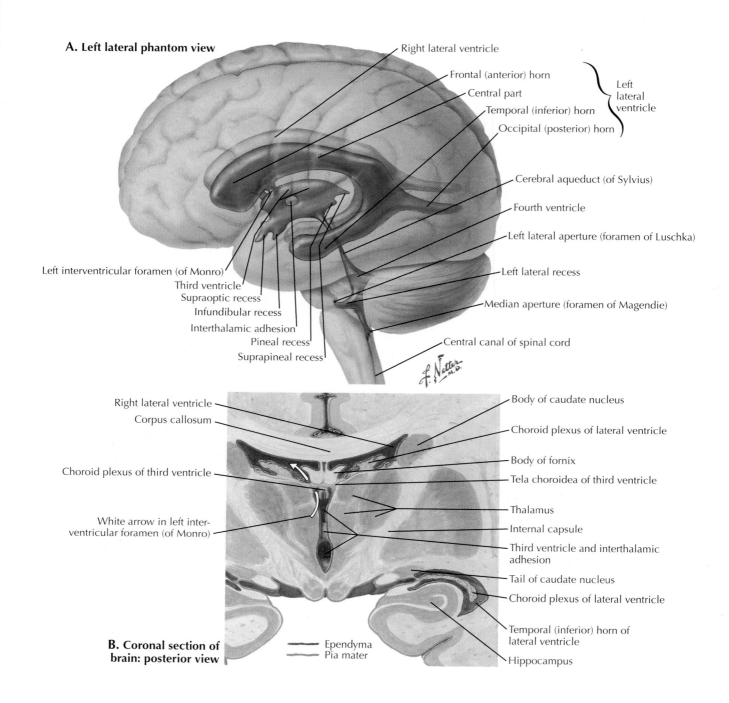

A. Left lateral phantom view

Right lateral ventricle

Frontal (anterior) horn

Central part

Temporal (inferior) horn

Occipital (posterior) horn

Left lateral ventricle

Cerebral aqueduct (of Sylvius)

Fourth ventricle

Left lateral aperture (foramen of Luschka)

Left lateral recess

Median aperture (foramen of Magendie)

Central canal of spinal cord

Left interventricular foramen (of Monro)

Third ventricle

Supraoptic recess

Infundibular recess

Interthalamic adhesion

Pineal recess

Suprapineal recess

Right lateral ventricle

Corpus callosum

Choroid plexus of third ventricle

White arrow in left inter-ventricular foramen (of Monro)

Body of caudate nucleus

Choroid plexus of lateral ventricle

Body of fornix

Tela choroidea of third ventricle

Thalamus

Internal capsule

Third ventricle and interthalamic adhesion

Tail of caudate nucleus

Choroid plexus of lateral ventricle

Temporal (inferior) horn of lateral ventricle

Hippocampus

B. Coronal section of brain: posterior view

Ependyma

Pia mater

8.47 VENTRICLES OF THE BRAIN

CSF is produced as an ultrafiltrate of blood in the choroid plexus of vessels in the ventricles of the brain, an interconnected series of chambers that develop from the lumen (central canal) of the neural tube. C-shaped left and right lateral ventricles connect via the interventricular foramina (of Monro) to a midline third ventricle in the middle of the thalamus. The third ventricle connects with the fourth ventricle via the cerebral aqueduct of Sylvius. CSF enters the subarachnoid space around the brain through a median foramen in the fourth ventricle, the foramen of Magendie, and bilateral foramina of Luschka.

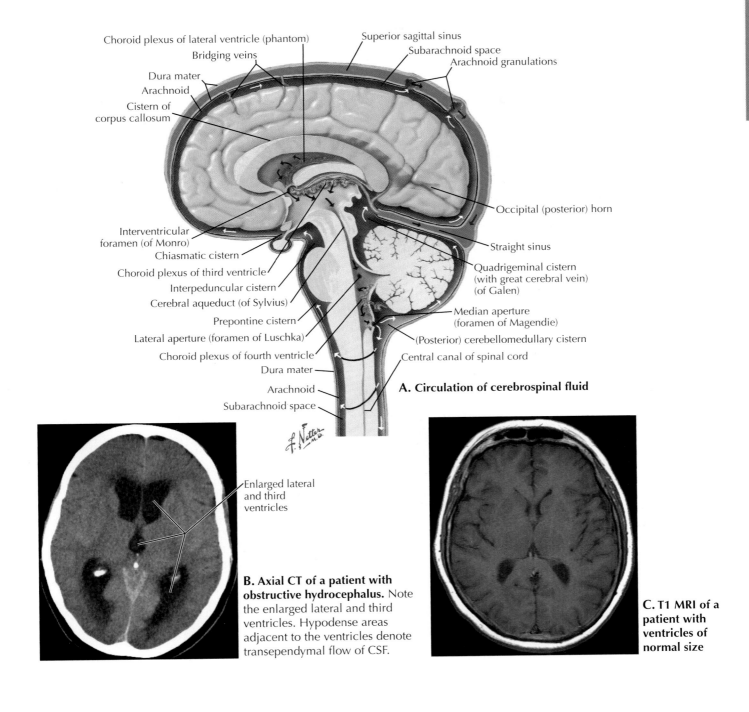

Choroid plexus of lateral ventricle (phantom)

Bridging veins

Dura mater

Arachnoid

Cistern of corpus callosum

Superior sagittal sinus

Subarachnoid space

Arachnoid granulations

Occipital (posterior) horn

Straight sinus

Interventricular foramen (of Monro)

Chiasmatic cistern

Choroid plexus of third ventricle

Interpeduncular cistern

Cerebral aqueduct (of Sylvius)

Prepontine cistern

Lateral aperture (foramen of Luschka)

Choroid plexus of fourth ventricle

Dura mater

Arachnoid

Subarachnoid space

Quadrigeminal cistern (with great cerebral vein) (of Galen)

Median aperture (foramen of Magendie)

(Posterior) cerebellomedullary cistern

Central canal of spinal cord

A. Circulation of cerebrospinal fluid

Enlarged lateral and third ventricles

B. Axial CT of a patient with obstructive hydrocephalus. Note the enlarged lateral and third ventricles. Hypodense areas adjacent to the ventricles denote transependymal flow of CSF.

C. T1 MRI of a patient with ventricles of normal size

8.48 CIRCULATION OF CEREBROSPINAL FLUID AND HYDROCEPHALUS

CSF passes sequentially from the lateral ventricles to the third ventricle to the fourth ventricle. From the fourth ventricle it enters the subarachnoid space around the brain and spinal cord through the median foramen of Magendie and lateral foramina of Luschka. CSF from the brain and spinal cord reenters the bloodstream by passing through tufts of arachnoid (granulations) that project into the dural venous sinuses. Obstructive, also known as *noncommunicating*, hydrocephalus is the accumulation of CSF within the ventricles caused by blockage of the foramina or cerebral aqueduct.

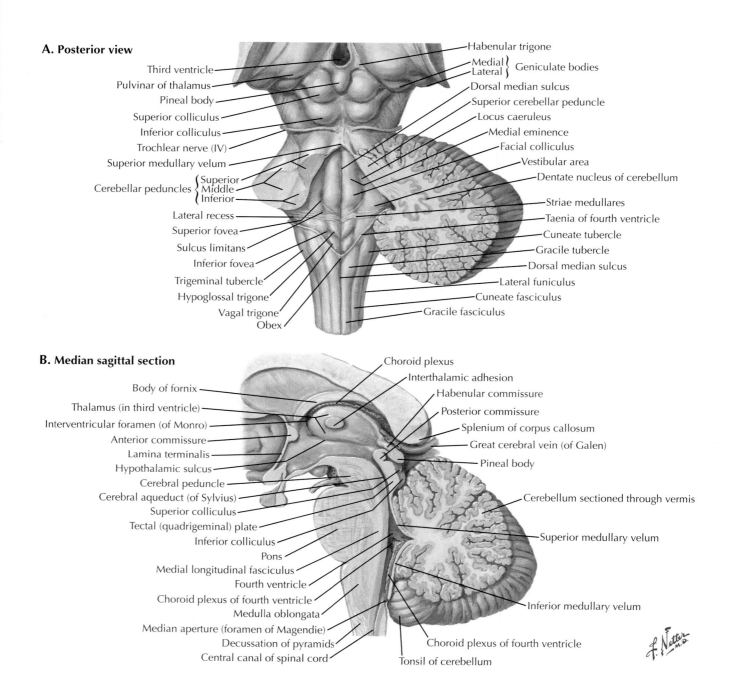

A. Posterior view

Third ventricle
Pulvinar of thalamus
Pineal body
Superior colliculus
Inferior colliculus
Trochlear nerve (IV)
Superior medullary velum
Cerebellar peduncles { Superior / Middle / Inferior }
Lateral recess
Superior fovea
Sulcus limitans
Inferior fovea
Trigeminal tubercle
Hypoglossal trigone
Vagal trigone
Obex

Habenular trigone
Medial } Lateral } Geniculate bodies
Dorsal median sulcus
Superior cerebellar peduncle
Locus caeruleus
Medial eminence
Facial colliculus
Vestibular area
Dentate nucleus of cerebellum
Striae medullares
Taenia of fourth ventricle
Cuneate tubercle
Gracile tubercle
Dorsal median sulcus
Lateral funiculus
Cuneate fasciculus
Gracile fasciculus

B. Median sagittal section

Body of fornix
Thalamus (in third ventricle)
Interventricular foramen (of Monro)
Anterior commissure
Lamina terminalis
Hypothalamic sulcus
Cerebral peduncle
Cerebral aqueduct (of Sylvius)
Superior colliculus
Tectal (quadrigeminal) plate
Inferior colliculus
Pons
Medial longitudinal fasciculus
Fourth ventricle
Choroid plexus of fourth ventricle
Medulla oblongata
Median aperture (foramen of Magendie)
Decussation of pyramids
Central canal of spinal cord

Choroid plexus
Interthalamic adhesion
Habenular commissure
Posterior commissure
Splenium of corpus callosum
Great cerebral vein (of Galen)
Pineal body
Cerebellum sectioned through vermis
Superior medullary velum
Inferior medullary velum
Choroid plexus of fourth ventricle
Tonsil of cerebellum

8.49 FOURTH VENTRICLE AND SECTIONS OF THE CEREBELLUM

In **A,** the right half of the cerebellum is cut in a coronal section. The left half of the cerebellum has been removed by cutting the cerebellar peduncles, opening up the fourth ventricle. The brainstem here is divided into left and right halves by the dorsal median sulcus. Each half is subdivided by the sulcus limitans into a medial eminence and hypoglossal and vagal trigones containing the motor nuclei of cranial nerves

and a lateral vestibular area containing the sensory nuclei of cranial nerves. In **B,** the diencephalon, brainstem, cerebellum, and ventricular system are cut in a midsagittal section. The slitlike third ventricle separates the two halves of the diencephalon. It is continuous with the narrow cerebral aqueduct of Sylvius in the midbrain and the triangular fourth ventricle between the pons and rostral medulla anteriorly and the cerebellum posteriorly.

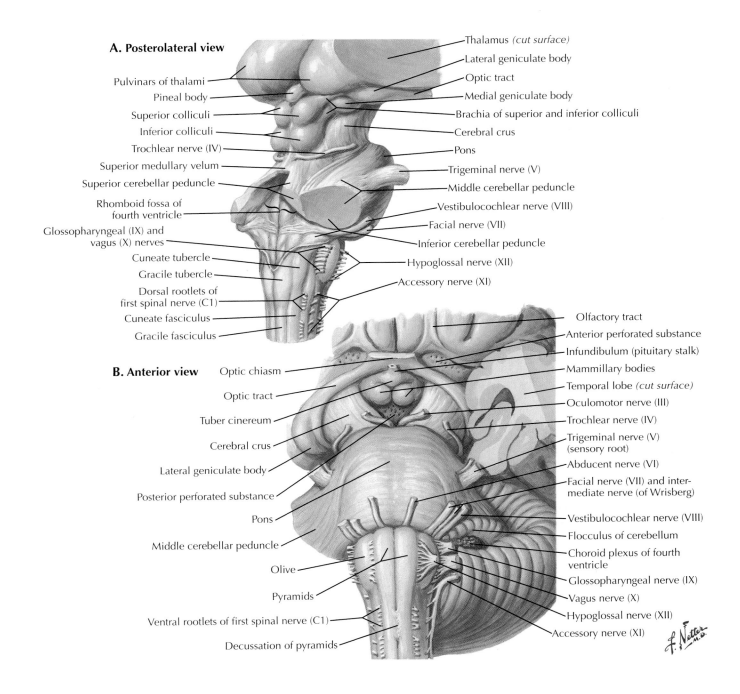

A. Posterolateral view

Pulvinars of thalami
Pineal body
Superior colliculi
Inferior colliculi
Trochlear nerve (IV)
Superior medullary velum
Superior cerebellar peduncle
Rhomboid fossa of fourth ventricle
Glossopharyngeal (IX) and vagus (X) nerves
Cuneate tubercle
Gracile tubercle
Dorsal rootlets of first spinal nerve (C1)
Cuneate fasciculus
Gracile fasciculus

Thalamus (cut surface)
Lateral geniculate body
Optic tract
Medial geniculate body
Brachia of superior and inferior colliculi
Cerebral crus
Pons
Trigeminal nerve (V)
Middle cerebellar peduncle
Vestibulocochlear nerve (VIII)
Facial nerve (VII)
Inferior cerebellar peduncle
Hypoglossal nerve (XII)
Accessory nerve (XI)

B. Anterior view

Optic chiasm
Optic tract
Tuber cinereum
Cerebral crus
Lateral geniculate body
Posterior perforated substance
Pons
Middle cerebellar peduncle
Olive
Pyramids
Ventral rootlets of first spinal nerve (C1)
Decussation of pyramids

Olfactory tract
Anterior perforated substance
Infundibulum (pituitary stalk)
Mammillary bodies
Temporal lobe (cut surface)
Oculomotor nerve (III)
Trochlear nerve (IV)
Trigeminal nerve (V) (sensory root)
Abducent nerve (VI)
Facial nerve (VII) and intermediate nerve (of Wrisberg)
Vestibulocochlear nerve (VIII)
Flocculus of cerebellum
Choroid plexus of fourth ventricle
Glossopharyngeal nerve (IX)
Vagus nerve (X)
Hypoglossal nerve (XII)
Accessory nerve (XI)

8.50 BRAINSTEM

In **A**, the cerebellum has been removed by cutting the cerebellar peduncles, opening up the rhomboid fossa of the fourth ventricle that overlies the posterior surface of the pons and the rostral medulla. The brainstem consists of, from inferior to superior, the medulla oblongata, pons, and midbrain. The tapering medulla is characterized by the pyramids and olive anteriorly and the gracile and cuneate fasciculi and tubercles posteriorly. The pyramidal decussation is the boundary between the medulla and the cervical spinal cord. The wide pons consists of a large anterior basal portion and a smaller posterior tegmentum in the floor of the rhomboid fossa. The short midbrain has the paired superior and inferior colliculi and their brachia posteriorly and the cerebral crus anteriorly. Cranial nerves III to XII arise from the brainstem. The trochlear (IV) nerve is the only one to leave the dorsal surface of the brainstem.

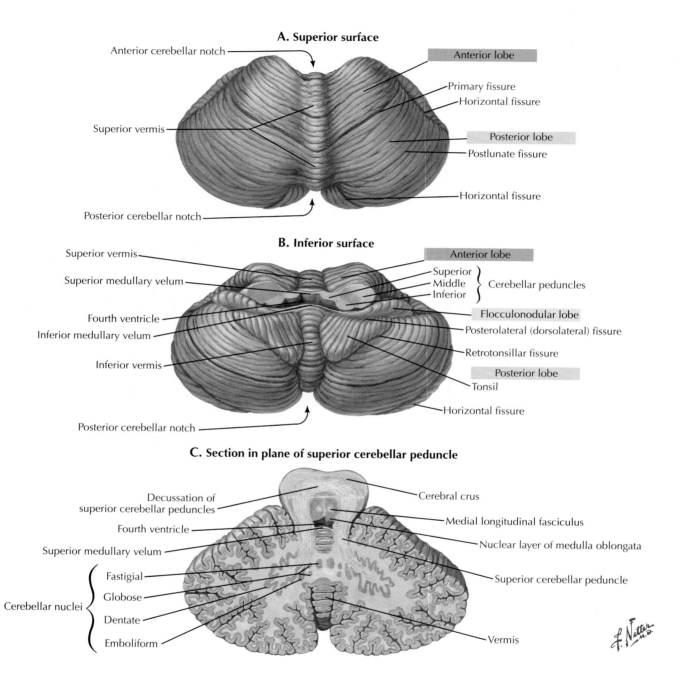

A. Superior surface

Anterior cerebellar notch

Anterior lobe

Primary fissure

Horizontal fissure

Superior vermis

Posterior lobe

Postlunate fissure

Horizontal fissure

Posterior cerebellar notch

B. Inferior surface

Superior vermis

Anterior lobe

Superior Middle Inferior } Cerebellar peduncles

Superior medullary velum

Flocculonodular lobe

Fourth ventricle

Posterolateral (dorsolateral) fissure

Inferior medullary velum

Retrotonsillar fissure

Inferior vermis

Posterior lobe

Tonsil

Horizontal fissure

Posterior cerebellar notch

C. Section in plane of superior cerebellar peduncle

Decussation of superior cerebellar peduncles

Cerebral crus

Fourth ventricle

Medial longitudinal fasciculus

Superior medullary velum

Nuclear layer of medulla oblongata

Fastigial

Globose

Superior cerebellar peduncle

Dentate

Cerebellar nuclei {

Emboliform

Vermis

8.51 CEREBELLUM

In these figures the cerebellum has been removed from the brainstem by cutting the superior, middle, and inferior cerebellar peduncles. The nerve fibers that make up the peduncles connect the cerebellum to the brainstem and thalamus. The cerebellum consists of a cortex or thin surface layer of gray matter that is extensively folded into thin, transverse, leaflike folia. White matter deep to the cortex is composed mostly of fibers going to or coming from the cortex. Four pairs of deep nuclei embedded in the white matter consist of neurons that project the cerebellar output to other portions of the brain. The dentate is the largest and most prominent. The cerebellum is divided into a narrow median vermis and large bilateral hemispheres. Two deep fissures divide the vermis and hemispheres into three lobes. The vermis and hemispheres can be further subdivided into lobules.

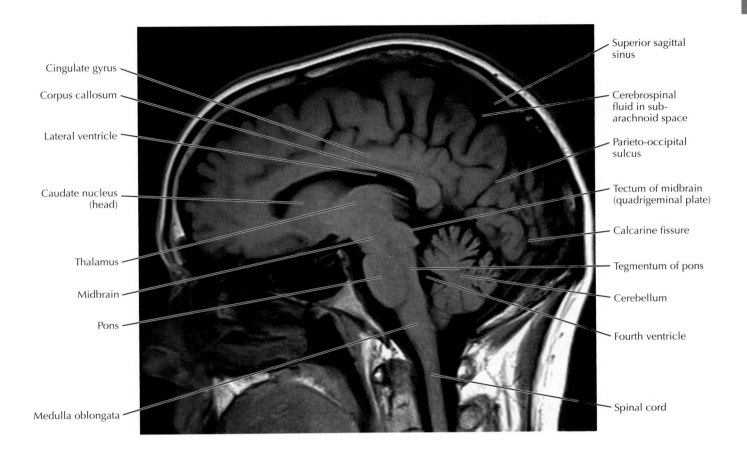

Cingulate gyrus

Corpus callosum

Lateral ventricle

Caudate nucleus (head)

Thalamus

Midbrain

Pons

Medulla oblongata

Superior sagittal sinus

Cerebrospinal fluid in sub-arachnoid space

Parieto-occipital sulcus

Tectum of midbrain (quadrigeminal plate)

Calcarine fissure

Tegmentum of pons

Cerebellum

Fourth ventricle

Spinal cord

8.52 T1 SAGITTAL MRI NEAR THE MIDLINE

This section is just off the midline lateral to the falx cerebri. More of the thalamus and a lateral ventricle are seen. The strategy for looking for pathology just lateral to the midline usually stems from the pathology that is also commonly seen in the midline, which may stretch laterally. For example, abnormalities in the corpus callosum, as can be seen in multiple sclerosis, may be off the midline. Sometimes pituitary or optic nerve abnormalities may also be seen off the midline. The basal ganglia and thalami are seen in the parasagittal plane, which allows the neuroradiologist to assess for changes to the brain as a result of hypertension affecting the small arteries that penetrate these structures.

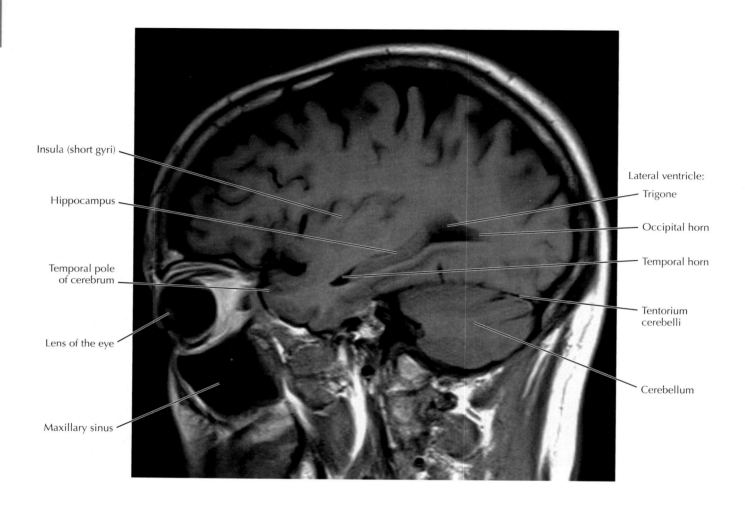

Insula (short gyri)

Hippocampus

Temporal pole
of cerebrum

Lens of the eye

Maxillary sinus

Lateral ventricle:

Trigone

Occipital horn

Temporal horn

Tentorium
cerebelli

Cerebellum

8.53 T1 SAGITTAL MRI THROUGH THE TEMPORAL LOBE

This is a parasagittal plane through the middle of the orbit, maxillary sinus, and cerebral hemisphere. The optic nerve and apex of the orbit are medial to the plane. The section is through the trigone of a lateral ventricle, including the occipital horn and full extent of the temporal horn in the middle of the temporal lobe of the cerebrum. The contours of the anterior, middle, and posterior cranial fossae are seen containing the frontal lobe of the cerebrum, temporal lobe, and cerebellum, respectively. The trigeminal (semilunar) ganglion and three divisions of the trigeminal nerve are medial to the plane of section. The dura mater of the tentorium cerebelli separates the cerebellum from the overlying occipital lobe of the cerebrum.

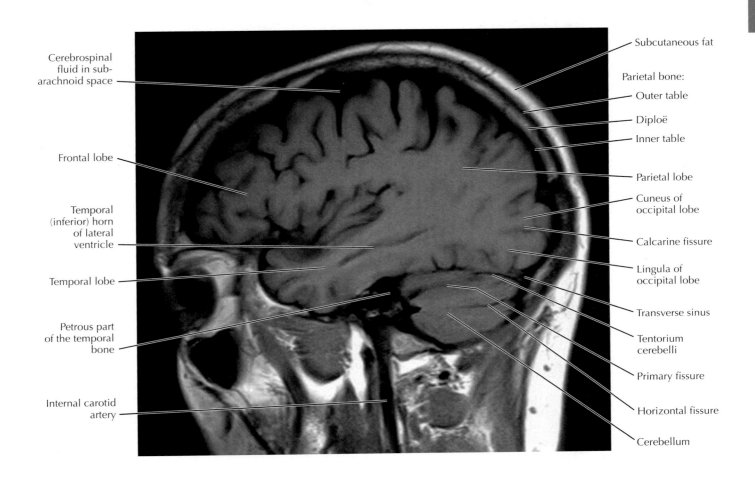

Cerebrospinal fluid in sub-arachnoid space

Frontal lobe

Temporal (inferior) horn of lateral ventricle

Temporal lobe

Petrous part of the temporal bone

Internal carotid artery

Subcutaneous fat

Parietal bone:

Outer table

Diploë

Inner table

Parietal lobe

Cuneus of occipital lobe

Calcarine fissure

Lingula of occipital lobe

Transverse sinus

Tentorium cerebelli

Primary fissure

Horizontal fissure

Cerebellum

8.54 T1 SAGITTAL MRI THROUGH THE TEMPORAL LOBE (CONT'D)

This section captures the internal carotid artery entering the carotid canal in the petrous part of the temporal bone inferior to the temporal lobe of the cerebrum. Recall that, with a T1-weighted MRI pulse sequence, fluid (including blood), bone, and air all appear dark. Attaching to the petrous posteriorly is the tentorium cerebelli between the cerebellum and occipital lobe. The transverse sinus is at the intersection of the tentorium cerebelli and the occipital bone on either side of the midline. Labeled in this section are the layers of the parietal bone—inner and outer tables of compact bone surrounding the more intense signal from the fatty diploë. It is hard to distinguish the inner table of bone from the underlying cerebrospinal fluid in the subarachnoid space.

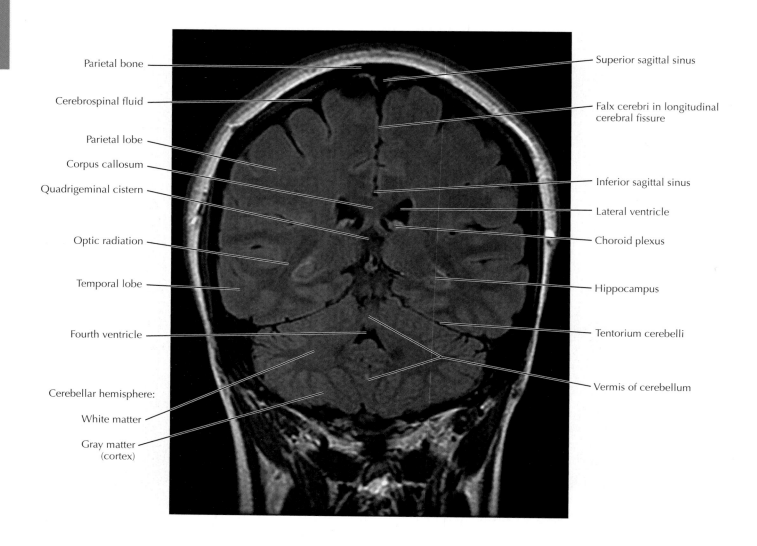

Parietal bone

Cerebrospinal fluid

Parietal lobe

Corpus callosum

Quadrigeminal cistern

Optic radiation

Temporal lobe

Fourth ventricle

Cerebellar hemisphere:

White matter

Gray matter
(cortex)

Superior sagittal sinus

Falx cerebri in longitudinal
cerebral fissure

Inferior sagittal sinus

Lateral ventricle

Choroid plexus

Hippocampus

Tentorium cerebelli

Vermis of cerebellum

8.55 T2 FLAIR CORONAL MRI THROUGH THE CEREBELLUM

The brain must be visualized in all three planes to evaluate the extent of a pathological process. This T2 fluid attenuation inversion recovery (FLAIR) MRI is a coronal section through the cerebellum, parietal lobes, and posterior aspect of the temporal lobes. This FLAIR pulse sequence on MRI is T2 based, but the normally T2 bright signal of fluid is suppressed on FLAIR imaging because of the application of an inversion pulse, which nulls the MRI signal from fluid. This is the reason that CSF appears dark on FLAIR imaging. In addition, white matter appears darker than gray matter. Also seen in this section are the lateral ventricles, fourth ventricle, and quadrigeminal cistern behind the third ventricle. The superior and inferior sagittal sinuses are seen in the superior and inferior margins of the falx cerebri.

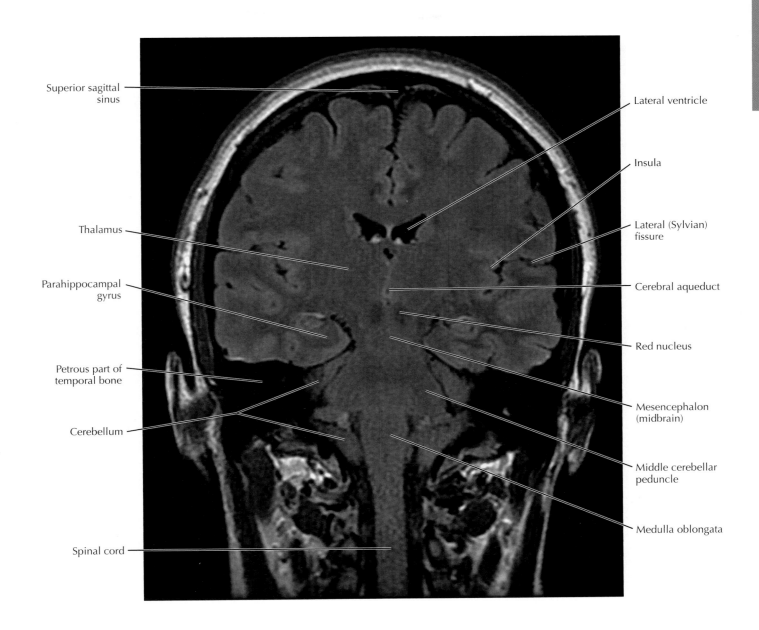

Superior sagittal sinus

Thalamus

Parahippocampal gyrus

Petrous part of temporal bone

Cerebellum

Spinal cord

Lateral ventricle

Insula

Lateral (Sylvian) fissure

Cerebral aqueduct

Red nucleus

Mesencephalon (midbrain)

Middle cerebellar peduncle

Medulla oblongata

8.56 T2 FLAIR CORONAL MRI THROUGH THE BRAINSTEM

FLAIR is a standard sequence that is obtained with most neurological MRIs. It is not requested for a particular suspected pathology because it is always done. It is most helpful because it highlights pathology with associated edema. The FLAIR sequence suppresses the fluid signal from CSF but not from edematous pathology such as edema surrounding a tumor or abscess. T1 images have black CSF but do not show edema with the same sensitivity as FLAIR images would. This section is just anterior to the cerebellum through the midbrain, medulla oblongata, and spinal cord. It is in between the third and fourth ventricles and through the cerebral aqueduct that connects them. The petrous part of the temporal bone is black; it contributes to the floor of the middle cranial fossa containing the temporal lobe.

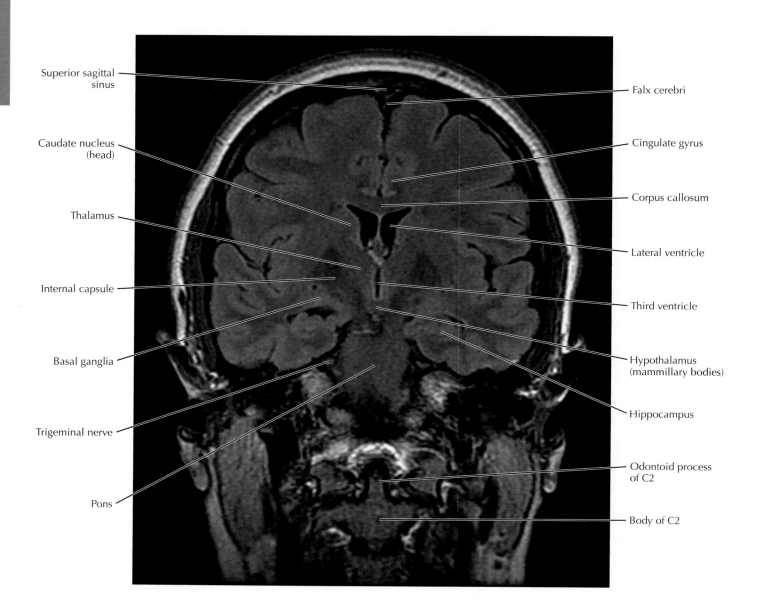

Superior sagittal sinus

Caudate nucleus (head)

Thalamus

Internal capsule

Basal ganglia

Trigeminal nerve

Pons

Falx cerebri

Cingulate gyrus

Corpus callosum

Lateral ventricle

Third ventricle

Hypothalamus (mammillary bodies)

Hippocampus

Odontoid process of C2

Body of C2

8.57 T2 FLAIR CORONAL MRI THROUGH THE PONS AND THIRD VENTRICLE

The body and odontoid process of the second cervical vertebra indicate that this section is just anterior to the foramen magnum and vertebral canal. The temporal lobe of the cerebrum connects with the parietal lobe above. The section is through the middle of the third ventricle with the thalamus and basal ganglia on either side. It is also through the pons at the level of cranial nerves exiting the brainstem. Here, the cisternal segment of the trigeminal (V) nerve is seen passing toward Meckel's cave in the middle cranial fossa. All of the coronal sections contain the corpus callosum connecting the left and right cerebral hemispheres just superior to the lateral ventricles. They also show the internal capsule of white matter sending information to and from the cerebral hemispheres.

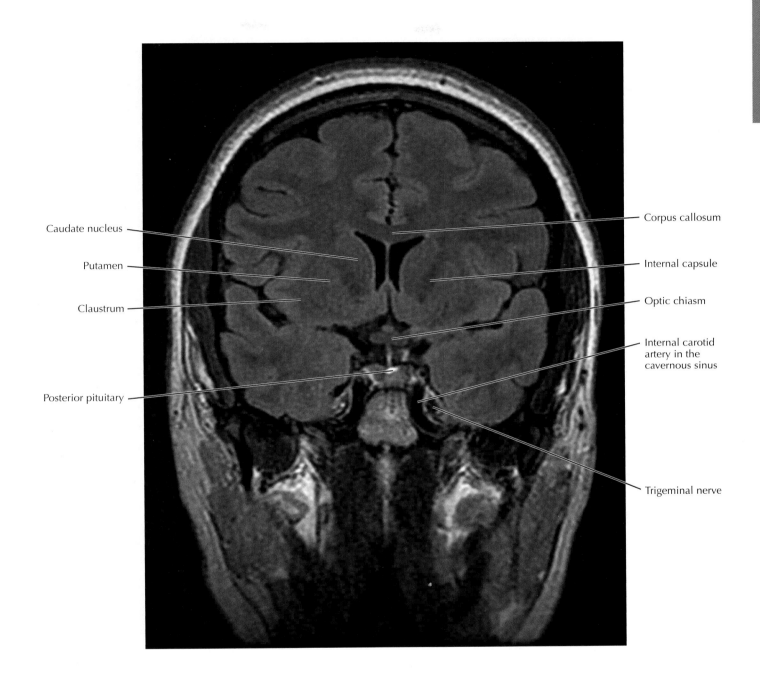

Caudate nucleus

Putamen

Claustrum

Posterior pituitary

Corpus callosum

Internal capsule

Optic chiasm

Internal carotid artery in the cavernous sinus

Trigeminal nerve

8.58 T2 FLAIR CORONAL MRI THROUGH THE OPTIC CHIASM

Continuing anteriorly, this section is through the posterior lobe of the pituitary gland (neurohypophysis) near the junction of the occipital and sphenoid bones in the midline. The continuity between the temporal and parietal lobes diminishes. The internal carotid artery enters the cavernous sinus from the carotid canal at the apex of the petrous part of the temporal bone on either side, just medial to the trigeminal nerve. Superior to the pituitary gland is the optic chiasm. The internal capsule courses between the caudate nucleus and putamen.

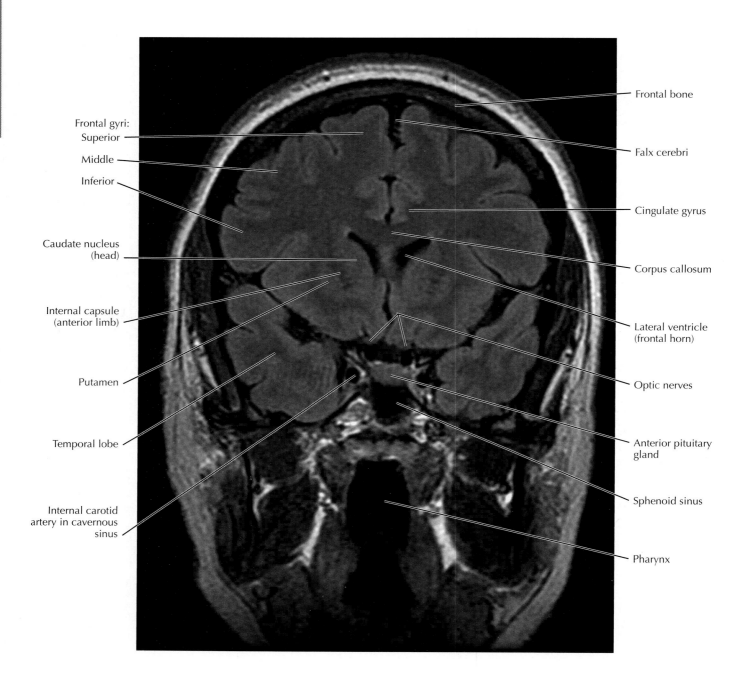

Frontal bone

Frontal gyri:
Superior

Middle

Inferior

Falx cerebri

Cingulate gyrus

Caudate nucleus
(head)

Corpus callosum

Internal capsule
(anterior limb)

Lateral ventricle
(frontal horn)

Putamen

Optic nerves

Temporal lobe

Anterior pituitary
gland

Internal carotid
artery in cavernous
sinus

Sphenoid sinus

Pharynx

8.59 T2 FLAIR CORONAL MRI THROUGH THE TEMPORAL LOBES

In this section the temporal lobes are now discrete and closer to the temporal poles. The section is through the anterior lobe of the pituitary gland (adenohypophysis), sphenoid sinus, and pharynx. Many important structures surround the body of the sphenoid bone. On either side of the sphenoid bone the internal carotid artery continues anteriorly through the cavernous sinus, a dural sinus that receives blood from the ophthalmic veins of the orbits and veins from deep in the brain. Also passing through the sinus with the internal carotid artery are cranial nerves III, IV, VI, and the first two divisions of the trigeminal nerve (V). The optic nerves are visible in this section, which is just anterior to the optic chiasm. The heads of the caudate nuclei are seen indenting the lateral ventricles.

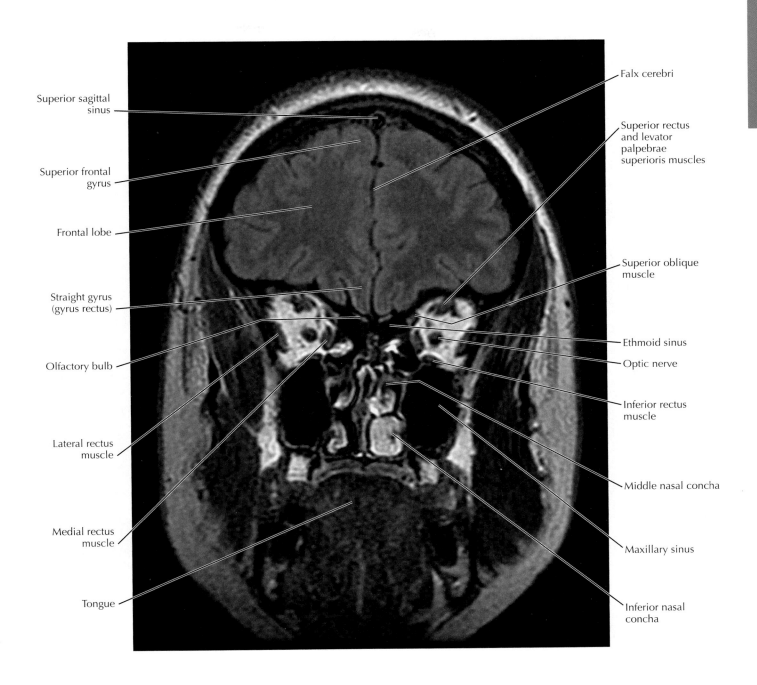

Superior sagittal sinus

Superior frontal gyrus

Frontal lobe

Straight gyrus (gyrus rectus)

Olfactory bulb

Lateral rectus muscle

Medial rectus muscle

Tongue

Falx cerebri

Superior rectus and levator palpebrae superioris muscles

Superior oblique muscle

Ethmoid sinus

Optic nerve

Inferior rectus muscle

Middle nasal concha

Maxillary sinus

Inferior nasal concha

8.60 T2 FLAIR CORONAL MRI THROUGH THE FRONTAL LOBES

The posterior aspects of the orbits and maxillary sinuses indicate that the plane of section is anterior to the temporal lobes; only the frontal lobes of the brain are visible. They are separated by the falx cerebri that is visible in all of the coronal sections of the brain. Just inferior to the frontal lobes near the midline are the olfactory bulbs resting on the cribriform plate of the ethmoid bone. The dark between the orbits is from air within the ethmoid sinus. Seen within the fat in each orbit are the optic nerve and extraocular muscles: the inferior rectus, medial rectus, lateral rectus, and superior rectus just below the levator palpebrae superioris muscle.

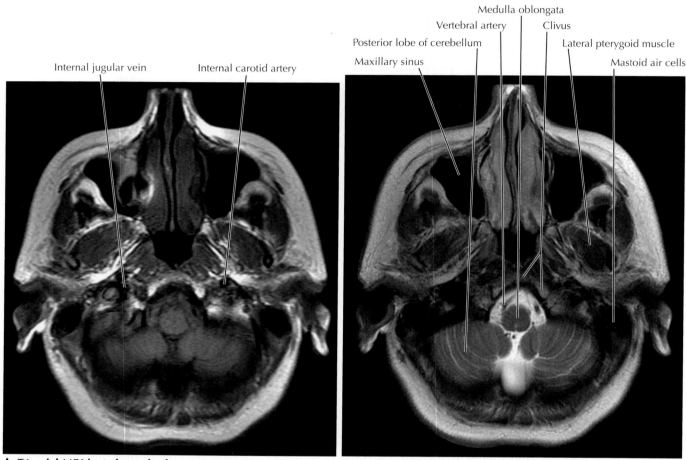

Internal jugular vein Internal carotid artery

Medulla oblongata
Vertebral artery Clivus
Posterior lobe of cerebellum Lateral pterygoid muscle
Maxillary sinus Mastoid air cells

A. T1 axial MRI just above the foramen magnum

B. T2 axial MRI at the same level in the same patient

8.61 T1 AND T2 AXIAL MRI THROUGH THE MEDULLA

This next series of MR images are axial T1-weighted (**A**) and T2-weighted (**B**) sections from the same subject. This section is through the medulla oblongata and inferior part of the cerebellum just superior to the foramen magnum. The vertebral arteries are easily seen entering the skull through the foramen magnum because the CSF that surrounds them is bright on the T2-weighted sequence (**B**). Pathology at this level may also involve cranial nerves IX, X, XI, and XII. The spinal accessory nerve (XI) exits the cervical spinal cord, ascends through the foramen magnum, and then exits the skull through the jugular canal to innervate the trapezius and sternocleidomastoid muscles. Rootlets of the glossopharyngeal (IX), vagus (X), and hypoglossal (XII) nerves exit the brainstem just superior to the foramen magnum.

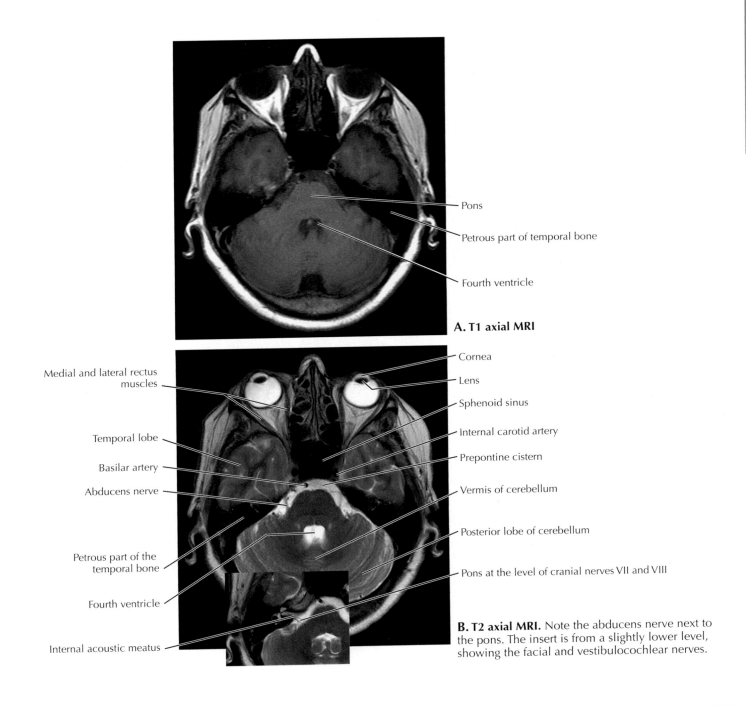

Pons

Petrous part of temporal bone

Fourth ventricle

A. T1 axial MRI

Cornea

Lens

Sphenoid sinus

Internal carotid artery

Prepontine cistern

Vermis of cerebellum

Posterior lobe of cerebellum

Pons at the level of cranial nerves VII and VIII

Medial and lateral rectus muscles

Temporal lobe

Basilar artery

Abducens nerve

Petrous part of the temporal bone

Fourth ventricle

Internal acoustic meatus

B. T2 axial MRI. Note the abducens nerve next to the pons. The insert is from a slightly lower level, showing the facial and vestibulocochlear nerves.

8.62 T1 AND T2 AXIAL MRI THROUGH THE CEREBELLUM, TEMPORAL LOBES, AND EYE

This section through the orbit and eye highlights the differences between T1- and T2-weighted MRI. Fluid is dark in T1 (**A**) and bright in T2 (**B**); note the vitreous humor of the eye and the CSF. White matter is lighter than gray matter in T1; the reverse is true for T2. Bone, connective tissue, and air have low signal (are dark) in both T1 and T2. Fat is bright in both but a bit lighter here in T1 compared with T2. This section is

through the pons, fourth ventricle, and middle of the cerebellum, and the inferior aspect of the temporal lobes is visible. The vertebral arteries have joined to form the basilar artery anterior to the brainstem. Sections through the pons contain cranial nerves, and it is important to look around the brainstem for tumors and other pathology involving these nerves. For example, this level is typical for identifying a vestibular schwannoma. Compare the abducens nerve in **B** with cranial nerves VII and VIII in the insert from a slightly lower level.

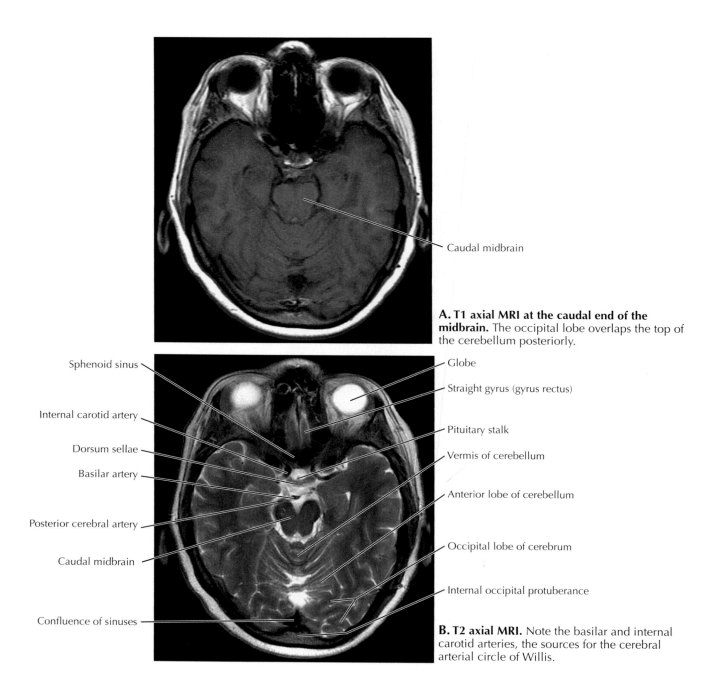

Caudal midbrain

A. T1 axial MRI at the caudal end of the midbrain. The occipital lobe overlaps the top of the cerebellum posteriorly.

Sphenoid sinus

Internal carotid artery

Dorsum sellae

Basilar artery

Posterior cerebral artery

Caudal midbrain

Confluence of sinuses

Globe

Straight gyrus (gyrus rectus)

Pituitary stalk

Vermis of cerebellum

Anterior lobe of cerebellum

Occipital lobe of cerebrum

Internal occipital protuberance

B. T2 axial MRI. Note the basilar and internal carotid arteries, the sources for the cerebral arterial circle of Willis.

8.63 T1 AND T2 AXIAL MRI THROUGH THE UPPER CEREBELLUM

This plane of section is through the temporal lobes, top of the cerebellum, and inferior aspect of the occipital lobes, where they overlap the cerebellum posteriorly. The confluence of sinuses, also known as the *torcular herophili*, is seen at the level of the tentorium cerebelli, although most of the tentorium is just out of the plane. The section is also through the stalk of the pituitary gland and caudal aspect of the midbrain near the level of the cerebral arterial circle (of Willis). The internal carotid arteries are anterior, and the basilar artery and posterior cerebral arteries are seen posteriorly. The latter are the termini of the basilar artery. A search strategy would include a careful assessment of the arteries for normal anatomical variants, aneurysms, calcifications, and other types of pathology.

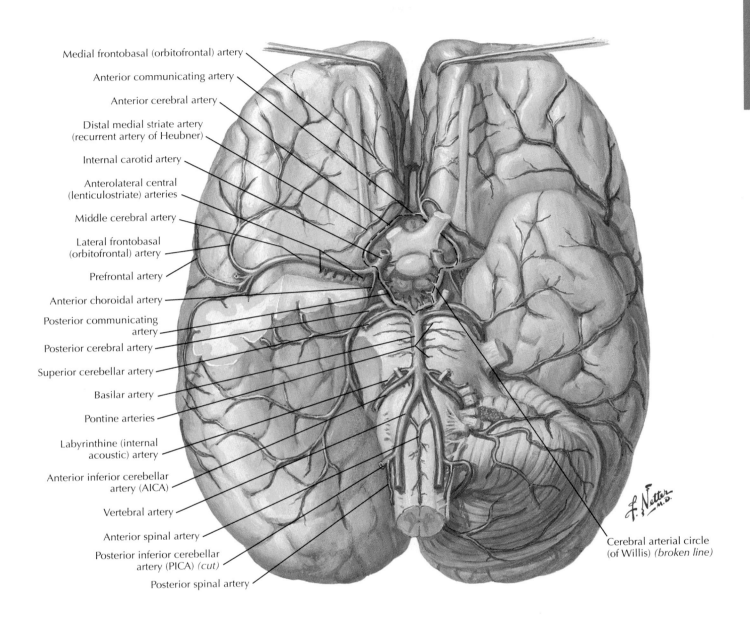

Medial frontobasal (orbitofrontal) artery

Anterior communicating artery

Anterior cerebral artery

Distal medial striate artery
(recurrent artery of Heubner)

Internal carotid artery

Anterolateral central
(lenticulostriate) arteries

Middle cerebral artery

Lateral frontobasal
(orbitofrontal) artery

Prefrontal artery

Anterior choroidal artery

Posterior communicating
artery

Posterior cerebral artery

Superior cerebellar artery

Basilar artery

Pontine arteries

Labyrinthine (internal
acoustic) artery

Anterior inferior cerebellar
artery (AICA)

Vertebral artery

Anterior spinal artery

Posterior inferior cerebellar
artery (PICA) (cut)

Posterior spinal artery

Cerebral arterial circle
(of Willis) (broken line)

8.64 ARTERIES OF THE BRAIN: INFERIOR VIEW

The brain receives its blood supply from the vertebral and internal carotid arteries. The vertebral arteries merge at the pontomedullary junction to form the basilar artery that divides into the posterior cerebral arteries at the top of the pons. The posterior vertebrobasilar circulation supplies the brainstem, cerebellum, occipital lobes, and the inferior and medial surfaces of the temporal lobes. The internal carotid arteries continue as the middle cerebral arteries and give off the smaller anterior cerebral arteries. The anterior internal carotid circulation supplies the frontal and parietal lobes and the lateral surface of the temporal lobes. The anterior and posterior circulations both contribute to the circle of Willis, and both supply the choroid plexus in the lateral ventricles. The circle of Willis surrounds the optic chiasm and the inferior surface of the hypothalamus.

A. Vessels dissected out: inferior view

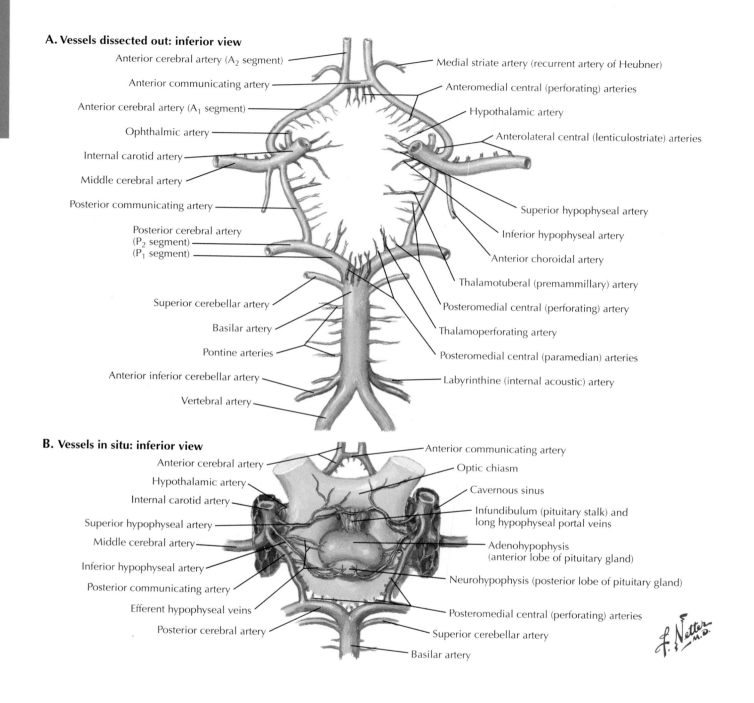

Anterior cerebral artery (A₂ segment)

Anterior communicating artery

Anterior cerebral artery (A₁ segment)

Ophthalmic artery

Internal carotid artery

Middle cerebral artery

Posterior communicating artery

Posterior cerebral artery
(P₂ segment)
(P₁ segment)

Superior cerebellar artery

Basilar artery

Pontine arteries

Anterior inferior cerebellar artery

Vertebral artery

Medial striate artery (recurrent artery of Heubner)

Anteromedial central (perforating) arteries

Hypothalamic artery

Anterolateral central (lenticulostriate) arteries

Superior hypophyseal artery

Inferior hypophyseal artery

Anterior choroidal artery

Thalamotuberal (premammillary) artery

Posteromedial central (perforating) artery

Thalamoperforating artery

Posteromedial central (paramedian) arteries

Labyrinthine (internal acoustic) artery

B. Vessels in situ: inferior view

Anterior cerebral artery

Hypothalamic artery

Internal carotid artery

Superior hypophyseal artery

Middle cerebral artery

Inferior hypophyseal artery

Posterior communicating artery

Efferent hypophyseal veins

Posterior cerebral artery

Anterior communicating artery

Optic chiasm

Cavernous sinus

Infundibulum (pituitary stalk) and
long hypophyseal portal veins

Adenohypophysis
(anterior lobe of pituitary gland)

Neurohypophysis (posterior lobe of pituitary gland)

Posteromedial central (perforating) arteries

Superior cerebellar artery

Basilar artery

8.65 CEREBRAL ARTERIAL CIRCLE (OF WILLIS)

Arteries that form the circle of Willis are, from anterior to posterior, the unpaired anterior communicating artery and the paired anterior cerebral, internal carotid, posterior communicating, and posterior cerebral arteries (**A**). The circle of Willis surrounds the optic tracts and the inferior surface of the hypothalamus (**B**). Small perforating or ganglionic arteries arise from the circle of Willis and supply deep structures in the diencephalon and cerebral hemispheres. The hypophyseal arteries that supply the pituitary gland (hypophysis) are branches of the internal carotid arteries rather than direct branches from the circle of Willis (**B**). Hypophyseal veins drain into the cavernous sinus. Hypophyseal portal veins lie in the infundibulum (pituitary stalk).

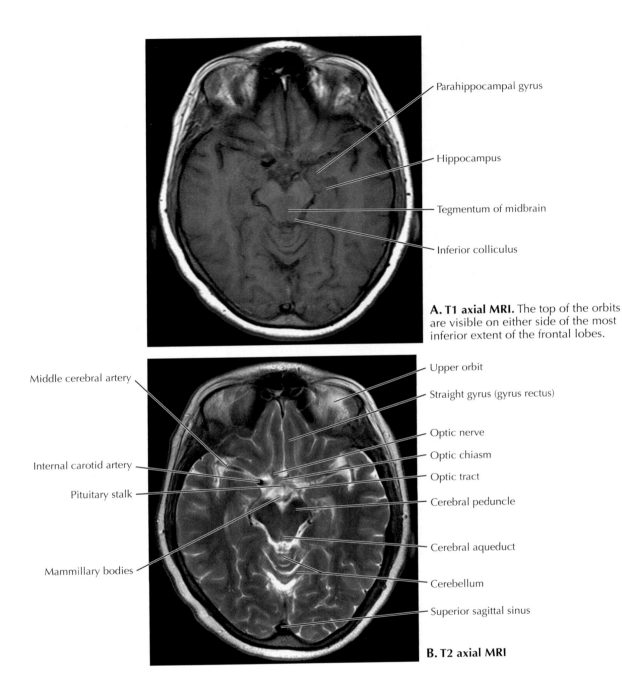

Parahippocampal gyrus

Hippocampus

Tegmentum of midbrain

Inferior colliculus

A. T1 axial MRI. The top of the orbits are visible on either side of the most inferior extent of the frontal lobes.

Middle cerebral artery

Internal carotid artery

Pituitary stalk

Mammillary bodies

Upper orbit

Straight gyrus (gyrus rectus)

Optic nerve

Optic chiasm

Optic tract

Cerebral peduncle

Cerebral aqueduct

Cerebellum

Superior sagittal sinus

B. T2 axial MRI

8.66 T1 AND T2 AXIAL MRI THROUGH THE OPTIC CHIASM

The cerebellum is nearly out of the plane of section, and more of the occipital lobes are seen. The most inferior aspects of the frontal lobes are visible between the orbits. The section captures the optic chiasm and mammillary bodies, the stalk of the pituitary gland, and the origin of the middle cerebral arteries from the internal carotid arteries. The plane is below the third and lateral ventricles and above the fourth ventricle anterior to the cerebellum. It transects the cerebral aqueduct through which CSF passes from the third to fourth ventricle. Although none of the ventricles are normally visible at this level, in a patient with hydrocephalus the enlarged temporal horns of the lateral ventricles may be seen. Their presence would aid in making the diagnosis.

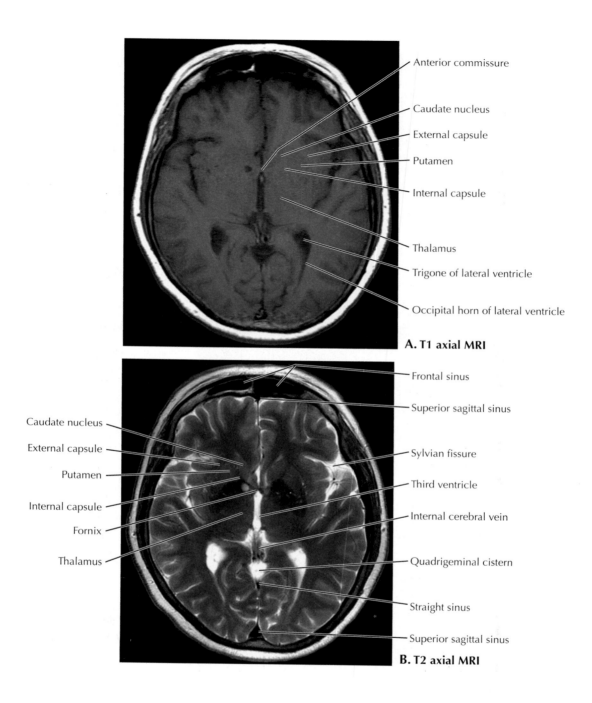

A. T1 axial MRI

- Anterior commissure
- Caudate nucleus
- External capsule
- Putamen
- Internal capsule
- Thalamus
- Trigone of lateral ventricle
- Occipital horn of lateral ventricle

B. T2 axial MRI

- Frontal sinus
- Superior sagittal sinus
- Sylvian fissure
- Third ventricle
- Internal cerebral vein
- Quadrigeminal cistern
- Straight sinus
- Superior sagittal sinus
- Caudate nucleus
- External capsule
- Putamen
- Internal capsule
- Fornix
- Thalamus

8.67 T1 AND T2 AXIAL MRI THROUGH THE THALAMUS AND THIRD VENTRICLE

This section is through the third ventricle flanked on either side by the thalamus. The trigone and occipital horn of the lateral ventricles are visible. Anterior to the thalamus are the caudate nucleus and putamen of the basal ganglia. The anterior limb of the internal capsule passes between the caudate nucleus and putamen. The posterior limb is lateral to the thalamus. The section is near the top of the cerebellum. Most of the tentorium cerebelli is out of the plane, although the straight sinus within it at the intersection of the falx cerebri is cut obliquely (**B**). The internal cerebral veins are also seen just before they join the great cerebral vein of Galen, which forms the straight sinus when it joins the inferior sagittal sinus. The superior sagittal sinus is seen just before it joins the straight sinus to form the transverse sinuses.

A. Horizontal sections through cerebrum

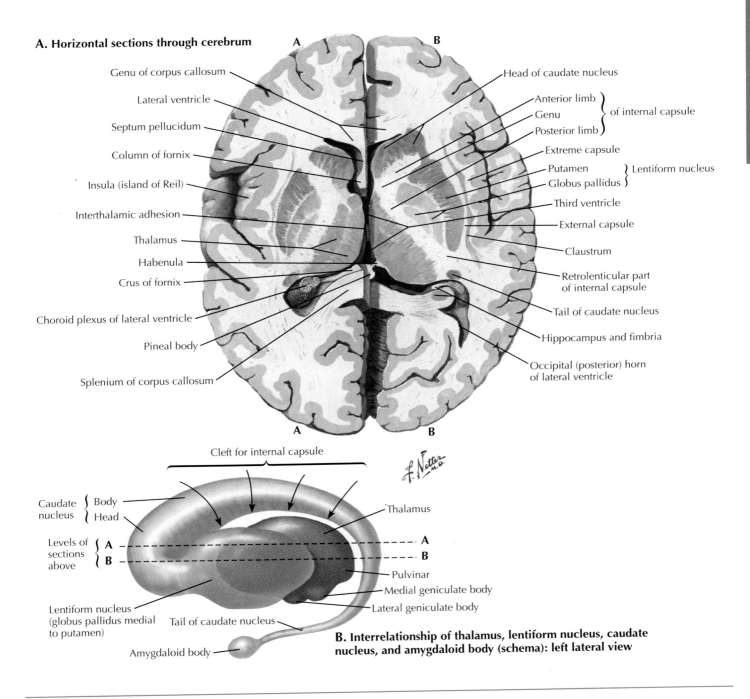

Genu of corpus callosum

Lateral ventricle

Septum pellucidum

Column of fornix

Insula (island of Reil)

Interthalamic adhesion

Thalamus

Habenula

Crus of fornix

Choroid plexus of lateral ventricle

Pineal body

Splenium of corpus callosum

Head of caudate nucleus

Anterior limb ⎰
Genu   ⎬ of internal capsule
Posterior limb ⎱

Extreme capsule

Putamen   ⎱ Lentiform nucleus
Globus pallidus ⎰

Third ventricle

External capsule

Claustrum

Retrolenticular part of internal capsule

Tail of caudate nucleus

Hippocampus and fimbria

Occipital (posterior) horn of lateral ventricle

Cleft for internal capsule

Caudate ⎰ Body
nucleus ⎱ Head

Levels of ⎰ A
sections ⎱ B
above

Lentiform nucleus
(globus pallidus medial to putamen)

Tail of caudate nucleus

Amygdaloid body

Thalamus

A
B

Pulvinar

Medial geniculate body

Lateral geniculate body

B. Interrelationship of thalamus, lentiform nucleus, caudate nucleus, and amygdaloid body (schema): left lateral view

8.68 TRANSVERSE (AXIAL) SECTION OF THE BRAIN AT THE LEVEL OF THE BASAL NUCLEI

Two levels of horizontal sections (**A** and **B**) through the cerebrum illustrate the relationships of the basal nuclei (ganglia), the thalamus, and the internal capsule. Embedded in the white matter of each cerebral hemisphere is a large mass of gray matter, the corpus striatum, which makes up most of the basal nuclei. The corpus striatum consists of the caudate nucleus and the lentiform (lenticular) nucleus that is further subdivided into the putamen laterally and the pale globus pallidus medially. The **C**-shaped caudate nucleus is named for its resemblance to a long tail as it follows the curvature of the lateral ventricle from the frontal lobe into the temporal lobe. In **B,** the caudate nucleus is seen to be continuous with the putamen. They are also functionally related and referred to as the striatum. Although the tail of the caudate nucleus ends at the amygdala in the temporal lobe, the two are not functionally related. The internal capsule, a **V**-shaped area of white matter, separates the lentiform nucleus laterally from the caudate nucleus and the thalamus medially. It consists of projection fibers connecting the cortex with subcortical structures.

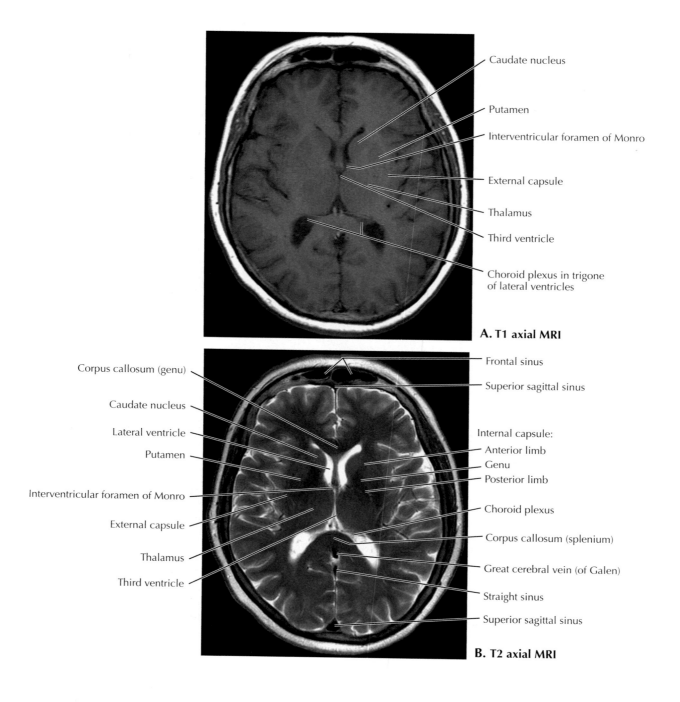

Caudate nucleus

Putamen

Interventricular foramen of Monro

External capsule

Thalamus

Third ventricle

Choroid plexus in trigone of lateral ventricles

A. T1 axial MRI

Corpus callosum (genu)

Caudate nucleus

Lateral ventricle

Putamen

Interventricular foramen of Monro

External capsule

Thalamus

Third ventricle

Frontal sinus

Superior sagittal sinus

Internal capsule:

Anterior limb

Genu

Posterior limb

Choroid plexus

Corpus callosum (splenium)

Great cerebral vein (of Galen)

Straight sinus

Superior sagittal sinus

B. T2 axial MRI

8.69 T1 AND T2 AXIAL MRI THROUGH THE THALAMUS AND LATERAL VENTRICLES

This plane of section is near the middle of the cerebrum through the frontal, parietal, and occipital lobes. The frontal sinus is prominent anteriorly within the frontal bone. The section is at the top of the third ventricle between the left and right thalamus at the level of the interventricular foramina of Monro on each side that communicate with the lateral ventricles. Choroid plexus is visible in the trigone of the lateral ventricles posteriorly. The superior sagittal sinus is visible both anteriorly and posteriorly in the falx cerebri between the cerebral hemispheres. The great cerebral vein of Galen approaches the straight sinus in the tentorium cerebelli, although most of the tentorium is below the plane of section between the occipital lobes and cerebellum.

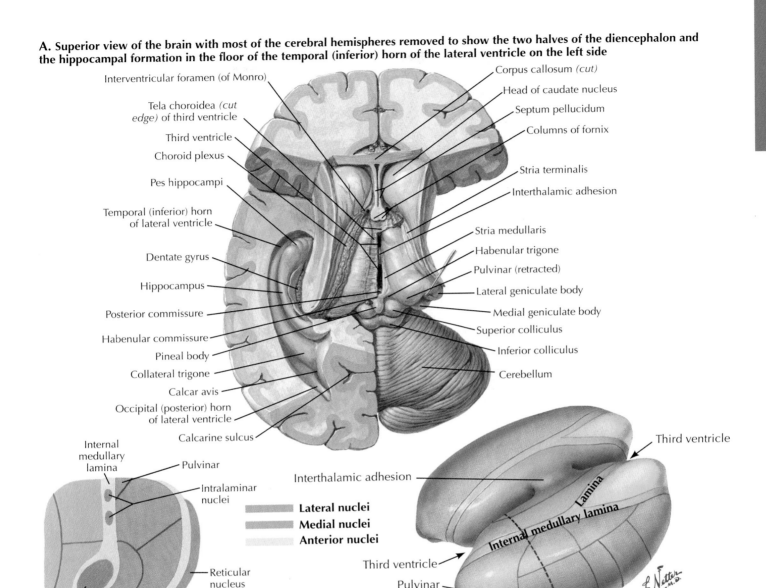

A. Superior view of the brain with most of the cerebral hemispheres removed to show the two halves of the diencephalon and the hippocampal formation in the floor of the temporal (inferior) horn of the lateral ventricle on the left side

Interventricular foramen (of Monro)

Tela choroidea *(cut edge)* of third ventricle

Third ventricle

Choroid plexus

Pes hippocampi

Temporal (inferior) horn of lateral ventricle

Dentate gyrus

Hippocampus

Posterior commissure

Habenular commissure

Pineal body

Collateral trigone

Calcar avis

Occipital (posterior) horn of lateral ventricle

Calcarine sulcus

Corpus callosum *(cut)*

Head of caudate nucleus

Septum pellucidum

Columns of fornix

Stria terminalis

Interthalamic adhesion

Stria medullaris

Habenular trigone

Pulvinar (retracted)

Lateral geniculate body

Medial geniculate body

Superior colliculus

Inferior colliculus

Cerebellum

Internal medullary lamina

Pulvinar

Intralaminar nuclei

Lateral nuclei
Medial nuclei
Anterior nuclei

Reticular nucleus

External medullary lamina

Centromedian nucleus

C. Schematic section through thalamus (at level of broken line shown in **B**)

Third ventricle

Interthalamic adhesion

Internal medullary lamina

Third ventricle

Pulvinar
Lateral geniculate body
Medial geniculate body

B. Schematic representation of thalamus (external medullary lamina and reticular nuclei removed)

8.70 THALAMUS

The vascular tela choroidea forms the roof of the third ventricle between the two halves of the diencephalon and extends laterally to form the choroid plexus of each lateral ventricle. Lying inferior to the roof of the third ventricle at the back of the thalamus is the epithalamus, consisting of the stria medullaris, the habenula, and the pineal gland (body). Posterior and inferior to the diencephalon are the paired superior and inferior colliculi of the midbrain. The internal medullary lamina, a vertical sheet of white matter, divides the thalamus into medial and lateral groups of nuclei and bifurcates anteriorly to enclose the anterior nuclei. The external medullary lamina separates the lateral nuclei from the thin reticular nucleus. The interthalamic adhesion (massa intermedia) is a bridge of gray matter extending across the third ventricle connecting the two halves of the thalamus. Most of the thalamic nuclei form reciprocal connections with specific motor, sensory, or limbic areas of cortex. The intralaminar, midline, and reticular nuclei have diffuse or nonspecific connections with widespread areas of cortex.

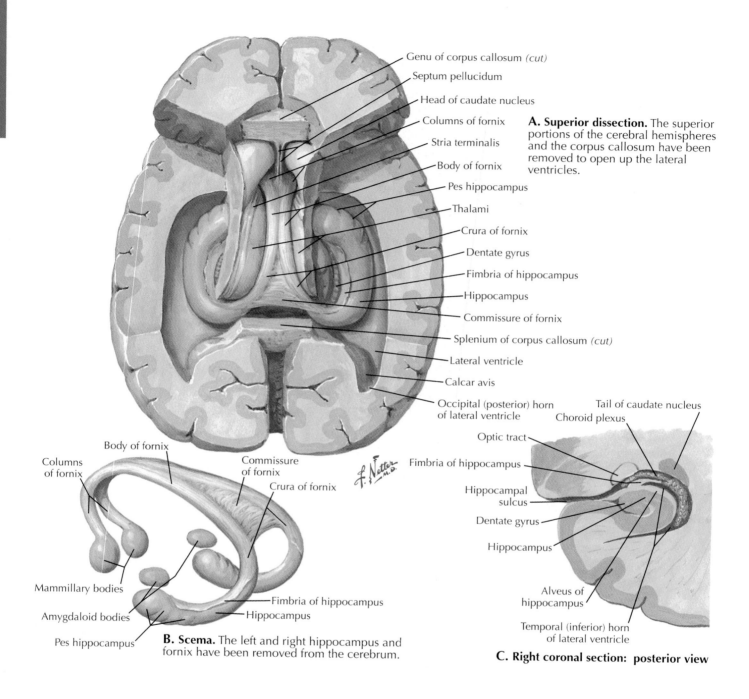

Genu of corpus callosum *(cut)*

Septum pellucidum

Head of caudate nucleus

Columns of fornix

Stria terminalis

Body of fornix

Pes hippocampus

Thalami

Crura of fornix

Dentate gyrus

Fimbria of hippocampus

Hippocampus

Commissure of fornix

Splenium of corpus callosum *(cut)*

Lateral ventricle

Calcar avis

Occipital (posterior) horn of lateral ventricle

A. Superior dissection. The superior portions of the cerebral hemispheres and the corpus callosum have been removed to open up the lateral ventricles.

Body of fornix

Columns of fornix

Commissure of fornix

Crura of fornix

Mammillary bodies

Amygdaloid bodies

Fimbria of hippocampus

Hippocampus

Pes hippocampus

B. Scema. The left and right hippocampus and fornix have been removed from the cerebrum.

Tail of caudate nucleus

Choroid plexus

Optic tract

Fimbria of hippocampus

Hippocampal sulcus

Dentate gyrus

Hippocampus

Alveus of hippocampus

Temporal (inferior) horn of lateral ventricle

C. Right coronal section: posterior view

f. Netter M.D.

8.71 HIPPOCAMPUS AND FORNIX

Bulging into the floor of each temporal horn of a lateral ventricle is the hippocampus (**A** and **B**), a curved, elongated ridge of three-layered archicortex that is continuous with the fornix (**B**). With the adjacent, curving parahippocampal gyrus (not labeled) it resembles the head and body of a seahorse (Gr., hippocampus). Its expanded anterior end resembles a foot with toes and is termed the *pes hippocampus*. Axons leave the hippocampus as the alveus that becomes the fimbria and then the C-shaped fornix that arches anteriorly over the thalamus. The small dentate gyrus medial to the fimbria resembles a row of teeth. Most of the fibers in the columns of fornix synapse in the mammillary body of the hypothalamus. The hippocampus consolidates short-term memories into long-term memories but does not store them.

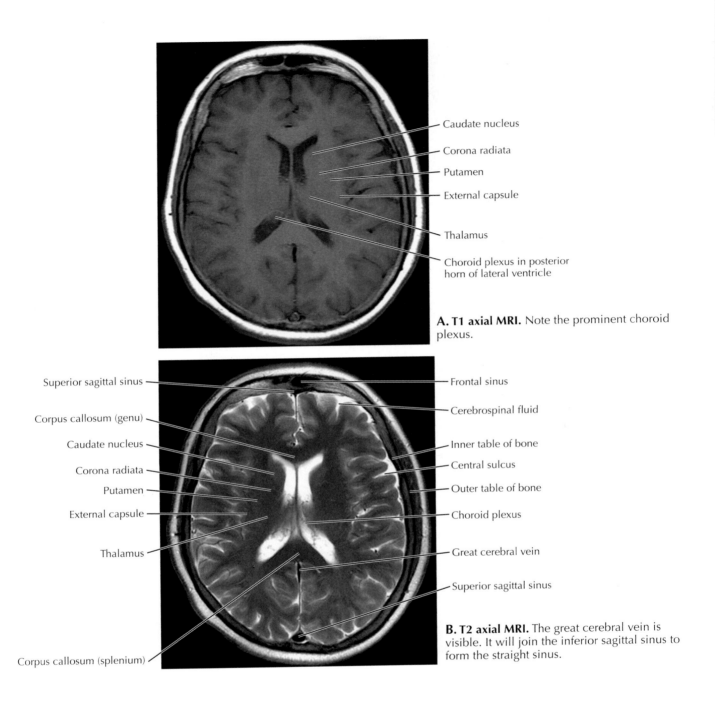

Caudate nucleus

Corona radiata

Putamen

External capsule

Thalamus

Choroid plexus in posterior
horn of lateral ventricle

A. T1 axial MRI. Note the prominent choroid
plexus.

Superior sagittal sinus

Corpus callosum (genu)

Caudate nucleus

Corona radiata

Putamen

External capsule

Thalamus

Corpus callosum (splenium)

Frontal sinus

Cerebrospinal fluid

Inner table of bone

Central sulcus

Outer table of bone

Choroid plexus

Great cerebral vein

Superior sagittal sinus

B. T2 axial MRI. The great cerebral vein is
visible. It will join the inferior sagittal sinus to
form the straight sinus.

8.72 T1 AND T2 AXIAL MRI THROUGH THE LATERAL VENTRICLES

The lateral ventricles are prominent features in this plane of section. An extensive choroid plexus is visible. Anterior and posterior to the lateral ventricles are the genu and splenium of the corpus callosum, respectively. The great cerebral vein is still seen. The plane is near the top of the frontal sinus, and bright signal of the fatty diploë between the inner and outer tables of compact bone is prominent all around the calvarium. With T1 (**A**), the inner table of bone cannot be distinguished from the CSF in the subarachnoid space. Both appear dark. Note the small size of the superior sagittal sinus near its origin anteriorly compared with its large size near its termination posteriorly as it approaches the confluence of sinuses.

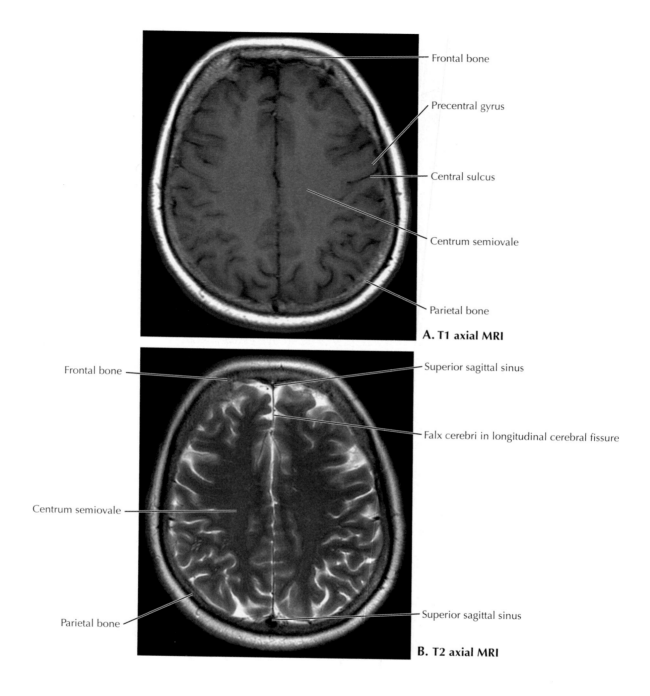

A. T1 axial MRI

B. T2 axial MRI

8.73 T1 AND T2 AXIAL MRI THROUGH THE MIDDLE OF THE CEREBRAL HEMISPHERES

This section is through the frontal and parietal lobes just above the occipital lobe. In the interior of the cerebral hemispheres above the lateral ventricles and corpus callosum is the centrum semiovale, the white matter tracts that pass to and from the internal capsule and corpus callosum. Part of the search for lesions, masses, stroke, and other pathology is the evaluation for symmetry of the two hemispheres and the contour of the falx cerebri for possible shift of midline structures. For example, bleeding or a tumor on one side of the brain increases the volume of that hemisphere. Midline structures push the falx cerebri toward the normal side.

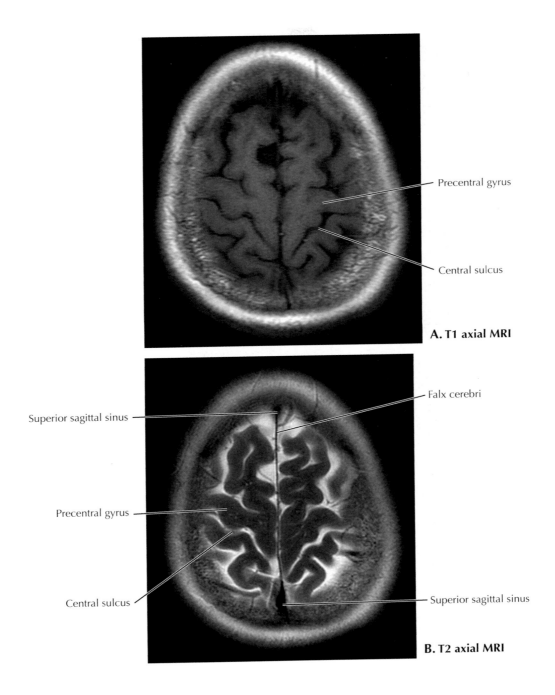

Precentral gyrus

Central sulcus

A. T1 axial MRI

Superior sagittal sinus

Falx cerebri

Precentral gyrus

Central sulcus

Superior sagittal sinus

B. T2 axial MRI

8.74 T1 AND T2 AXIAL MRI THROUGH THE THALAMUS AND LATERAL VENTRICLES

A section through the high convexities of the cerebral hemispheres shows the gyri of the frontal and parietal lobes. The falx cerebri is in sharp contrast to the bright cerebrospinal fluid on the T2-weighted MRI (**B**). The profile of the superior sagittal sinus has a more oblique section because the sinus has a more horizontal orientation near the top of the skull. The curving frontal and parietal bones at the top of the calvarium are also sectioned obliquely, and the inner and outer tables of compact bone do not present sharp profiles because of an imaging phenomenon known as *partial volume averaging*.

GLOSSARY

Activity The strength of a radioactive source, formally the number of atoms that decay and emit radiation in 1 second. Areas of increased activity observed in nuclear images are called "hot spots" and are caused by increased regional uptake of the radiotracer by the tissue, which in turn leads to a greater number of observed radioactive decay events.

Angiography X-ray, computed tomography (CT), or magnetic resonance (MR) examination designed to highlight blood vessels. Frequently a contrast agent is injected into a blood vessel (artery or vein) to opacify the vascular system. Time-of-flight MR angiography does not need a contrast agent to be administered.

Anteroposterior (AP) projection An x-ray obtained in which the x-ray beam passes through the patient from anterior to posterior before striking the detector plate that is placed posterior to the patient. Usually taken with portable x-ray machines on sicker patients who cannot stand up for the more standard posteroanterior (PA) projection (see below).

Aortic knob The contour of the arch of the aorta as seen against the left lung field on a chest x-ray.

Arteriogram Imaging study of arteries.

Atelectasis Collapse of an anatomical structure, frequently used to describe collapse of a lung, lobe, or part of a lobe.

Attenuation Reduction of x-rays or other signal (e.g., in ultrasound) reaching a detector as a result of absorption or scatter by tissues and structures in the body.

Axial Transverse/horizontal plane.

Catheter Specially designed tubes of varying sizes placed into the body to accomplish a specific task. Catheters may be used for injecting contrast into vessels or other body parts, removing urine from the bladder or fluid from body cavities, measuring intracardiac pressure, and other clinical procedures.

Cerebrospinal fluid (CSF) The fluid that bathes the brain and spinal cord in the subarachnoid space. CSF is produced by the choroid plexus of vessels within the brain ventricles.

Collimation Restricting x-rays to the area of the body to be imaged, with lead-lined shutters below the source of the x-ray beam.

Contrast media Suspensions of high-molecular-weight substances such as iodine or barium introduced orally, rectally, or into the bloodstream to assist in imaging specific structures. They make blood vessels, hollow organs, and organs in general more visible by increasing their attenuation of an x-ray beam. Gadolinium is the most common contrast agent for magnetic resonance imaging (MRI) studies.

Computed radiography (CR) Similar to conventional radiography (plain films), except that the image is captured on a digital detector plate rather than film.

Computed tomography (CT) Radiographical planes in the body (tomograms) reconstructed by computer from data collected using an x-ray beam and array of detectors that move around a patient passing through the machine on a horizontal table.

Computed tomography angiography (CTA) The study of blood vessels in serial CT planes.

Coronal A plane passing from right to left, perpendicular to the transverse plane, and separating anterior from posterior.

Costodiaphragmatic recess A potential space in each pleural cavity in which the costal pleura reflects against the diaphragmatic pleura around the dome of the hemidiaphragm. The inferior lobe of each lung does not extend into the costodiaphragmatic recess.

Costophrenic angle/sulcus A radiological term for the costal and diaphragmatic (phrenic) pleura that surround the most inferior margin of the lower lobes of the lungs. Blunting of this normally sharp angle on an x-ray may indicate the pooling of fluid (pleural effusion) or blood (hemothorax).

Cross section A section through the body in the axial (transverse) plane.

Decubitus Position in which patient is lying on one side (e.g., a right lateral decubitus view to look for an effusion layering).

Density A descriptor of the gray-scale appearance of structures or tissues in an x-ray–based examination. By convention, dense items such as bone or metal are white, and lucent items such as air or fat appear dark.

Diffusion-weighted imaging (DWI) An MRI sequence designed to identify the reduced brownian motion of water molecules that is seen in the setting of stroke, abscess, or high-grade tumor.

Echo Reflection of sound waves at an interface of tissues/structures with different acoustic properties.

Echocardiogram Ultrasound images of the heart.

Echoic/echogenicity Descriptors used with ultrasound examinations to describe the gray-scale appearance of tissues/structures when compared to each other (something more echogenic looks white, and something decreased in echogenicity looks darker; fluid is anechoic [no echoes—totally black]).

Edema ("a swelling") The accumulation of excessive fluid in cells and tissues.

Effusion ("pouring out") A pathologic collection of fluid (e.g., in pleural spaces, pericardial cavity, joint spaces).

Endoscopic retrograde cholangiopancreatography (ERCP) X-ray imaging of the biliary tract and pancreatic duct system obtained by the direct retrograde injection of contrast directly into the common bile and pancreatic ducts. The injection is facilitated by using an endoscope.

Endoscopy Viewing the interior of the body with a small camera on a catheter introduced into the gastrointestinal (GI) tract. (Laparoscopy refers to looking into the abdominal/pelvic cavities with a camera; arthroscopy is looking into a joint with a camera.)

FLAIR (fluid attenuation inversion recovery) Typically a T2-weighted MRI sequence in which CSF is suppressed by a special pulse and therefore appears dark. Pathologic edema is not suppressed.

Fluoroscopy A continuous beam of x-rays generating real-time images viewed on a monitor. It can be used to guide procedures, to guide the taking of images, or to monitor the motion of structures such as the diaphragm or portions of the GI tract.

Free air Air in the abdominal cavity introduced by surgery or the rupture of a hollow organ (viscus).

French Name of the scale used to measure the outer diameter of catheters. The size in French divided by π gives the measurement in millimeters.

Gantry Outer housing of a CT or an MRI machine.

Gating Coordinating image collection with a physiological parameter, usually respiration or the heartbeat, using an electrocardiogram (ECG) for the latter.

Helical CT CT in which the x-rays are recorded in a spiral fashion as the patient moves through the gantry. It was called *spiral CT* when the technique was first developed.

Hemothorax Bloody fluid in the pleural cavity.

Hounsfield Scale of densities (attenuation units) in CT from −1000 (black for air) to +3095 (white for bone), with 0 calibrated for the density of water. Named after Sir Godfrey Hounsfield, the British scientist who developed the first practical CT scanner and was awarded the Nobel Prize in Medicine in 1979.

Hydrothorax Fluid in the pleural cavity.

Intra-arterial (IA) Administration of a medicine or contrast media directly into the arteries.

Intravenous (IV) Administration of a medicine or contrast media directly into the veins.

Kerley lines Dilated lymphatic vessels seen on chest x-rays in the periphery of the lungs as small, parallel, horizontal lines.

Lateral projection X-ray view from the side, usually of the chest. This is most frequently a left lateral, with the left side against the detector, to decrease heart magnification.

Lymphangiogram Imaging study of lymphatic vessels using an injected contrast material that is absorbed by lymphatic capillaries.

Maximum intensity projection (MIP) A computer method for visualizing three-dimensional data on a screen where only the voxels with the highest intensity, usually contrast in blood vessels, are displayed. The sense of depth is created by changing perspectives, which gives the appearance of rotation.

Meniscus A crescent shape. The "meniscus sign" in an x-ray refers to the curving interface of fluid against a lung.

Millisievert A unit of measurement of the effective radiation dose that factors in the dose absorbed, the type of radiation, its biological effect, and the sensitivities of different tissues to different types of radiation.

MRA Magnetic resonance angiography.

MRV Magnetic resonance venography.

Myelography Imaging study of the spinal cord and nerve roots using the injection of special contrast into the subarachnoid space.

Nuclear imaging Images that are created by radiation emanating from the body following administration of a radiotracer. The molecules are introduced into the body, usually by IV injection, and after an appropriate amount of time their emissions are measured with a gamma camera.

Oblique projection An x-ray view at an angle to one of the standard three planes (sagittal, coronal, axial).

Orthogonal projection An x-ray view in one of the standard three planes (sagittal, coronal, axial).

PACS Picture Archiving and Communication System consisting of hardware, software, and protocol standards in a digital environment to address all aspects of the use of medical images, from capture, viewing, tagging, and storing to sharing, incorporating reports, and monitoring/managing the workloads of radiologists.

Pantomography A method to display the maxillary and mandibular dental arches in a single x-ray image (also known as Panorex).

Plain film A traditional x-ray; more and more images are digitally acquired now using special detector plates instead of x-ray film.

Pneumothorax Air in the pleural cavity introduced from a ruptured bleb near the surface of the lung, from a medical procedure such as a thoracentesis, or from penetrating trauma to the thoracic wall. (see Tension pneumothorax)

Positron emission tomography (PET) Physiological nuclear medicine study using radioactively tagged glucose to look for sites of increased glucose metabolism. Very high glucose metabolism is usually associated with malignancies.

Posteroanterior (PA) projection Standard chest x-ray view in which the x-ray beam passes from posterior to anterior through the patient. This places the heart close to the image detector to minimize cardiac enlargement from the divergent x-ray beam.

Prone Face-down position (on a table).

Proton density (PD) An MRI sequence that reflects the relative distribution of water and is intermediate in weighting between T1 and T2.

Radiolucent Descriptor term for things that look blacker because of increased x-ray exposure on the image detector (decreased attenuation).

Radiopaque Descriptor term for things that look brighter because of decreased x-ray exposure on the image detector (increased attenuation).

Radiopharmaceutical A molecule tagged with a radioactive substance used in nuclear imaging studies. Also called a *radiotracer* or *radioactive tracer*.

Radiotracers Radioactively tagged molecules engineered to image very specific functions.

Retrograde The opposite from the physiological direction of flow, which is known as *antegrade* or *anterograde* (e.g., contrast introduced into a duct as in ERCP).

Roentgen (or Röntgen) A unit of measure for exposure to x-rays named after Wilhelm Conrad Röntgen, who first described the properties of x-rays late in the 19th century.

Sagittal A plane passing from anterior to posterior in a vertical orientation, perpendicular to the transverse plane and separating right from left.

Scotty dog In an oblique x-ray of the vertebral column, the Scotty dog shape outlined by the transverse process, pedicle, pars interarticularis, articular processes, and spinous process. The neck of the Scotty dog is where fractures of the pars interarticularis are seen.

Scout On x-ray studies, the initial x-ray used as a control before barium or some other contrast agent is introduced. In CT, a quick, planar image of the body used to determine the range of sections to be obtained in the examination (aka a topogram or localizer).

Signal intensity Description of the brightness of structures in MRI. This is similar to the use of the terms *density* and *attenuation* in plain x-rays and *CT* and *activity* in nuclear medicine.

Silhouette sign In chest x-rays, the loss of the contour of an organ (e.g., the heart) or structure where it abuts an abnormality of similar density.

Single photon emission computed tomography (SPECT) A way of creating cross-sectional images from nuclear medicine data. It is the most common nuclear imaging technique for evaluating perfusion and function of the left ventricle.

Sternal angle An anatomical landmark where the manubrium joins the body of the sternum. It marks the level of the bifurcation of the trachea and great vessels of the heart at the T4 vertebral level.

STIR Short tau inversion recovery; an MRI sequence that is designed to suppress signal from fat.

Supine Face-up position.

Susceptibility weighted imaging (SWI) An MRI sequence designed to identify subtle hemorrhage.

T1 An MRI sequence based on the relaxation time of hydrogen ion spin along an axis parallel to the magnetic field. It is used for general anatomical study.

T2 An MRI sequence based on the relaxation time of hydrogen ion spin along an axis perpendicular to the magnetic field. It is useful for the study of pathology because fluid appears bright white (e.g., in edema, effusion, cysts).

Target Tungsten source of the x-ray beam.

Tension pneumothorax A medical emergency in which air is introduced into the pleural cavity from trauma to the thoracic wall. The opening acts as a one-way valve during inspiration and expiration, spreading air around the lung, causing it to collapse. There is a shift of mediastinal structures to the side opposite the pneumothorax.

Tesla A unit of strength of the magnet in MRI devices; named after Nikola Tesla, a Serbian-American electrical engineer (1856-1953).

Tomogram A thin radiographical image in one plane.

Ultrasonography Real-time imaging of the body using sound waves from a transducer/receiver probe, coupled with an acoustic gel, that is moved on the skin over the area of interest.

Venography Imaging study of veins.

View The orientation of an image described by the direction of x-rays passing through the body.

Volume rendering A computer method for visualizing three-dimensional data on a screen with CT or MRI in which specific structures such as blood vessels or bones are digitally reconstructed, with color, shading, highlights, and other effects added to enhance the three-dimensional effect.

Voxel A volume element or volumetric pixel that is the three-dimensional correlate of the two-dimensional pixel.

Window Vernacular for CT image display settings. Windows are defined by two values, the level and width on the Hounsfield scale. These are chosen to optimally view different structures to best advantage (e.g., bone windows, lung windows, soft tissue windows).

INDEX

Page numbers followed by "f" indicate figures.

A

Abdomen
  bony framework of, 35f, 78
  colon. *See* Colon
  computed tomography of
    bony framework, 78, 78f
    contrast-enhanced, 79, 79f-81f
    magnetic resonance imaging versus, 80, 80f
  foregut arteries of, 97, 97f
  hiatal hernia, 94, 94f
  hindgut arteries of, 98, 98f
  magnetic resonance imaging of, 80, 80f
  midgut arteries of, 98, 98f
  pathology of, 101, 101f
  peritoneum of, 100, 100f
  retroperitoneum of, 100, 100f
  stomach. *See* Stomach
Abdominal aorta, 82f, 85f-91f, 93f, 97f, 109f, 113f
Abdominal cavity
  anatomy of, 82
  free air in, 101
Abducent nerve, 221f-222f, 235f, 247f
Abductor digiti minimi muscle, 179f
Abductor hallucis muscle, 179f
Abductor pollicis brevis muscle, 138f
Abductor pollicis brevis tendon, 138f
Abductor pollicis longus muscle, 138f, 145f
Abductor pollicis longus tendon, 138f
Accessory hemiazygos vein, 40f
Accessory nerve, 235f
Accessory process, 20f
Acetabular fossa, 116f, 150f
Acetabular labrum, 150f, 152f
Acetabular ligament, 150f
Acetabular margin, 105f, 149f
Acetabular notch, 149f
Acetabulum, 104, 104f, 106f, 111f, 149f, 151f
Achilles tendon, 170f-171f, 180f
Acromial angle, 122f

Acromioclavicular joint, 123, 125f
Acromion, 122, 122f, 124f-125f
Adductor brevis muscle, 156f-157f
Adductor canal, 158
Adductor longus muscle, 154f, 156f-158f
Adductor magnus muscle, 153, 154f-158f
Adductor magnus tendon, 156f
Adductor tubercle, 162f
Adenohypophysis, 250f
Adrenal glands, 82f
Airway studies, 46, 46f
Ala, sacral, 21f, 106f
Alar fascia, 202f
Alar folds, 160f
ALARA principle, 6
Alveolar artery, 201f, 206f
Alveolar process, 186f, 217f
Alveolar vein, 206f
Alveus, 256f
Ampulla of Vater, 96f
Amygdaloid bodies, 256f
Anal canal, 107f
Anatomical neck, 122f-123f
Anatomical snuffbox, 138f
Anconeus muscle, 138f
Angiography, 13
  computed tomography. *See* Computed tomography angiography
  digital subtraction. *See* Digital subtraction angiography
  left coronary artery, 52, 52f
  magnetic resonance. *See* Magnetic resonance angiography
  maximum intensity projection, 13
  volume-rendering algorithms, 13
Angular artery, 201f
Ankle. *See also* Foot
  magnetic resonance imaging of, 179-180, 179f-180f
  x-rays of, 178, 178f
Annular ligament, 134, 134f
Anorectal junction, 115f
Ansa cervicalis, 200f
Anserine bursa, 160f

Antebrachial vein, 139f
Anterior axillary computed tomography, 39, 39f
Anterior axillary magnetic resonance imaging, 39, 39f
Anterior cerebellar notch, 236f
Anterior cerebral artery, 225, 225f-226f, 249f-250f
Anterior choroidal artery, 249f
Anterior circumflex humeral artery, 128f, 130f
Anterior circumflex humeral vein, 128f
Anterior commissure, 230f-231f, 234f, 252f
Anterior communicating artery, 225f, 249f-250f
Anterior cranial fossa, 194
Anterior cruciate ligament, 161f-162f, 162, 164, 164f
Anterior ethmoidal foramen, 188f, 194f
Anterior fontanelle, 195f
Anterior humeral line, 135
Anterior inferior cerebellar artery, 225f, 249f-250f
Anterior inferior iliac spine, 78f, 104f-105f, 149f
Anterior intercavernous sinus, 220f
Anterior interosseous artery, 128f, 139f
Anterior interosseous nerve, 139f
Anterior jugular vein, 200f
Anterior longitudinal ligament, 24f, 105f, 203f, 219f
Anterior nasal spine, 186f, 189f
Anterior perforated substance, 235f
Anterior scalene muscle, 37f-38f, 40f-41f, 201f-202f
Anterior spinal artery, 249f
Anterior superior iliac spine, 78f, 104f-105f, 149f, 154
Anterior tibial artery, 166f, 169, 169f, 172f, 174f
Anterior tibial recurrent artery, 166f
Anterior ulnar recurrent artery, 128f

Anteroposterior view, 64, 64f
   breast implants on, 67f
   hand, 142, 142f
   shoulder, 123, 123f
   skull, 187, 187f
   wrist, 142, 142f
Aorta
   abdominal, 82f, 85f-91f, 93f, 97f, 109f, 113f
   ascending, 38f-39f, 50f, 53f, 61f
   atherosclerotic calcifications of, 73
   computed tomography of, 82f, 91, 91f, 101f
   descending, 37f, 40f, 46f, 49f, 61f-62f, 88f
   echocardiography of, 54f
   general images of, 83f
   magnetic resonance imaging of, 26f, 49f, 167f
   posteroanterior x-ray of, 36f
   sagittal section of, 91, 91f
   thoracic, 40f, 49f, 84f, 86f
Aortic arch
   angiogram of, 226f
   computed tomography of, 37f, 46f
   general images of, 35f, 40f, 47f, 58f, 60f
Aortic sinus, 50f, 53f
Aortic valve, 38f, 50f
Appendix, 95f
Aqueduct of Sylvius, 230f-233f, 241f
Arachnoid granulations, 192, 192f, 223, 233f
Arachnoid mater, 22, 22f-23f, 223f-224f, 233f
Arcades, 98
Archiving and communication system, 15, 15f
Arcuate eminence, 227f
Arcuate ligament, 58f, 161f
Arcuate line, 78f, 104f-105f, 149f
Arm. See also Hand; Humerus; Radius; Ulna; Wrist
   cross section of, 131f
   magnetic resonance imaging of, 132, 132f
   muscles of, 130, 130f
Arteriae rectae, 98f
Arteries. See also specific artery
   brain, 225, 225f, 249, 249f
   foregut, 97, 97f
   hand, 129f
   hindgut, 98, 98f
   knee joint, 166, 166f
   midgut, 98, 98f
   neck, 200, 200f, 225, 225f
   oral region, 201, 201f
   pharyngeal region, 201, 201f
   thigh, 166, 166f
Arteriovenous shunt, 222
Articular cartilage, 150f, 164f
Articular facets, 197f-198f
Articular tubercle, 189f, 193f
Articularis genus muscle, 156f, 160f
Arytenoid cartilage, 205f

Arytenoid muscle, 203f, 218f
Ascending aorta, 38f-39f, 50f, 53f, 61f
Ascending colon, 87f-90f, 95f, 99f, 101f, 109f-110f, 113f
Ascending palatine artery, 201f
Ascending pharyngeal artery, 201f
Ascites, 85, 101, 101f
Asterion, 189f
Atelectasis, 75, 75f
Atherosclerotic calcifications, 73
Atlantoaxial joint, 198f
Atlantooccipital joint, 198f
Atlantooccipital membrane, 203f
Atlas (C1) vertebra
   anatomy of, 191, 191f, 197f-198f, 198, 209f, 218f-219f
   axial computed tomography of, 207, 207f
   trauma to, 199, 199f
Atria, 50, 50f. See also Left atrium; Right atrium
Atrial appendage, 50f
Atrioventricular branch, of right coronary artery, 51f
Atrioventricular nodal branch, of right coronary artery, 51f
Auditory tube, 209, 209f-210f, 215f, 218f, 227f
Auricle, 227f
Auricular artery, 201f, 225f
Auricular cartilage, 210f
Auriculotemporal nerve, 201f
Automatic intracardiac defibrillator, 66
Avascular necrosis, 152
Axial computed tomography
   C1 vertebra, 207, 207f
   C2 vertebra, 207, 207f
   cervical vertebrae, 202-204, 202f-204f
   epidural hematoma, 224f
   hydrocephalus, 233f
   male pelvis, 115, 115f
   neck, 202, 202f
   urinary bladder, 116f, 118, 118f
Axial magnetic resonance imaging
   knee joint, 165, 165f
   lateral ventricle, 254, 254f, 257, 257f, 259, 259f
   medulla, 246, 246f
   temporal lobe, 247, 247f
   thalamus, 252, 252f, 254, 254f, 259, 259f
Axillary artery
   digital subtraction angiography of, 129f
   fluoroscopic imaging of, 11f
   general images of, 37f-38f, 128f, 130f
Axillary fossa, 59f
Axillary lymph nodes, 37f
Axillary vein, 37f-38f
Axis (C2) vertebra, 191, 191f, 198, 198f, 203f, 207, 207f, 209f, 218f
   anatomy of, 191, 191f, 197f-198f, 198, 209f, 218f-219f, 242f
   axial computed tomography of, 207, 207f
   fracture of, 199f

Axis (C2) vertebra (Continued)
   odontoid process of, 242f
   trauma to, 199, 199f
Azygos vein, 37f, 41f, 49f, 60f-62f, 84f

B

Back. See also Spinal cord
   vertebrae. See Vertebrae
   vertebral column, 18, 18f
Bacterial pneumonia, 76
Basal ganglia, 242f
Basal nuclei, 253, 253f
Basilar artery, 219f, 225f-226f, 247f-250f, 249
Basilar venous plexus, 220f
Basilic vein, 131f, 139f
Biceps brachii muscle
   general images of, 122, 122f, 125f, 130, 130f
   magnetic resonance imaging of, 132f
Biceps brachii tendon, 127f, 130f, 134f, 137f
Biceps femoris muscle, 155f-159f, 159, 170f-171f
Biceps femoris tendon, 160f, 169f
Bicipital aponeurosis, 130f, 137f
Bile ducts, 96, 96f
Bladder. See Urinary bladder
Blood oxygen level–dependent contrast imaging. See BOLD imaging
"Blow-out" fractures, 188
Body. See specific body
BOLD imaging, 16, 16f
Bone(s). See also specific bone
   elbow, 133, 133f
   foot, 176-177, 176f-177f
   hand, 141, 141f
   thoracic wall, 68, 69f
   wrist, 141, 141f
Bone window, 5f, 30f, 216, 216f
Bowel. See Large intestine; Small intestine
Brachial artery, 11f, 128, 128f-129f, 131f, 137f
Brachial plexus, 38f, 40f-41f, 200f
Brachial vein, 131f
Brachialis muscle, 130f-131f, 134f, 136f
Brachiocephalic trunk, 39f, 47f, 59f, 225f
Brachiocephalic vein, 38f-41f, 43f, 47f, 59f
Brachioradialis muscle, 130f-131f, 136f-138f, 137, 140f
Brachioradialis tendon, 139f
Brain. See also Cerebellum; Cerebrum; Pons
   arteries of, 225, 225f, 249, 249f
   basal nuclei level of, 253, 253f
   coronal section of, 232f
   magnetic resonance imaging of, 231, 231f
   midsagittal section of, 230, 230f
   transverse section of, 253, 253f
   ventricles of, 232, 232f. See also Fourth ventricle; Lateral ventricle; Third ventricle

Brainstem
  fluid attenuation inversion recovery
    magnetic resonance imaging of,
    241, 241f
  general images of, 205f, 235, 235f
Breast implants, 67f
Breasts. *See also* Mammary glands
  contours of, 36f
  metastases to, 10f
Bregma, 192f
Bridging veins, 223f, 233f
Broad ligament, 109f
Bronchial arteries, 40f-41f
Bronchopulmonary lymph nodes, 40f
Bronchus
  inferior lobe, 37f
  intermediate, 37f
  main, 37f, 40f-41f, 43f, 46f, 49f, 61f
  upper lobe, 37f, 46f
Buccinator muscle, 196f, 201f, 206, 206f,
    208f, 212f, 217f
Buccopharyngeal fascia, 202f-203f
Bulbar conjunctiva, 213f
Bulbospongiosus muscle, 114f, 117f
Bulbourethral gland, 114f, 117f

C
C1 vertebra
  anatomy of, 191, 191f, 197f-198f, 198,
    209f, 218f-219f
  axial computed tomography of, 207,
    207f
  trauma to, 199, 199f
C2 vertebra
  anatomy of, 191, 191f, 197f-198f, 198,
    209f, 218f-219f, 242f
  axial computed tomography of, 207,
    207f
  fracture of, 199f
  odontoid process of, 242f
  trauma to, 199, 199f
Calcaneal tendon, 170f-171f
Calcaneal tuberosity, 170f, 177f
Calcaneus, 176f-180f
Calcar, 153f
Calcar avis, 255f-256f
Calcarine fissure, 237f
Calcarine sulcus, 230f, 255f
Calcific atherosclerosis, 101f
Calcified granuloma, 39f
Calvaria, 192, 192f, 223f
Capitate, 141f-144f, 143
Capitulum, 122f, 133f
Cardiac impression, 40f-41f
Cardiac notch
  of left lung, 35f
  of stomach, 92f
Cardiomyopathy, 73f
Carotid body, 225f
Carotid canal, 193f-194f
Carotid sheath, 202-203, 202f
Carpal bones, 141f, 143, 143f
Carpometacarpal joints, 141
Cartilage. *See specific cartilage*

Cauda equina
  anatomy of, 23, 23f, 25f, 88f
  magnetic resonance imaging of, 27f, 29f
Caudal midbrain, 248f
Caudate nucleus, 232f, 237f, 242f-244f,
    252-253, 252f-257f
Cavernous sinus, 221f-222f, 222, 225f,
    243f-244f, 244
Cecal junction, 110f
Cecum, 95f, 109f, 113f
Celiac arteriogram, 2f, 97, 97f
Celiac ganglia, 85f
Celiac trunk, 82, 82f, 86f-87f, 91f, 97, 97f
Central artery, 250f
Central canal, 232, 232f-234f
Central sulcus of Rolando, 230f, 257f-259f
Centrum semiovale, 258f
Cephalic vein, 38f, 131f-132f, 139f
Cerebellar hemisphere, 240f
Cerebellar notch, 236f
Cerebellar nuclei, 236f
Cerebellar peduncle, 234f-235f, 241f
Cerebellomedullary cistern, 233f
Cerebellum
  general images of, 224f, 234, 234f, 236,
    236f-239f, 246f-247f
  magnetic resonance imaging of
    axial, 247-248, 247f-248f, 251f
    fluid attenuation inversion recovery,
    240, 240f
Cerebral aqueduct of Sylvius, 230f-233f, 241f
Cerebral artery, 223f, 225, 225f-226f
Cerebral crus, 235f-236f
Cerebral fissure, 240f
Cerebral hemispheres, 223f, 230, 230f, 258,
    258f
Cerebral peduncle, 230f, 251f
Cerebral vein of Galen, 220, 220f-221f,
    230f, 233f-234f, 252, 254, 254f, 257,
    257f
Cerebral veins, 219f-220f, 220, 223, 223f
Cerebrospinal fluid (CSF), 26f-27f, 192,
    219f, 223-224, 231-233, 233f, 237f,
    239f-240f, 251, 257f
Cerebrum, 230, 230f
Cervical artery, 225f
Cervical nerves, 25f
Cervical parietal pleura, 35f, 40f-41f
Cervical sympathetic ganglion, 206f
Cervical vertebrae
  anatomy of, 18, 18f, 197, 197f, 202f
  axial computed tomography of,
    202-204, 202f-204f
  cross section of, 202, 202f
  trauma to, 199, 199f
Chest x-ray
  anteroposterior view, 64, 64f
  evaluation of, 63, 63f
  expiration view, 64, 64f
  inspiration view, 64, 64f, 73
  lateral, 42, 42f
  left lateral decubitus position, 64, 64f
  posteroanterior, 36, 36f
  upper abdomen in, 71, 71f

Chiasmatic cistern, 233f
Choana, 209f
Choledochal stone, 96f
Cholesteatoma, 229, 229f
Choroid plexus, 224f, 230f, 232, 232f,
    234f-235f, 240f, 253f-257f, 255
Ciliary body, 214f
Cingulate gyrus, 230f-231f, 237f, 242f, 244f
Cingulate sulcus, 230f
Circle of Willis, 248-250, 249f-250f
Circumflex branch, of left coronary artery,
    52f
Circumflex scapular artery, 128f
Claustrum, 243f, 253f
Clavicle, 19f, 35f-36f, 39f, 41f, 43f, 68,
    122f-124f, 126f, 200f, 205f
Clitoris, 107f, 117f
Clivus, 194f, 197f, 199f, 246f
Coccygeal nerve, 25f
Coccyx, 18, 18f, 25f, 78f, 104f, 115f-116f
Cochlea, 227f-228f, 228
Cochlear duct, 227f
Cochlear nerve, 229f
Cochlear window, 227f
Cold spots, 10
Colic artery, 91f, 97f-98f
Colic flexure, 83f, 89f, 92f
Collateral circulation, 167f
Collateral ligaments
  fibular, 161f-162f, 171f
  lateral, 160, 160f-161f, 165
  medial, 160, 160f-161f, 165, 165f
  radial, 134, 134f
  tibial, 160, 161f-162f, 169f
  ulnar, 134, 134f
Collateral trigone, 255f
Colles' fascia, 117f
Colles fracture, 142
Colon
  ascending, 87f-90f, 95f, 99f, 101f,
    109f-110f, 113f
  computed tomography of, 81f-82f, 86f,
    95f
  descending, 83f, 86f-87f, 90f, 95f, 99f,
    109f-110f, 113f
  diverticulum of, 95f
  general images of, 83f
  haustra of, 86, 95f
  sigmoid, 95f, 109f, 111f, 113f
  splenic flexure of, 85f
  transverse, 83f, 86f-88f, 91f, 95f, 101f
Colonography, computed tomography,
    95
Color Doppler ultrasound, 12f, 54f
Common bile duct, 83f, 86f-88f, 96,
    96f-97f
Common carotid artery
  general images of, 200f-203f, 201, 205f,
    207, 207f, 225f
  left, 38f, 47f, 59f, 226f
  right, 226f
Common extensor tendon, 138f
Common femoral artery, 115f
Common femoral vein, 115f

Common fibular nerve, 155f-156f, 159f-160f, 169-171, 170f-171f
Common hepatic artery, 83f, 85f, 97f
Common hepatic duct, 85f, 96f
Common iliac artery, 99f, 110f, 167f, 175f
Common iliac vein, 110f
Common interosseous artery, 128f-129f, 139f
Communicating artery, 225f
Communicating vein, 200f
Computed tomography
    abdomen
        bony framework, 78, 78f
        contrast studies, 79, 79f
    advantages of, 6, 6f
    airway studies, 46, 46f
    anterior axillary, 39, 39f
    atelectasis, 75f
    axial
        C1 vertebra, 207, 207f
        C2 vertebra, 207, 207f
        cervical vertebrae, 202-204, 202f-204f
        epidural hematoma, 224f
        hydrocephalus, 233f
        male pelvis, 115, 115f
        neck, 202, 202f
        urinary bladder, 116f, 118, 118f
    C2 fracture, 199f
    contrast-enhanced
        abdominal imaging studies with, 79, 79f, 81f
        advantages of, 6
        example of, 4f
    cross-sectional views
        L1-L2, 88, 88f
        L3-L4, 90, 90f
        T3, 59, 59f
        T7, 62, 62f
        T8, 49, 49f
        T10, 84, 84f
        T12, 85-86, 85f-86f
        T12-L1, 87, 87f
        T3-T4, 60, 60f
        T4-T5, 61, 61f
    cystogram, 119, 119f
    disadvantages of, 6, 6f
    ear, 228, 228f
    heart, 53, 53f
    hiatal hernia, 94, 94f
    Hounsfield scale, 5, 5f
    large intestine, 95, 95f
    laryngeal mass, 205f
    L1-L2 cross section, 88, 88f
    L3-L4 cross section, 90, 90f
    mathematical algorithms used with, 4
    multidetector, 4
    orbit, 214, 214f
    osteoporosis, 30, 30f
    overview of, 4, 4f
    paranasal sinuses, 212f
    pelvis, 104f-105f, 108, 108f, 111f
        female, 107, 107f
        male, 114-115, 114f-115f

Computed tomography (Continued)
    single-photon emission, 55-56
        description of, 10
        examinations using, 55f
        left ventricle, 55f
        long-axis views, 55-56
        principles of, 55-56
        radiotracer tracers used with, 55-56
        reversible defect, 55f
        short-axis views, 55-56
    T3-T4 cross section, 60, 60f
    T4-T5 cross section, 61, 61f
    T3 cross section, 59, 59f
    T7 cross section, 62, 62f
    T8 cross section, 49, 49f
    T10 cross section, 84, 84f
    T12 cross section, 85-86, 85f-86f
    thorax, 43
    T12-L1 cross section, 87, 87f
    upper gastrointestinal studies, 93, 93f
    uses of, 6
Computed tomography angiography (CTA)
    description of, 13-14, 13f
    inferior mesenteric artery, 99, 99f
    leg, 174, 174f
    superior mesenteric artery, 99, 99f
    upper extremity, 129
Computed tomography colonography, 95
Condylar canal, 194f
Confluence of sinuses, 220f-221f, 221, 248f
Conjunctiva, 213f
Conus arteriosus, 50f
Conus medullaris, 23, 23f, 25f, 88f
Coracoacromial ligament, 125f
Coracobrachialis muscle
    general images of, 122, 122f, 130, 130f-131f
    magnetic resonance imaging of, 132f
Coracoclavicular ligament, 125f
Coracohumeral ligament, 125f
Coracoid process, 36f, 122, 122f-125f, 130f
Cornea, 213f-214f, 247f
Corona radiata, 257
Coronal suture, 186f, 189, 189f-191f, 195f
Coronary artery
    general images of, 50f
    left, 47f, 52, 52f-53f
    right, 47f, 51, 51f, 53f
Coronary sinus, 37f-38f, 49f, 62f
Coronary sulcus, 47f
Coronoid fossa, 122f
Coronoid process
    of elbow, 133f, 135f-136f
    of mandible, 189f, 191f, 196f, 210f
Corpus callosum, 230, 230f-233f, 237f, 242f-244f, 253f-257f
Corpus cavernosum, 114f, 118f
Corpus luteum, 112f
Corpus spongiosum, 114f, 117f-118f
Corpus striatum, 253
Cortical veins, 221f
Costal cartilage, 35f, 59f, 61f, 68f, 84f-85f

Costal facets, 197f
Costal pleura, 40f
Costocervical trunk, 225f
Costodiaphragmatic recess of pleural cavity, 35f-38f, 40f-41f, 84f-85f, 89f
Costomediastinal recess of pleural cavity, 35f
Cowper's gland, 114f, 117f
Cranial base
    inferior view of, 193, 193f
    superior view of, 194, 194f
Cranial fossa, 194f
Cribriform plate, 190f, 194, 194f, 209f, 245
Cricoid cartilage, 58f, 203f, 205f, 218f
Crista galli, 187f-188f, 190f, 194f
Cruciate ligaments, 160, 160f-162f, 162, 164-165, 164f-165f
Cuboid, 176f-178f, 180f-181f
Cuneate funiculus, 234f-235f
Cuneate tubercle, 234f-235f
Cuneiform bones, 176f-177f, 181f
Cuneus, 230f, 239f
Cystic artery, 97f
Cystic duct, 85f, 96f
Cystogram, 119, 119f

D
De Quervain's syndrome, 145
Decussation of pyramids, 234f-236f
Deep cervical artery, 225f
Deep cervical fascia, 203f
Deep cervical muscles, 202f-203f
Deep external pudendal artery, 166f
Deep femoral artery, 166, 166f
Deep fibular nerve, 172f
Deep inguinal ring, 113f
Deep palmar arch, 129, 129f
Deltoid muscle, 38f, 125f, 130f-131f
Deltoid tuberosity, 122f
Dens, 197f
Dens of axis, 191f, 197f-198f, 207f-209f, 218f-219f
Dentate gyrus, 255f-256f, 256
Dentate nucleus, 234f
Denticulate ligament, 22f-23f
Descending aorta, 37f, 40f, 46f, 49f, 61f-62f, 88f
Descending colon, 83f, 86f-87f, 90f, 95f, 99f-110f, 113f
Diaphragm
    anatomy of, 82, 82f
    aortic opening of, 82f
    central tendon of, 58f, 91f
    crus of, 58f, 84f, 86f-89f
    dome of, 35f
    general images of, 38f, 69, 69f, 92f
    openings of, 58f, 82f
Diencephalon, 255f
Digastric muscle, 196f, 200f, 204, 204f, 217f
Digastric tendon, 206f
Digital imaging and communications in medicine, 15

Digital subtraction angiography
celiac trunk, 97f
description of, 14, 14f
lower extremity, 175, 175f
neck, 226, 226f
upper extremity, 129
Diploë, 239f
Dislocation of humeral head, 68f
Distal medial striate artery, 249f
Distal radioulnar joint, 143f-145f, 145
Diverticulitis, 95
Diverticulum, 95f, 111f
Dorsal digital nerves, 169f
Dorsal median sulcus, 234f
Dorsal root ganglion, 22f
Dorsum sellae, 194f, 248f
Ductus deferens, 113f
Duodenojejunal flexure, 83f, 93f
Duodenum, 83f, 86f, 88f-89f, 91f-92f, 96f
Dura mater, 22, 22f-23f, 223f, 233f, 238
Dural venous sinuses, 220-222, 220f-222f

E

Ear
computed tomography of, 228, 228f
external, 227, 227f
inner, 227, 227f
middle, 227, 227f
pathology of, 229, 229f
Echocardiography, 54, 54f, 57, 57f
Edema
interstitial, 76f
magnetic resonance imaging of, 8f
Eighth rib, 49f
Ejaculatory ducts, 116f
Elbow
bones of, 133, 133f
description of, 133
joints of, 134, 134f
x-rays of, 135, 135f
Emissary vein, 223f
Endolymphatic duct, 228f
Endometrial cavity, 111f-112f
Endoscopic retrograde
cholangiopancreatography, 96, 96f
Epicondylitis, 136
Epidural fat, 26f
Epidural hematoma, 6f, 224, 224f
Epidural space, 23
Epiglottis, 197f, 203f-204f, 218f-219f
Epiphyseal plate, 152f
Epitympanic recess, 227f-229f, 228
Erector spinae muscle, 84f, 90f
Esophageal plexus, 41f, 49f
Esophagogastric junction, 38f, 84f
Esophagus
abdominal portion of, 92f
anatomy of, 37, 37f-38f, 40f-41f, 72f, 82, 218f-219f
dilation of, 72f
fluoroscopic imaging of, 11f
general images of, 49f, 82f, 91f, 202f
Ethmoid sinuses, 187

Ethmoidal air cells, 187f-188f, 190f, 209, 209f, 211, 211f-212f, 214f, 217f
Ethmoidal bone, 186, 186f, 188f-190f, 194, 194f-195f
Ethmoidal bulla, 209f
Ethmoidal foramen, 188f
Expiration view, 64, 64f
Extensor carpi radialis brevis muscle, 138f, 145f
Extensor carpi radialis brevis tendon, 138f
Extensor carpi radialis longus muscle, 131f, 138f, 145f
Extensor carpi radialis longus tendon, 138f
Extensor carpi ulnaris muscle, 138f-140f, 145f
Extensor carpi ulnaris tendon, 138f-139f
Extensor digiti minimi muscle, 138f, 145f
Extensor digiti minimi tendon, 138f
Extensor digitorum longus muscle, 160f, 169f, 173f, 179
Extensor digitorum longus tendon, 171f
Extensor digitorum muscle, 138f, 145f
Extensor digitorum tendons, 138f, 169f
Extensor hallucis longus muscle, 169f, 171f, 173f
Extensor hallucis longus tendon, 169f, 171f
Extensor indicis tendon, 138f
Extensor pollicis brevis muscle, 138f
Extensor pollicis longus muscle, 138f, 145f
Extensor retinaculum, 138f
External acoustic meatus, 189f, 193f-195f, 227, 227f-228f
External capsule, 252f-254f, 257f
External carotid artery, 200f, 204f, 206, 206f-208f, 225, 225f-226f
External ear, 227, 227f
External iliac artery, 99f, 111f, 167f, 175f
External iliac vein, 111f
External jugular vein, 38f, 200f
External medullary lamina, 255
External oblique aponeurosis, 90f
External oblique muscle, 87f, 90f
External occipital protuberance, 189f-191f, 193f
External pudendal artery, 166f
Extraocular muscles, 213, 213f
Eye, 247, 247f
Eyeball, 211f-212f, 214f
Eyelid, 213f

F

Facets
articular, 197f-198f
costal, 197f
thoracic vertebrae, 19, 19f
Facial artery, 200f-201f, 206f, 225f
Facial colliculus, 234f
Facial mass, 215, 215f
Facial nerve, 206, 206f, 221f, 227-228, 227f, 229f, 235f
Facial vein, 200f, 206f
Falciform ligament, 85f, 92f
Fallopian tube, 107f, 109f
False pelvis, 104f

Falx cerebri, 217f, 220, 220f-221f, 223f-224f, 240f, 242f, 244f-245f, 254, 258f-259f
Fascia lata, 154f, 156f
Female pelvis
computed tomography of, 107, 107f-108f
contents of, 109, 109f
lower, 111, 111f
magnetic resonance imaging of, 108f
male pelvis versus, 113
midsagittal section of, 107, 107f
upper, 110, 110f
x-rays of, 106, 106f
Femoral artery, 115f-116f, 154, 156f-157f, 166, 166f, 175f
Femoral nerve, 116f, 154, 154f, 156f
Femoral vein, 115f-116f, 154f, 156f-157f
Femur
anatomy of, 153, 153f
condyles of, 163f
diaphysis of, 151f
greater trochanter of, 78f, 106f, 115f, 150f-151f, 153, 153f, 155f
head of, 105f-106f, 111f, 115f-116f, 150, 150f-152f, 153
lateral epicondyle of, 153f, 160f
lesser trochanter of, 78f, 106f, 150f-151f, 153, 153f
magnetic resonance imaging of, 165f
medial epicondyle of, 153f, 160f
neck of, 116f, 150f-152f, 153
physiology of, 153
shaft of, 153
Fibrous pericardium, 40f-41f
Fibula, 160f, 162f-163f, 168, 168f, 171f, 178f, 181f
Fibular artery, 166, 166f, 170f, 172f-174f
Fibular collateral ligament, 161f-162f, 171f
Fibular nerve, 169f, 172f
Fibular notch, 168f
Fibular vein, 172f-173f
Fibularis brevis muscle, 169f, 171, 171f, 173f
Fibularis brevis tendon, 170f-171f
Fibularis longus muscle, 160f, 171, 171f, 173f
Fibularis longus tendon, 170f-171f
Fibularis tertius muscle, 171
Fibularis tertius tendon, 171f
Fifth metacarpal, 138f
Fifth metatarsal, 171f, 176f
First rib, 35f-36f, 40f-41f
Flexor carpi radialis muscle, 130f, 136f-137f, 139f
Flexor carpi radialis tendon, 145f
Flexor carpi ulnaris muscle, 137f-140f
Flexor carpi ulnaris tendon, 139f, 145f
Flexor digitorum brevis muscle, 179f
Flexor digitorum longus muscle, 173f
Flexor digitorum longus tendon, 170f
Flexor digitorum profundus tendon, 145f
Flexor digitorum superficialis muscle, 136f-137f, 145f

Flexor digitorum superficialis tendon, 145f
Flexor hallucis longus muscle, 173f, 177f
Flexor hallucis longus tendon, 170f
Flexor pollicis longus tendon, 145f
Flexor retinaculum, 145f
"Floating" ribs, 68
Flocculonodular lobe, 236f
Fluid attenuation inversion recovery
    (FLAIR) magnetic resonance imaging
    brainstem, 241, 241f
    cerebellum, 240, 240f
    description of, 9, 9f
    frontal lobe, 245, 245f
    optic chiasm, 243, 243f
    pons, 242, 242f
    temporal lobes, 244, 244f
    third ventricle, 242, 242f
Fluoroscopy, 11
    equipment used in, 11f
    hiatal hernia, 94f
    principles of, 11
Foley catheter, 119, 119f
Fontanelles, 195, 195f
Foot. *See also* Ankle
    bones of, 176-177, 176f-177f
    x-rays of, 181, 181f
Foramen cecum, 194f, 203f, 218f
Foramen lacerum, 193f-194f
Foramen magnum, 190f, 193f-194f, 197f,
    199f, 230
Foramen of Luschka, 232, 232f-233f
Foramen of Magendie, 232, 232f-234f
Foramen of Monro, 230f, 232, 232f-234f,
    254, 254f-255f
Foramen of Winslow, 85f, 92f
Foramen ovale, 193f-194f, 194
Foramen rotundum, 194, 194f
Foramen spinosum, 193f-194f, 194
Foramen transversarium, 197f, 207f
Forearm. *See also* Radius; Ulna
    cross section of, 139, 139f
    extensor compartment of, 138, 138f
    flexor compartment of, 137, 137f
    magnetic resonance imaging of, 140,
        140f
    middle, 140f
    muscles of, 137-138, 137f-138f
    proximal, 140f
Fornix, 230, 230f-232f, 234f, 252f, 255f-
    256f, 256
Fossa. *See specific fossa*
Fossa ovalis, 38f
Fourth ventricle, 224f, 230f-237f, 232, 234,
    240f, 247f
Fovea capitis, 152, 152f
Frontal bone, 186, 186f, 190f, 192f,
    194f-195f, 244f, 258f
Frontal crest, 194f
Frontal gyrus, 230f, 244f-245f
Frontal lobe, 245, 245f
Frontal process, 186f, 189f
Frontal sinus, 187f-188f, 190, 190f-191f,
    203f, 209f, 211, 211f-212f, 217f-218f,
    252f, 254f, 257f

Frontal suture, 195f
Frontobasal artery, 249f

G
Galea aponeurotica, 223f
Gallbladder
    anatomy of, 96, 96f
    body of, 96f
    computed tomography of, 81f
    fundus of, 96f
    general images of, 35f, 85f-86f, 92f
    magnetic resonance imaging of, 86f
Gallstones, 96, 96f, 101f
Gastric antrum, 85f, 93f, 101f
Gastric artery, 83f, 85f, 97f
Gastric folds, 84f
Gastric fundus, 84f, 93f-94f, 99f
Gastric vein, 85f
Gastrocnemius muscle, 155f, 160f, 164f,
    169f-171f, 170, 173f
Gastroduodenal artery, 87f, 97f
Gastroepiploic artery, 97f
Gastroesophageal junction, 82f, 94f, 99f
Gastro-omental artery, 97f
Gastrosplenic ligament, 85f
Genial tubercle, 196f
Genicular artery, 166, 166f
Geniculate body, 234f-235f, 253f, 255f
Genioglossus muscle, 203f, 206, 206f-207f,
    217f-218f
Geniohyoid muscle, 203f, 217f-218f
Gerdy's tubercle, 162f
Gerota's fascia, 89f
Glabella, 186f, 189f, 191f
Gland. *See specific gland*
Glans penis, 114f
Glenohumeral ligament, 125f-126f
Glenoid cavity of scapula, 122f, 125f
Glenoid fossa, 123f-124f, 126f-127f
Glenoid labrum, 125f
Globus pallidus, 253f
Glossopharyngeal nerve, 201f, 221f, 235f
Gluteal aponeurosis, 155f
Gluteal lines, 149f
Gluteal tuberosity, 153f
Gluteus maximus muscle, 110f, 155, 155f,
    157, 157f
Gluteus medius muscle, 110f, 154f-155f,
    155
Gluteus minimus muscle, 154f-155f, 155
Gouty arthritis, 181
Gracile fasciculus, 235f
Gracile tubercle, 234f-235f
Gracilis muscle, 154f-156f, 158f-159f, 170f
Gracilis tendon, 160f
Gradient recalled magnetic resonance
    imaging, 9, 9f
Granular foveola, 192f, 223f
Gray matter, 8f, 240f
Gray rami communicantes, 22f-23f
Great auricular nerve, 200f
Great cerebral vein of Galen, 220, 220f-
    221f, 230f, 233f-234f, 252, 254, 254f,
    257, 257f

Great saphenous nerve, 172f
Great saphenous vein, 156f, 158, 158f,
    172f
Greater curvature of stomach, 92f
Greater omentum, 88f, 90f, 92f
Greater palatine foramen, 193f
Greater petrosal nerve, 194f
Greater sciatic foramen, 104f-105f
Greater sciatic notch, 78f, 149f
Greater thoracic splanchnic nerve,
    40f-41f
Greater trochanter of the femur, 78f, 106f,
    150f-151f, 153, 153f, 155f
Greater tubercle, 123f, 125f
Greater wing of sphenoidal bone, 186f-
    190f, 188, 193f-195f
Gyrus rectus, 245f, 248f, 251f

H
Habenula, 253f
Habenular commissure, 230f, 234f, 255f
Habenular trigone, 234f, 255f
Halo device, 66f
Hamate, 141f-144f
Hamstring muscles, 154f-155f, 155, 158,
    158f
Hamulus, 193f
Hand. *See also* Wrist
    anteroposterior x-ray of, 142, 142f
    arteries of, 129f
    bones of, 141, 141f
Hangman's fracture, 199, 199f
Hard palate, 203f, 217f, 219f
Hartmann's pouch, 96f
Haustra, 95f
Head
    of femur, 105f-106f, 111f, 115f-116f,
        150, 150f-152f, 153
    of humerus, 122f-124f, 126f-127f
    of pancreas, 83, 83f, 87, 99f, 101f
    of radius, 133, 133f, 135f-136f
Head vascular imaging studies, 226, 226f
Heart
    anterior view of, 47, 47f
    apex of, 47f, 62f
    atria of, 50, 50f. *See also* Left atrium;
        Right atrium
    base of, 47f
    border of, 35f
    cardiomyopathy of, 73f
    chambers of, 48, 48f, 54f. *See also* Left
        atrium; Left ventricle; Right
        atrium; Right ventricle
    computed tomography of, 6f, 30f, 53,
        53f, 73
    coronal magnetic resonance imaging of,
        47f
    echocardiography of, 54, 54f, 57, 57f
    enlargement of, 73f
    interventricular septum of, 43f, 49f-50f,
        50
    lateral x-ray of, 48, 48f
    magnetic resonance imaging of, 47f, 53,
        53f

Heart (*Continued*)
  margins of, 48, 48f
  posterior view of, 47, 47f
  posteroanterior x-ray of, 48, 48f
  ventricles of, 50, 50f. *See also* Left
    ventricle; Right ventricle
Heart valve replacements, 73f
Helicotrema, 227f
Hemiazygos vein, 49f, 61f
Hemidiaphragm, 36f, 42f, 71, 71f
Hepatic artery, 83f, 97f
Hepatic duct, 96f
Hepatic flexure, 89f, 93f
Hepatic vein, 84f-85f
Hepatoduodenal ligament, 86f, 92f
Hepatogastric ligament, 92f
Hepatopancreatic ampulla, 96f
Hernia, 94, 94f
Herniated disk, 28-29, 28f-29f
Hiatal hernia, 94, 94f
Hill-Sachs deformity, 123
Hip adductors, 152f, 153
Hip bone
  anatomy of, 149, 149f
  fracture of, 152
Hip joint
  anatomy of, 150, 150f
  imaging studies of, 152, 152f
  magnetic resonance imaging of, 152,
    152f
  osteoarthritis of, 151
  subchondral cysts of, 151
  x-ray of, 151, 151f
Hip pain, 151
Hippocampal sulcus, 256f
Hippocampus, 232f, 240f, 242f, 251f, 253f,
  256, 256f
Hook of hamate, 141f-143f, 143, 145f
Hospital information systems, 15
Hot spots, 10
Hounsfield scale, 5, 5f
Humerus
  anatomy of, 122, 122f
  diaphysis of, 123f-124f
  dislocation of, 68f
  general images of, 42f, 131f, 134f-135f
  head of, 122f-124f, 126f-127f
  surgical neck of, 122f-123f
Hydatid of Morgagni, 112f
Hydrocephalus, 233, 233f
Hyoepiglottic ligament, 203f
Hyoglossus muscle, 206f
Hyoid bone, 197f, 199f-200f, 200, 203f-
  204f, 204, 206f, 218f-219f
Hypoglossal canal, 193f-194f
Hypoglossal nerve, 201f, 206f, 235f
Hypoglossal trigone, 234f
Hypophyseal arteries, 250, 250f
Hypophyseal fossa, 194f
Hypophysis, 209f, 212f, 221f-222f, 230f
Hypothalamic artery, 250f
Hypothalamic sulcus, 230f, 234f
Hypothalamus, 242f
Hysterosalpingogram, 112, 112f

I
Ileal artery, 98f
Ileocecal valve, 110f
Ileocolic artery, 98f
Ileum, 88f, 90f
Iliac artery, 99f
Iliac bone, 110f
Iliac crest, 24f, 78f, 89f, 104f-105f, 149f,
  155f
Iliac fossa, 104f-105f
Iliacus muscle, 110f
Iliofemoral ligament, 150, 150f
Iliolumbar ligament, 24f
Iliopectineal bursa, 150f
Iliopsoas muscle, 111f, 153, 154f, 156f
Iliopubic eminence, 78f, 105f, 149f-150f
Iliotibial band, 157f-158f
Iliotibial band syndrome, 165
Iliotibial tract, 155f-156f, 159f-161f, 165f,
  169f-171f
Ilium
  general images of, 106f, 110f
  wing of, 78f, 104f, 149f
Incisive canal, 203f, 209f, 218f
Incisive fossa, 193f
Incus, 227f-228f
Inferior alveolar artery, 201f, 206f
Inferior alveolar vein, 206f
Inferior angle of scapula, 62f
Inferior articular facet, 198f
Inferior articular process, 19f-21f, 24f
Inferior cerebellar peduncle, 235f
Inferior colliculus, 230f, 234f-235f, 251f,
  255f
Inferior fovea, 234f
Inferior gemellus muscle, 155f
Inferior hypophyseal artery, 250f
Inferior labial artery, 201f
Inferior labrum, 126f
Inferior medullary velum, 230f, 234f, 236f
Inferior mesenteric artery
  anatomy of, 98, 98f
  angiogram of, 99, 99f
Inferior nasal concha, 186f-188f, 190f,
  209f-211f, 217f, 245f
Inferior nasal meatus, 209f, 217f
Inferior oblique muscle, 213f
Inferior orbital fissure, 188f-189f
Inferior petrosal sinus, 190f, 194f, 220f
Inferior phrenic artery, 97f
Inferior pubic ramus, 105f, 117f, 149f-151f
Inferior rectal artery, 98f
Inferior rectus muscle, 213f, 245f
Inferior sagittal sinus, 220, 220f, 240f
Inferior subtendinous bursa, 160f
Inferior thyroid artery, 201f, 225f
Inferior thyroid vein, 200f
Inferior ulnar collateral artery, 128f, 130f
Inferior vena cava
  computed tomography of, 39f, 82f, 93f,
    101f
  general images of, 38f, 41f, 82f-90f, 109f,
    113f
  posteroanterior x-ray of, 36f

Inferior vertebral notch, 20f
Infraglenoid tubercle, 122, 122f
Infrahyoid fossa, 202f
Infraorbital artery, 201f
Infraorbital foramen, 186f, 188f-189f
Infraorbital groove, 188f
Infraorbital nerve, 213f
Infrapatellar bursa, 164f
Infrapatellar fat pads, 160f-161f, 164f
Infrapatellar synovial fold, 160f-161f
Infraspinatus fossa, 122, 122f
Infraspinatus muscle, 125f
Infratemporal fossa, 189f
Infundibular recess, 232f
Infundibulum, 235f, 250, 250f
Inguinal ligament, 154f
Inguinal ring, 113f
Inner ear, 227, 227f
Inspiration view, 64, 64f, 73
Insula, 238f, 241f
Interatrial septum, 62f
Intercavernous sinus, 220f
Intercondylar eminence, 163f
Intercondylar fossa, 153f
Intercondylar tubercle, 168f
Intercostal muscles, 37f-38f
Intercostal nerve, 40f
Intercostal vein, 40f-41f
Interior acoustic meatus, 194f
Intermediate bronchus, 37f
Intermediate nerve, 221f, 235f
Intermetacarpal joints, 143f
Intermuscular septum, 130f, 154f, 156f,
  173f
Internal acoustic artery, 249f
Internal acoustic meatus, 198f, 227f-229f,
  247f
Internal capsule, 232f, 242f-244f, 252f-
  254f, 253
Internal carotid artery, 194f, 201f, 204f,
  206f-208f, 214f, 221f-222f, 222, 225,
  225f, 228f, 239f, 243f-244f, 244,
  246f-249f, 251f
Internal cerebral vein, 219f-220f, 220, 252f
Internal iliac artery, 98f-99f
Internal jugular vein, 38f, 200f, 202f-206f,
  203, 208f, 210f, 221f, 227f, 246f
Internal medullary lamina, 255
Internal oblique muscle, 90f
Internal obturator muscle, 115f
Internal occipital protuberance, 194f, 248f
Internal pudendal artery, 116f
Internal pudendal vein, 116f
Internal thoracic artery, 40f-41f, 60f-61f
Internal thoracic vein, 60f-61f
Internal urethral sphincter, 117f
Interosseous border, 168f
Interosseous ligament, 139f
Interosseous membrane, 139, 139f-140f,
  145f, 166f, 173f
Interosseous nerve, 139f
Interpeduncular cistern, 233f
Interspinous ligament, 24, 24f
Interstitial edema, 76f

Interthalamic adhesion, 230f, 232f, 234f, 253f, 255, 255f
Intertrochanteric crest, 150f, 153f
Intertrochanteric line, 150f, 153f
Intertubercular sulcus, 122f
Intertubercular tendon, 125f
Interventricular branch
    of left coronary artery, 52f
    of right coronary artery, 51f
Interventricular foramen, 230f, 232, 232f-234f, 255f
Interventricular septum, 43f, 49f-50f, 50, 62f
Interventricular sulcus, 47f, 62f
Intervertebral disk
    anatomy of, 19f, 21f, 26f-27f
    herniation of, 28-29, 28f-29f
    T12-L1, 87f
    T3-T4, 60f
Intervertebral foramen, 19f-21f, 24f, 26f, 42f, 197f
Intestine. See Large intestine; Small intestine
Ischial spine, 104, 104f-105f, 149f-150f
Ischial tuberosity, 78f, 104, 104f-105f, 149f-151f, 155f
Ischioanal fossa, 116f-117f
Ischiocavernous muscle, 117f
Ischiofemoral ligament, 150, 150f
Ischium, 106f, 115f, 149f, 151f

J

Jaw. See Mandible
Jejunal artery, 98f
Jejunum
    computed tomography of, 82f, 85f
    general images of, 83f, 86f-88f, 90f
Joint. See specific joint
Jones fracture, 181
Jugular bulb, 198f, 221f, 227, 227f, 229, 229f
Jugular foramen, 190f, 194f, 221f
Jugular fossa, 193f
Jugular notch, 35f, 68f
Jugular vein, 200f

K

Kerley B lines, 73f, 76f
Kidneys
    anatomy of, 89, 89f
    computed tomography of, 37f, 43f, 46f, 82f, 89f, 93f, 101f
    general images of, 83f, 86f-88f, 92f
    ptotic, 89
Knee/knee joint, 160
    anatomy of, 160-161, 161f
    arteries of, 166, 166f
    axial magnetic resonance imaging of, 165, 165f
    coronal magnetic resonance imaging of, 165, 165f
    effusion of, 163
    interior of, 161, 161f
    ligaments of, 161f-162f, 162, 164, 164f

Knee/knee joint (Continued)
    magnetic resonance imaging of, 164-165, 164f-165f
    osteoarthritis of, 163
    sagittal section of, 164, 164f
    x-ray of, 163, 163f
Kyphosis, 18

L

Labial artery, 201f
Labium majus, 107f
Labium minus, 107f
Labyrinthine artery, 249f-250f
Lacrimal bone, 186f, 188f-189f, 195f
Lacrimal gland, 213, 213f
Lacrimal sac fossa, 188f
Lambda, 187f, 189, 189f, 191f-192f
Lambdoid suture, 187f, 189, 189f, 191f-192f, 195f
Lamina terminalis, 230f, 234f
Large intestine. See also Colon; Rectum
    computed tomography of, 95, 95f
    imaging studies of, 95, 95f
    posteroanterior x-ray of, 36f
Laryngeal artery, 201f, 225f
Laryngeal inlet, 203f
Laryngopharynx, 203f-204f, 218f
Larynx
    anatomy of, 203, 203f
    mass in, 205f
    tumor of, 205, 205f
Lateral antebrachial cutaneous nerve, 131f
Lateral circumflex femoral artery, 154f, 166f
Lateral collateral ligament, 160, 160f-161f, 165
Lateral condyle, 122f, 153f
Lateral cuneiform, 181f
Lateral epicondyle
    of femur, 153f, 160f
    of humerus, 122f, 133, 133f-136f
Lateral epicondylitis, 136
Lateral femoral cutaneous nerve, 154f, 156f
Lateral funiculus, 234f
Lateral genicular artery, 166, 166f
Lateral geniculate body, 235f, 253f, 255f
Lateral horn, 22f
Lateral malleolus, 168, 168f-171f, 178f-179f
Lateral meniscus, 160f, 162f, 164f
Lateral palpebrae superioris muscle, 213f
Lateral palpebral ligament, 213f
Lateral patellar retinaculum, 160f
Lateral plantar artery, 174f
Lateral pterygoid muscle, 196f, 210f, 215f, 246f
Lateral pterygoid plate, 210f
Lateral rectus muscle, 213f-214f, 245f, 247f
Lateral supracondylar line, 153f
Lateral supracondylar ridge, 122f, 133f
Lateral sural cutaneous nerve, 170f
Lateral thoracic artery, 128f

Lateral ventricle
    axial magnetic resonance imaging of, 254, 254f, 257, 257f, 259, 259f
    general images of, 224f, 231f, 237f-238f, 240f-242f, 244f, 253f, 256f
Lateral x-ray
    cervical vertebrae, 197, 197f
    evaluation of, 63, 63f
    heart, 48, 48f
    lungs, 45, 45f
    normal, 63f
    thorax, 42, 42f
Latissimus dorsi muscle, 84f, 130f
Latissimus dorsi tendon, 130f-131f
Left atrium
    computed tomography of, 37f, 39f, 43f, 46f
    echocardiography of, 54f
    general images of, 62f
    lateral x-ray of, 48, 48f
    magnetic resonance imaging of, 43f, 53f
    posteroanterior x-ray of, 48, 48f
Left auricle, 37f, 47f, 53f
Left coronary artery, 47f, 52, 52f-53f
Left lung, 35f, 40, 40f, 43f-45f, 44, 60f, 93f
Left ventricle, 38f
    computed tomography of, 39f, 43f, 46f
    echocardiography of, 54f
    general images of, 47f, 49f, 62f
    lateral x-ray of, 48, 48f
    magnetic resonance imaging of, 39f, 49f, 53f
    posteroanterior x-ray of, 36f, 48, 48f
    single-photon emission computed tomography of, 55f
Leg. See also Ankle; Femur; Fibula; Foot; Thigh; Tibia
    computed tomography angiography of, 174, 174f
    cross section of, 172, 172f
    fascial compartments of, 172, 172f
    magnetic resonance angiography of, 174, 174f
    muscles of, 169-171, 169f-171f
Lens, 213f-214f, 238f, 247f
Lenticulostriate arteries, 249f-250f
Lentiform nucleus, 253, 253f
Lesser curvature of stomach, 92f
Lesser omentum, 83f, 85f, 91f-92f
Lesser palatine foramen, 193f
Lesser petrosal nerve, 194f
Lesser saphenous vein, 172f
Lesser sciatic foramen, 104f-105f
Lesser sciatic notch, 78f, 149f
Lesser trochanter of the femur, 78f, 106f, 150f-151f, 153, 153f
Lesser wing of sphenoidal bone, 186f-188f, 188, 190f, 194, 194f
Levator ani muscle, 116f-117f
Levator palpebrae superioris, 214f, 245f
Levator scapulae muscle, 202f-203f, 207f
Levator veli palatini muscle, 210f
Ligament. See specific ligament
Ligament of ovary, 107f, 109f, 112f

Ligamentum flavum, 24, 24f
Linea alba, 85f, 90f, 109f, 113f
Linea aspera, 153f, 158f
Lingual artery, 201f, 206f, 225f
Lingual nerve, 206f
Lingual tonsil, 203f, 218f-219f
Lingula, 40f, 196f
Lisfranc joint, 181f
Liver
    computed tomography of, 37f, 39f, 46f,
        81f-82f, 89f, 91f, 99f, 101f
    general images of, 35f, 38f, 85f, 91f
    lobes of, 92f
    magnetic resonance imaging of, 39f, 86f
    metastases of, 6f, 81f
Local area network, 15
Locus caeruleus, 234f
Longitudinal cerebral fissure, 258f
Longus capitis muscle, 207f, 210f
Longus colli muscle, 202f
Lordosis, 18, 199f
Lower extremity. *See also* Leg; Pelvis;
        Thigh
    digital subtraction angiography of, 175,
        175f
    vascular studies of, 174, 174f
Lumbar disk herniation, 28-29, 28f-29f
Lumbar nerves, 25f
Lumbar spine
    L1-L2 cross section, 88, 88f
    L3-L4 cross section, 90, 90f
    T12-L1 cross section, 87, 87f
Lumbar vertebrae
    anatomy of, 18, 18f, 20-21, 20f-21f,
        23f-24f
    spondylolisthesis of, 32, 32f
Lumbosacral region
    ligaments of, 24, 24f
    T2-weighted magnetic resonance
        imaging of, 27f
Lunate, 141f-144f, 143
Lung
    alveolar opacities in, 76, 76f
    anatomy of, 44, 44f
    apex of, 35f
    atelectasis of, 75, 75f
    bronchus. *See* Bronchus
    collapsed, 69f
    fissure of, 60f-61f
    general images of, 23f, 38f
    interstitial opacities in, 76, 76f
    lateral x-ray of, 45, 45f
    left, 35f, 40, 40f, 43f-45f, 44, 60f, 93f
    lobes of, 45, 45f
    oblique fissure of, 60f-61f
    opacities in, 76, 76f
    pneumonia of, 76f
    posteroanterior x-ray of, 45, 45f
    right, 41, 41f, 44, 44f-45f, 60f, 93f, 96f
    silhouette sign, 3, 3f, 74, 74f
Lung mass, 72f
Lung window, 5f, 61f
Lunotriquetral ligament, 144
Lymphadenopathy, 81f

M

Magnetic resonance angiography
    description of, 13-14, 13f-14f, 129
    leg, 174, 174f
    with maximum intensity projection,
        167, 167f
    technique for, 167
    thigh, 167, 167f
Magnetic resonance
        cholangiopancreatography, 96
Magnetic resonance imaging
    abdomen, 80, 80f
    advantages of, 8, 8f
    ankle, 179-180, 179f-180f
    anterior axillary, 39, 39f
    arm, 132, 132f
    brain, 231, 231f
    cardiac indications for, 57f
    cavernous sinus, 222f
    cerebellum, 240, 240f, 247-248,
        247f-248f
    cerebral hemispheres, 258, 258f
    cholesteatoma, 229f
    concept map of, 7f
    disadvantages of, 8, 8f
    distal radioulnar joint, 145f
    fluid attenuation inversion recovery, 9,
        9f
        brainstem, 241, 241f
        cerebellum, 240, 240f
        frontal lobe, 245, 245f
        optic chiasm, 243, 243f
        pons, 242, 242f
        temporal lobes, 244, 244f
        third ventricle, 242, 242f
    forearm, 140, 140f
    gradient recalled, 9, 9f
    heart, 47f, 53, 53f
    herniated disk, 29, 29f
    hip joint, 152, 152f
    knee joint, 164, 164f
    lateral ventricle, 254, 254f, 257, 257f,
        259, 259f
    medulla, 246, 246f
    metastases, 31, 31f
    neck, 219, 219f
    optic chiasm, 243, 243f, 251, 251f
    orbit, 214, 214f
    overview of, 7, 7f
    paranasal sinuses, 212f
    pelvis, 108f
        female, 111f
        male, 115, 115f
    prostate gland, 115f
    proton density, 9f
    pulse sequences, 9, 9f
    shoulder, 123
    spondylolisthesis, 32, 32f
    STIR, 31, 31f
    T8, 49, 49f
    temporal lobe, 237-239, 237f-239f
    thalamus, 252, 252f, 254, 254f, 259, 259f
    thigh, 157-159, 157f-159f
    third ventricle, 242, 242f, 252, 252f

Magnetic resonance imaging (*Continued*)
    thoracic spine metastases, 31, 31f
    thorax, 43
    T1-weighted
        abdominal studies, 80f
        ankle, 179-180, 179f-180f
        brain, 231, 231f
        cerebral hemispheres, 258, 258f
        description of, 9
        distal radioulnar joint, 145f
        forearm, 140, 140f
        head, 219, 219f
        herniated disk, 29f
        hip joint, 152f
        illustration of, 7f, 9f
        lateral ventricle, 257, 257f, 259, 259f
        medulla, 246, 246f
        neck, 219, 219f
        optic chiasm, 251, 251f
        temporal lobe, 237-238, 237f-238f
        thalamus, 259, 259f
        thigh, 157-159, 157f-159f
        thoracic spine metastases, 31f
        uses of, 8
        vertebral column, 26f
        wrist joint, 144, 144f
    T2-weighted
        abdominal studies, 80f
        ankle, 179-180, 179f-180f
        biliary duct system, 96, 96f
        cerebral hemispheres, 258, 258f
        description of, 9
        elbow, 136f
        female pelvis, 111f
        head, 219, 219f
        hip joint, 152f
        illustration of, 7f, 9f
        knee joint, 164-165, 164f-165f
        lateral ventricle, 257, 257f, 259, 259f
        medulla, 246, 246f
        neck, 219, 219f
        optic chiasm, 251, 251f
        prostate gland, 115, 115f
        shoulder joint, 126, 126f
        thalamus, 259, 259f
        thoracic spine metastases, 31f
        uses of, 8
        vertebral column, 27f
        wrist joint, 144, 144f
    urinary bladder, 115, 115f
    uses of, 8, 8f
    vertebral column, 26, 26f-27f
Magnetic resonance venogram, 220f
Major calyx, 88f
Major duodenal papilla, 96f
Male pelvis
    axial computed tomography of, 115,
        115f
    computed tomography of, 108f,
        114-115, 114f-115f
    contents of, 113, 113f
    female pelvis versus, 113
    magnetic resonance imaging of, 108f,
        115, 115f

Male pelvis (Continued)
    midsagittal section of, 114, 114f
    x-rays of, 106, 106f
Malleus, 227f-228f
Mammary glands. See also Breasts
    computed tomography of, 60f
    contours of, 36f
    lateral chest x-ray of, 42f
Mammillary body, 230, 231f, 235f, 251f,
    256f
Mammillary process, 20f
Mandible, 186f
    anatomy of, 196, 196f, 203f, 218f-219f
    angle of, 187f, 191f, 196f
    body of, 189f, 191f, 196, 196f, 217f
    condyle of, 189, 191f, 194f, 196, 196f
    coronoid process of, 189f, 191f, 196f,
        210f
    neck of, 210f
    ramus of, 187f, 191f, 196, 196f, 199f,
        206f-208f
    styloid process of, 189f, 193f, 195f, 205f,
        210f
Mandibular foramen, 196f
Mandibular fossa, 189f, 193, 193f, 195f
Mandibular nerve, 221f
Mandibular notch, 189, 196f
Manubriosternal junction, 61f
Manubrium, 59f, 68f, 203f, 218f-219f
Marginal artery, 98f
Marginal branch, of left coronary artery,
    52f
Marginal sulcus, 230f
Masseter muscle, 196f, 206-207, 206f-208f,
    210f
Masseteric artery, 201f
Mastoid air cells, 188f, 191f, 194f, 210f,
    227-228, 227f-228f, 246f
Mastoid antrum, 228f, 229
Mastoid fontanelle, 195f
Mastoid foramen, 194f
Mastoid process, 189f, 193f, 198f, 205f
Maxilla, 186f, 188f-191f, 193f, 195f, 207f,
    209f, 217f
Maxillary artery, 201f, 225f-226f
Maxillary nerve, 221f-222f
Maxillary sinus
    anatomy of, 187f-188f, 191f, 194f,
        209f-212f, 210-211, 214f, 217f,
        238f, 245f-246f
    fracture of, 216, 216f
    mucous retention cyst of, 215, 215f
Maxillary tuberosity, 189f
Maximum intensity projection, 13, 167,
    167f
Medial antebrachial cutaneous nerve,
    130f-131f
Medial brachial cutaneous nerve,
    130f-131f
Medial circumflex femoral artery, 152f,
    166f
Medial collateral ligament, 160, 160f-161f,
    165, 165f
Medial condyle, 122f, 153f

Medial cuneiform, 181f
Medial eminence, 234f
Medial epicondyle
    of femur, 153f, 160f
    of humerus, 122f, 130f, 133, 133f-136f,
        138f
Medial epicondylitis, 136
Medial genicular artery, 166, 166f
Medial geniculate body, 235f, 253f, 255f
Medial longitudinal fasciculus, 234f, 236f
Medial malleolus, 168, 168f-170f,
    178f-179f
Medial meniscus, 160, 160f-162f, 165f
Medial patellar retinaculum, 160f-161f
Medial plantar artery, 174f
Medial pterygoid muscle, 196f, 206,
    206f-208f, 210f, 215f
Medial rectus muscle, 213f-214f, 245f, 247f
Medial retinaculum, 165, 165f
Medial striate artery, 250f
Medial supracondylar line, 153f
Medial supracondylar ridge, 122f, 133f
Medial sural cutaneous nerve, 170f
Median antebrachial vein, 139f
Median aperture, 232f-234f
Median nerve, 130f-131f, 137f, 139,
    139f-140f, 145, 145f
Median sacral artery, 98f
Median umbilical fold, 109f, 113f
Median umbilical ligament, 91f, 109f, 113f
Mediastinal lymph node, 59f
Mediastinal window, 5f, 61f
Mediastinum
    anatomy of, 72
    left lateral view of, 40, 40f, 43f
    right lateral view of, 41, 41f
    T8 cross-sectional view of, 49, 49f
Medulla
    axial magnetic resonance imaging of,
        246, 246f
    general images of, 199f
Medulla oblongata, 210f, 230f-231f,
    236f-237f, 241f, 246f
Medullary velum, 230f, 234f
Membranous septum, 50f
Meniscofemoral ligament, 161f-162f
Meniscus, 160, 160f-161f
Meniscus sign, 64f
Mental foramen, 186f, 189f, 196f
Mental protuberance, 186f, 196f
Mental spine, 196f
Mental tubercle, 186f, 196f
Mesencephalon, 230, 231f, 241f
Mesenteric artery. See Inferior mesenteric
    artery; Superior mesenteric artery
Mesometrium, 112f
Mesosalpinx, 112f
Mesovarium, 112f
Metacarpal bones, 138f, 141f-142f
Metacarpophalangeal joint, 141
Metastases
    breasts, 10f
    liver, 81f
    thoracic spine, 31, 31f

Metatarsal bones, 176f-177f, 181f
Metencephalon, 230
Methylene-diphosphonate, 10
Metopic suture, 195f
Microadenoma, 222f
Midbrain, 231f, 237f
Midcarpal joint, 143f
Middle cerebellar peduncle, 235f, 241f
Middle cerebral artery, 225, 225f-226f, 249,
    249f-251f
Middle colic artery, 83f, 91f, 97f-98f
Middle colic vein, 83f
Middle cranial fossa, 194, 194f
Middle cuneiform, 181f
Middle ear, 227, 227f
Middle genicular artery, 166, 166f
Middle meningeal artery, 191f, 194, 194f,
    201f, 221f, 223-224, 223f-224f, 226f
Middle nasal concha, 186, 186f, 188f, 190f,
    209f, 211f, 217f, 245f
Middle nasal meatus, 209f, 211f, 217f
Middle rectal artery, 98f
Middle scalene muscle, 37f, 201f-202f
Middle thyroid vein, 200f
Mitral valve, 38f, 49f-50f, 54f, 62f
Molars, 187f
Mucous retention cyst, 215, 215f
Multimodal image guidance, 16, 16f
Muscle. See specific muscle
Musculocutaneous nerve, 130f-131f
Myelencephalon, 230
Mylohyoid groove, 196f
Mylohyoid line, 196f
Mylohyoid muscle, 200f, 203f-204f, 204,
    206, 206f-207f, 217f-218f

N
Nasal bone, 186f, 189f-190f, 195f
Nasal cavity
    general images of, 217f
    lateral wall of, 209, 209f
    midsagittal section of, 218, 218f
    in transverse plane, 210, 210f
Nasal concha, 186, 186f, 188f, 190f, 211f,
    217f, 245f
Nasal meatus, 209f, 211f, 217f
Nasal septal cartilage, 210f
Nasal septum, 187f-188f, 190f, 194f, 203f,
    211f-212f, 217f-218f
Nasal spine, 186f, 189f
Nasal vestibule, 209f-210f
Nasion, 186f
Nasogastric tube, 66f, 71f
Nasolacrimal duct, 209, 209f
Nasopharynx, 203f, 207f-210f, 215f,
    218f-219f, 222f, 227, 227f
Navicular bone, 176f-178f, 180f-181f
Navicular fossa, 114f
Neck
    arteries of, 200, 200f, 225, 225f
    axial computed tomography of, 202,
        202f
    cross section of, 202, 202f

Neck *(Continued)*
  magnetic resonance imaging of, 219, 219f
  midsagittal section of, 218-219, 218f-219f
  muscles of, 200, 200f
  vascular imaging studies of, 226, 226f
  veins of, 200, 200f
Nerve. *See specific nerve*
Nerve of Wrisberg, 221f, 235f
Neurocranium, 189-190
Neurofibromatosis, 67f
Neurohypophysis, 250f
Newborn skull, 195, 195f
Nose, 210, 210f
Notch. *See specific notch*
Nuclear medicine imaging, 10
  description of, 10
  whole-body scan, 10, 10f
Nuclear spin, 7
Nutrient foramen, 153f, 168f

O

Obex, 234f
Oblique popliteal ligament, 161f
Obturator artery, 116f, 150f, 152f, 166f
Obturator canal, 104f
Obturator crest, 149f
Obturator foramen, 78f, 105f-106f
Obturator groove, 149f
Obturator internus muscle, 116f-117f
Obturator membrane, 104f, 150f
Obturator nerve, 116f, 154, 156f
Obturator vein, 116f
Occipital artery, 201f, 225f-226f
Occipital bone, 189f-191f, 193f-195f, 209f
Occipital condyle, 190f, 193f, 197f-198f, 205f
Occipital horn, 238f
Occipital lobe, 239f
Occipital sinus, 194f, 220f
Oculomotor nerve, 221f-222f, 235f
Odontoid process, 197f, 242f
Olecranon, 133f, 135f-136f
Olecranon bursa, 134, 134f
Olecranon fossa, 122f
Olfactory bulbs, 217f, 245f
Olfactory tract, 235f
Olive, 235f
Omental appendices, 90f
Omental bursa, 85, 85f, 91f
Omental foramen, 85f, 92f
Omohyoid muscle, 200, 200f, 202f
Opacities, 76, 76f
Ophthalmic artery, 201f, 225f, 250f
Ophthalmic nerve, 221f-222f
Ophthalmic vein, 221f
Optic canal, 188f, 190f, 194f
Optic chiasm
  general images of, 211f, 222f, 230f, 235f, 250f
  magnetic resonance imaging of
    axial, 251, 251f
    fluid attenuation inversion recovery, 243, 243f

Optic foramen, 188f
Optic nerve, 211f, 213, 213f-214f, 221f, 244f-245f, 251f
Optic radiation, 240f
Optic tract, 235f, 251f, 256f
Oral cavity
  coronal section of, 217, 217f
  general images of, 203f
  midsagittal section of, 218, 218f
Oral region
  arteries of, 201, 201f
  mandible. *See* Mandible
  tongue. *See* Tongue
Orbicularis oris muscle, 206f
Orbit
  computed tomography of, 214, 214f
  coronal section of, 213, 213f, 217, 217f
  cross section of, 213, 213f
  fracture of, 216, 216f
  general images of, 211f
  magnetic resonance imaging of, 214, 214f
  pathology of, 215-216, 215f-216f
  upper, 251f
Orbital fat, 211f-212f, 217f
Orbital fissure, 187f
Orbital margin, 188f
Orbital plate, 186f, 189f
Orbitofrontal artery, 249f
Oropharynx, 203f, 208f, 218f-219f
Osteoarthritis
  of hip joint, 151
  of knee joint, 163
Osteonecrosis, 144
Osteophyte "lipping", 21f
Osteophytes, 123
Osteoporosis, 30, 30f
Oval window, 227f-228f
Ovarian follicles, 111f
Ovary, 111, 111f-112f

P

Palate
  hard, 203f, 217f, 219f
  soft, 203f, 207, 207f-209f, 218f-219f
Palatine artery, 201f
Palatine bone, 188f, 190f, 193f, 195f, 209f
Palatine foramen, 193f
Palatine glands, 203f, 218f-219f
Palatine process, 190f-191f, 209f
Palatine tonsil, 203f, 218f
Palatoglossus muscle, 206f
Palatopharyngeus muscle, 206f
Palmar aponeurosis, 137f, 145f
Palmar arch, 129, 129f
Palmar carpal ligament, 137f
Palmaris longus muscle, 137f
Palmaris longus tendon, 137f, 145f
Palpebral conjunctiva, 213f
Pancreas
  anatomy of, 83, 83f
  body of, 85f, 101f
  computed tomography of, 43f, 82f, 91f, 93f, 101f

Pancreas *(Continued)*
  general images of, 86f, 91f
  head of, 83, 83f, 87, 99f, 101f
  magnetic resonance imaging of, 86f
  neck of, 83f
  tail of, 83, 85f, 99f
  uncinate process of, 83f, 87f-88f, 91f
Pancreatic duct, 96, 96f
Pancreaticoduodenal artery, 97f-98f
Papillary muscle, 49f-50f, 62f
Paracentral lobule, 230f
Paracentral sulcus, 230f
Paracolic gutter, 90f, 109f, 113f
Paraesophageal hernia, 94f
Parahippocampal gyrus, 241f, 251f
Paranasal sinuses. *See also specific sinus*
  anatomy of, 2f, 187, 209f, 211, 211f
  computed tomography of, 212f
  coronal section of, 217, 217f
  magnetic resonance imaging of, 212f
  pathology of, 215-216, 215f-216f
Pararectal fossa, 109f, 113f
Pararenal fat, 88f-89f
Parietal bone, 186f, 189, 189f, 191f-195f, 239f-240f, 258f
Parietal foramen, 192f
Parietal lobe, 239f-240f
Parietal peritoneum, 85f, 90f-91f, 101, 109f, 113f
Parietal pleura, 35f, 40f-41f, 49f, 69
Parietooccipital sulcus, 230f-231f, 237f-238f
Parotid duct, 201f
Parotid gland, 200f, 205f-208f, 206, 210f, 227f
Pars interarticularis, 20f, 32f
Partial volume averaging, 259
Patella, 160f, 163f, 165f, 169f
Patellar anastomosis, 166f
Patellar ligament, 160, 160f-161f, 163f-164f, 169f, 171f
Patellar retinaculum, 160f-161f
Pathological imaging, 9
Pecten pubis, 104f-105f
Pectineal line, 78f, 104f, 153f
Pectineus muscle, 154f, 156f
Pectoralis major muscle, 38f, 59f, 130f-131f, 200f
Pectoralis major tendon, 131f
Pectoralis minor muscle, 38f, 59f, 122, 122f, 130f
Pedicle, 20f-21f, 24f
Pelvic brim, 104
Pelvic inlet, 106f
Pelvis
  bony framework of, 104-105, 104f-105f
  computed tomography of, 104f-105f, 108, 108f
  female
    computed tomography of, 107, 107f-108f
    contents of, 109, 109f
    lower, 111, 111f
    magnetic resonance imaging of, 108f

Pelvis (*Continued*)
male pelvis versus, 113
midsagittal section of, 107, 107f
upper, 110, 110f
x-rays of, 106, 106f
magnetic resonance imaging of, 108f
male
axial computed tomography of, 115, 115f
computed tomography of, 108f, 114-115, 114f-115f
contents of, 113, 113f
female pelvis versus, 113
magnetic resonance imaging of, 108f, 115, 115f
midsagittal section of, 114, 114f
x-rays of, 106, 106f
midsagittal section of, 104f
Penis, 114f, 117f-118f
Perforating arteries, 250f
Pericardial cavity, 49f
Pericardial reflection, 47f
Pericardial sinus, 62f
Pericranium, 223f
Perineal body, 114f
Perineal fascia, 117f
Perineal flexure, 116f
Perineal membrane, 114f, 117f
Periorbita, 213f
Peripancreatic fluid, 101f
Perirenal fat, 88f-89f, 101f
Peritoneal cavity, 93f
Peritoneal sac, 94f
Peritoneum, 89f, 117f
abdominal, 100, 100f
parietal, 85f, 90f-91f, 101, 109f, 113f
Peroneal artery, 166, 166f, 170f, 174f
Peroneal nerve, 172f
Perpendicular plate, 186f, 190f, 212f
Pes anserinus, 160f, 169f, 173, 173f
Pes hippocampus, 255f-256f, 256
Petrosal nerve, 194f
Petrosal sinus, 190f, 220f
Petrous part of temporal bone, 187, 187f-188f, 193, 193f-195f, 228f, 239f, 241f, 247f
Phalanges
of foot, 176f-177f, 181f
of hand, 141f-142f
Pharyngeal artery, 201f
Pharyngeal constrictor muscles, 58f, 201f, 203f, 206f, 218f
Pharyngeal raphe, 203f
Pharyngeal recess, 210f
Pharyngeal region, 201, 201f
Pharyngeal tonsil, 203f, 209f, 218f
Pharyngeal tubercle, 193f, 203f
Pharynx, 190f, 218, 218f, 244f
Phrenic nerve, 40f-41f, 60f, 200f-201f
Phrenoesophageal membrane, 94f
Pia mater, 22, 22f-23f, 223f
Picture archiving and communication system, 15, 15f
Pineal body, 230f, 234f-235f, 253f, 255f

Pineal recess, 232f
Piriformis muscle, 111f, 155f
Pisiform, 137, 141f, 143f, 145f
Pituitary gland, 219f, 221f-222f, 230f, 243, 243f-244f, 250f
Pituitary stalk, 235f, 248f, 250, 250f-251f
Plantar aponeurosis, 180, 180f
Plantar artery, 174f
Plantaris muscle, 170f
Plantaris tendon, 155f, 170f, 172f
Platysma muscle, 200f, 202f-203f
Pleura
costal, 40f
general images of, 23f
parietal, 35f, 40f-41f, 49f, 69
visceral, 69
Pleural cavity
costodiaphragmatic recess of, 35f-38f, 40f-41f, 84f-85f, 89f
costomediastinal recess of, 35f
general images of, 49f
Pleural effusion, 69
Pleural reflection, 35f
Pleural spaces, 69, 69f
Pneumonia, 76, 76f
Pneumothorax, 69f, 70
Pons
fluid attenuation inversion recovery magnetic resonance imaging of, 242, 242f
general images of, 230f-231f, 234f-235f, 237f, 247f
Pontine arteries, 249f-250f
Popliteal artery, 156f, 159f, 165f-167f, 166, 169, 170f, 175f
Popliteal vein, 156f, 159f, 165f, 170f
Popliteus muscle, 155f
Popliteus tendon, 160, 160f-162f, 162
Port-a-cath, 69f
Portal triad, 83f, 86f
Portal vein, 38f, 83f-86f, 93f, 96f, 99f, 101f
Posterior articular facet, 198f
Posterior auricular artery, 225f
Posterior cerebellar notch, 236f
Posterior cerebral artery, 225f-226f, 248f-249f
Posterior cervical triangle, 202f
Posterior circumflex humeral artery, 130f
Posterior clinoid process, 194f
Posterior commissure, 230f
Posterior communicating artery, 222f, 225f-226f, 249f-250f
Posterior cruciate ligament, 161f-162f, 162
Posterior ethmoidal foramen, 188f, 194f
Posterior fat pad, 180f
Posterior femoral cutaneous nerve, 156f
Posterior fontanelle, 195f
Posterior inferior cerebellar artery, 225f-226f, 249f
Posterior inferior iliac spine, 24f, 149f
Posterior intercavernous sinus, 220f
Posterior interosseous artery, 128f
Posterior interosseous nerve, 139f
Posterior longitudinal ligament, 24f

Posterior nasal spine, 193f
Posterior perforated substance, 235f
Posterior scalene muscle, 37f, 202f
Posterior spinal artery, 249f
Posterior superior cerebellar artery, 226f
Posterior superior iliac spine, 24f, 105f, 149f
Posterior tibial artery, 166f, 170, 170f, 172f, 174f
Posterior tibial recurrent artery, 166f
Posterior tibial vein, 170f, 172f
Posterior ulnar recurrent artery, 128f
Posteroanterior x-ray
atelectasis, 75f
evaluation of, 63, 63f-64f
heart chambers, 48, 48f
lungs, 45, 45f
normal, 63f
thorax, 36, 36f, 63, 63f-64f, 68f
Posterolateral branches, of right coronary artery, 51f
Pouch of Douglas, 107, 107f, 109f, 112f
Precentral gyrus, 258f-259f
Precuneus, 230f
Prefrontal artery, 249f
Prepatellar bursa, 164f
Prepontine cistern, 233f, 247f
Prepuce, 114f
Pretracheal fascia, 202f-203f
Prevertebral fascia, 203, 219f
Prevertebral fat, 26f
Profunda brachii artery, 128f, 130f-132f
Profunda femoris artery, 154f, 156f, 166f-167f, 175f
Promontory, 227f
Pronator quadratus muscle, 139f
Pronator teres muscle, 130f, 137, 137f, 139f
Proper hepatic artery, 85f-86f, 97f
Prosencephalon, 230
Prostate gland
computed tomography of, 114f-116f, 116, 118f
cross section of, 116, 116f
general images of, 91f, 114f
magnetic resonance imaging of, 115, 115f
Proton density magnetic resonance imaging, 9f
Psoas major muscle, 29f, 88f-89f, 110f
Psoas minor muscle, 90f
Pterion, 189f
Pterygoid muscles, 196f, 206, 206f-208f, 210f, 215f
Pterygoid process, 189f, 193, 193f
Pterygomandibular raphe, 196f, 206f
Pterygopalatine fossa, 189f, 211f
Pubic arch, 78f
Pubic bone, 91, 91f, 104, 107f
Pubic ramus, 78f, 104f, 149f-151f
Pubic symphysis, 78f, 105f-107f, 114f, 116f
Pubic tubercle, 104f-105f, 149f
Pubofemoral ligament, 150, 150f
Pudendal nerve, 116f

Pulmonary artery, 37f, 40f-42f, 46f, 61f
Pulmonary trunk, 38f-39f, 50f, 53f, 61f
Pulmonary veins
    computed tomography of, 37f, 39f, 46f, 53f
    general images of, 40f-41f, 43f, 47f, 49f
    inferior, 62f
Pulmonary vessels. *See also specific vessel*
    computed tomography of, 6f
    posteroanterior x-ray of, 36f
Pulse-echo concept, 12, 12f
Pulvinar, 255f
Putamen, 243f-244f, 252f-254f, 257f
Pyloric antrum, 93f
Pyloric canal, 86f, 93f
Pylorus, 92f-93f

Q

Quadrate ligament, 134f
Quadrate tubercle, 153f
Quadratus femoris muscle, 155f
Quadratus femoris tendon, 160f, 164f, 171f
Quadratus lumborum muscle, 89, 89f
Quadratus plantae, 179f
Quadrigeminal cistern, 233f, 240f, 252f
Quadrigeminal plate, 230f-231f, 234f, 237f

R

Radial artery
    digital subtraction angiography of, 129f
    fluoroscopic imaging of, 11f
    general images of, 130f, 139f, 145f
Radial collateral artery, 128f
Radial collateral ligament, 134, 134f
Radial fossa, 122f, 133f
Radial groove, 122f
Radial nerve, 131f, 137, 138f
Radial notch of ulna, 133f
Radial recurrent artery, 128f
Radial tilt, 142
Radial tuberosity, 135f
Radiocarpal joint, 141
Radiofrequency energy, 7
Radiotracer tracers, 55-56
Radius
    anteroposterior x-ray of, 142f
    fracture of, 142
    general images of, 135f, 139f-140f, 144f
    head of, 133, 133f, 135f-136f
    neck of, 133f
    styloid process of, 142f-143f
Rectal artery, 98f
Rectosigmoid junction, 111f
Rectouterine pouch, 107, 107f, 109f, 112f
Rectovesical pouch, 113f-114f
Rectum
    computed tomography of, 95f, 115f, 118f
    general images of, 91f, 107f, 109f, 113f-114f
Rectus abdominis muscle, 84f-85f, 90f
Rectus femoris muscle, 115f, 154f, 157f-158f

Rectus femoris tendon, 156f, 159, 159f-160f, 169f
Rectus muscle, 213f-214f, 245f, 247f
Recurrent artery of Heubner, 249f-250f
Recurrent interosseous artery, 128f
Recurrent laryngeal nerve, 59f-60f, 202f
Red nucleus, 241f
Renal artery, 88f-89f, 99f
Renal cortex, 87f
Renal fascia, 88f-89f, 89
Renal medulla, 87f
Renal pelvis, 88f
Renal vein, 86f, 88f-89f, 91f, 93f
Retention cyst, 215, 215f
Retinacular arteries, 152f
Retinacular foramina, 153f
Retrobulbar fat, 213f
Retromandibular vein, 200f, 206f-207f
Retroperitoneal fat, 90f
Retroperitoneum
    anatomy of, 100, 100f
    fluid in, 101, 101f
Retropharyngeal space, 199f, 202f-203f, 219f
Retrotonsillar fissure, 236f
Reversible defect, 55f
Rhomboid fossa, 235f
Ribs
    anatomy of, 68
    eighth, 49f
    first, 35f-36f, 40f-41f
    "floating",, 68
    seventh, 62f
    twelfth, 35f, 89f
Right atrium
    computed tomography of, 39f
    echocardiography of, 54f
    general images of, 38f, 47f, 62f
    lateral x-ray of, 48, 48f
    magnetic resonance imaging of, 49f
    posteroanterior x-ray of, 36f, 48, 48f
Right auricle, 47f, 53f
Right coronary artery, 47f, 51, 51f, 53f
Right lung, 41, 41f, 44, 44f-45f, 60f, 93f, 96f
Right ventricle, 38f
    color Doppler imaging of, 54f
    computed tomography of, 39f, 43f
    echocardiography of, 54f
    general images of, 49f
    lateral x-ray of, 48, 48f
    magnetic resonance imaging of, 39f, 43f
    posteroanterior x-ray of, 48, 48f
Round ligament
    of liver, 90f, 92f
    of uterus, 109f, 117f
Round window, 227f
Rugae, 84f, 92

S

Saccule, 227, 227f-228f
Sacral artery, 98f
Sacral foramina, 105f-106f

Sacral promontory, 78f, 105f, 107f, 109f, 113f
Sacroiliac joint, 32f, 106f
Sacrospinous ligament, 104f-105f, 155f
Sacrotuberous ligament, 104f-105f, 116f, 155f
Sacrum, 18, 18f, 78f, 106f
Sagittal sinus. *See* Inferior sagittal sinus; Superior sagittal sinus
Sagittal suture, 187f, 192, 192f, 195f
"Sail" sign, 135
Salivary glands, 206, 206f
Saphenous muscle, 156f
Saphenous nerve, 154f
Saphenous vein, 170f
Sartorius muscle, 154f-159f, 159, 169f
Sartorius tendon, 160f
Scala tympani, 227f
Scala vestibuli, 227f
Scalene muscles, 37f-38f, 40f-41f, 201f-202f
Scaphoid, 141f-144f, 142-143
Scapholunate ligament, 144
Scapula
    anatomy of, 122, 122f
    anteroposterior x-ray of, 123f
    body of, 124f
    coracoid process of, 36f
    description of, 68
    general images of, 59f, 61f-62f
    spine of, 122, 122f-123f
Sciatic nerve, 116f, 155, 155f-159f
Sclera, 213f-214f
Scoliosis, 68f
"Scotty dog" profile, 32f
Scrotum, 114f
Sella turcica, 190, 190f-191f, 194f, 209f, 212f, 218f
Semicircular canals, 227, 227f-228f
Semilunar hiatus, 209f, 211f
Semimembranosus muscle, 155f-159f, 170f
Semimembranosus tendon, 161f
Seminal colliculus, 117f
Seminal vesicle, 113f-115f
Semitendinosus muscle, 155f-159f, 159, 170f
Semitendinosus tendon, 160f
Septomarginal trabecula, 50f
Septum pellucidum, 230f, 253f, 256f
Serratus anterior muscle, 38f, 84f
Sesamoid bones, 141f, 176f, 181f
Seventh rib, 62f
Shoulder
    anatomy of, 125, 125f
    anteroposterior x-ray of, 123, 123f
    axial T1 arthrogram of, 127, 127f
    axillary view of, 124, 124f
    magnetic resonance imaging of, 123, 126
    T1 arthrogram of, 127, 127f
    x-rays of, 123-124, 123f-124f
    Y view x-rays of, 124, 124f
Sigmoid arteries, 98f

Sigmoid colon, 95f, 109f, 111f, 113f
Sigmoid mesocolon, 98f
Sigmoid sinus, 190f, 194f, 220f-221f, 222, 228f, 229
Silhouette sign, 3, 3f, 74, 74f
Single-photon emission computed tomography (SPECT), 55-56
  description of, 10
  examinations using, 55f
  left ventricle, 55f
  long-axis views, 55-56
  principles of, 55-56
  radiotracer tracers used with, 55-56
  reversible defect, 55f
  short-axis views, 55-56
Sinoatrial nodal branch, of right coronary artery, 51f
Sinus(es). See also specific sinus
  dural venous, 220-222, 220f-222f
  paranasal. See Paranasal sinuses; specific sinus
Sinus of Valsalva, 50f, 53f
Skull
  anterior view of, 186, 186f
  anteroposterior Caldwell view of, 188, 188f
  anteroposterior x-ray of, 187, 187f
  calvaria, 192, 192f, 223f
  lateral view of, 189, 189f
  lateral x-ray of, 191, 191f
  newborn, 195, 195f
SLAP lesion, 127
"Sliding" hiatal hernia, 94, 94f
Small intestine
  anatomy of, 90f
  computed tomography of, 81f, 93f, 99f, 101f, 110f-111f, 114f
  decompressed, 81f
  dilation of, 6f
  general images of, 91f
  magnetic resonance imaging of, 39f
  mesentery of, 91f
  obstruction of, 81f
Small lung cancer, 69f
Smith fracture, 142
Soft palate, 203f, 207, 207f-209f, 218f-219f
Soft tissue window, 5f
Soleus muscle, 155f, 169f-171f, 170, 173f
Spermatic cord, 115f-116f
Sphenoccipital synchondrosis, 203f, 218f
Sphenoethmoidal recess, 209, 209f
Sphenoid bone, 186f-187f, 189f-190f, 194f-195f, 210f
Sphenoid sinus, 190, 190f-191f, 194f, 203f, 209f, 211, 211f-212f, 214f-215f, 215, 218f-219f, 222f, 244f, 247f-248f
Sphenoidal fontanelle, 195f
Sphenopalatine artery, 201f
Sphenopalatine fossa, 189f
Sphincter urethrae muscle, 117f
Spinal artery, 249f
Spinal canal, 88f

Spinal cord
  diameter of, 25
  general images of, 199f, 207f
  magnetic resonance imaging of, 26f, 219f, 237f, 241f
Spinal membranes, 22, 22f
Spinal nerve
  cross section of, 202f
  groove for, 197f
  magnetic resonance imaging of, 26f
  origins of, 23
  ramus of, 22f
  roots of, 22f, 25, 25f
Spine. See Vertebrae; specific vertebrae
Spinous process, 19, 19f-21f, 24f, 197f, 219f
Spleen
  computed tomography of, 37f, 46f, 81f-82f
  general images of, 35f, 37f, 84f-86f, 92f
Splenic artery, 83f, 86f, 97f
Splenic flexure, 83f, 95f
Splenic vein, 83f, 86f-87f, 87
Splenorenal ligament, 85f
Spondylolisthesis
  computed tomography of, 6f
  magnetic resonance imaging of, 32, 32f
Squamocolumnar junction, 94f
Stapes, 227f
Sternal angle, 42f
Sternoclavicular joint, 35f, 59f
Sternocleidomastoid muscle, 200, 200f, 202f-203f, 203, 205f, 207f
Sternohyoid muscle, 200, 200f, 202f
Sternothyroid muscle, 200, 200f, 202f
Sternum, 30f, 49f, 58f, 68, 68f, 218f-219f
Stomach
  anatomy of, 92, 92f
  antrum of, 85f, 93f, 101f
  body of, 92f-93f
  computed tomography of, 39f, 43f, 81f-82f, 93f
  fluoroscopic imaging of, 11f
  fundus of, 84f, 92f-94f, 99f
  general images of, 35f, 37f-38f, 83f, 85f
  greater curvature of, 92f
  in situ image of, 92, 92f
  lesser curvature of, 92f
  magnetic resonance imaging of, 39f
  posteroanterior x-ray of, 36f
  pylorus of, 92f-93f
  rugae of, 84f, 92
Straight gyrus, 245f, 248f, 251f
Straight sinus, 219f-221f, 221, 230f, 233f, 252f, 254f
Stress fractures, 181
Stria medullaris, 230f, 234f, 255f
Stria terminalis, 255f-256f
Styloglossus muscle, 206f
Styloid process
  of mandible, 189f, 193f, 195f, 205f, 210f
  of radius, 142f-143f
Stylomandibular ligament, 196f
Stylomastoid foramen, 193f

Subarachnoid hematoma, 224f
Subarachnoid space, 233f, 237f, 239f
Subcallosal area, 230f
Subcallosal gyrus, 230f
Subchondral cysts, 151
Subclavian artery, 40f-41f, 59f, 128, 201f, 225f-226f
Subclavian vein, 40f-41f
Subclavius muscle, 38f, 40f-41f
Subdeltoid bursa, 125f
Subdural hematoma, 224, 224f
Sublingual gland, 206, 206f, 217f
Submandibular gland, 200f-201f, 204f, 206, 206f-207f
Submandibular lymph node, 206f
Submental vein, 200f
Subpopliteal recess, 161f
Subpubic angle, 106f
Subpulmonic fluid, 69
Subscapular artery, 128f
Subscapular fossa, 122f
Subscapularis muscle, 37f, 125f, 130f
Subscapularis tendon, 127f
Subtendinous bursa, 164f, 171f
Sulcus limitans, 234f
Superficial cortical veins, 221f
Superficial external pudendal artery, 166f
Superficial palmar arch, 129, 129f
Superficial temporal artery, 225f-226f
Superior articular facet, 19f, 197f-198f
Superior articular process, 20f
Superior cerebellar artery, 225f-226f, 249f-250f
Superior cerebellar peduncle, 234f-236f
Superior cerebral vein, 223f
Superior colliculus, 230f, 234f-235f, 255f
Superior constrictor muscle, 207f
Superior facial artery, 201f
Superior frontal gyrus, 245f
Superior gemellus muscle, 155f
Superior hypophyseal artery, 250f
Superior labial artery, 201f
Superior labrum, 126f
Superior laryngeal artery, 201f, 225f
Superior medullary velum, 230f, 234f, 236f
Superior mesenteric artery
  anatomy of, 83, 83f, 86f, 88f-89f, 91, 91f, 93f, 98, 98f
  angiogram of, 99, 99f
Superior mesenteric vein, 83, 83f, 87, 87f-89f, 101f
Superior nasal concha, 209f
Superior nasal meatus, 209f
Superior oblique muscle, 213f-214f, 245f
Superior orbital fissure, 187f-188f, 188, 194, 194f, 214f
Superior pancreaticoduodenal artery, 97f
Superior petrosal sinus, 190f, 194f, 220f-221f
Superior pubic ramus, 104f-105f, 149f-151f
Superior rectal artery, 98f
Superior rectus muscle, 213f-214f, 245f

Superior sagittal sinus, 192, 192f, 194f, 220-221, 220f-221f, 223, 223f-224f, 230f, 233f, 237f, 240f-242f, 245f, 251f-252f, 254, 254f, 257f-259f, 259
Superior thoracic artery, 128f
Superior thyroid artery, 200f-201f, 225f
Superior thyroid vein, 200f
Superior ulnar collateral artery, 128f, 130f-131f
Superior vena cava
    computed tomography of, 39f
    general images of, 38f, 41f, 47f, 49f-50f, 61f-62f
    magnetic resonance imaging of, 39f, 53f
Superior vermis, 236f
Superior vertebral notch, 20f
Supinator, 140f
Supraclavicular nerves, 200f
Supracondylar line, 153f
Supracondylar ridge, 122f
Supraduodenal artery, 97f
Supraglenoid tubercle, 122, 122f
Supramastoid crest, 189f
Supraoptic recess, 230f, 232f
Supraorbital artery, 201f
Supraorbital notch, 186f, 188f-189f
Suprapatellar bursa, 160f-161f, 163, 164f
Suprapatellar fat body, 164f
Suprapineal recess, 232f
Suprarenal glands, 35f, 83f, 85f-87f, 87, 89f
Suprascapular foramen, 125f
Suprascapular notch, 122f
Supraspinatus fossa, 122, 122f
Supraspinatus muscle, 37f, 126f
Supraspinatus tendon, 126f
Supraspinous ligament, 24, 24f
Suprasternal notch, 35f
Suprasternal space, 203f
Supratrochlear artery, 201f
Supraventricular crest, 50f
Sural cutaneous nerve, 170f
Surgical neck of humerus, 122f-123f
Suspensory ligament
    of ovary, 107f, 109f, 112f
    of penis, 114f
Sustentaculum tali, 176, 176f-178f, 181f
Sutural bone, 189f, 192f
Suture
    coronal, 186f, 189, 189f-191f, 195f
    frontal, 195f
    lambdoid, 187f, 189, 189f, 191f-192f, 195f
    metopic, 195f
    sagittal, 187f, 192, 192f, 195f
Swan-Ganz catheter, 66f
Sylvian fissure, 252f
Sympathetic ganglion, 23f
Sympathetic trunk, 40f, 90f, 202f, 210f
Synovial membrane, 152f, 160f

T

Talus, 176f-181f
Tarsal joint, 176f-177f
Tarsometatarsal joint, 176f-177f

Technetium-99m, 55-56
Tectal plate, 230f, 234f
Tectum of midbrain, 231f, 237f
Tegmen tympani, 227f-228f
Tegmentum, 251f
Tela choroidea, 232f, 255, 255f
Telencephalon, 230
Temporal artery, 210f, 225f-226f
Temporal bone
    anatomy of, 186f, 187, 189, 189f-190f, 193f-194f, 228, 228f
    pathology of, 229, 229f
    petrous part of, 187, 187f-188f, 193, 193f-195f, 228f, 239f, 241f, 247f
Temporal fossa, 189f
Temporal horn, 238f
Temporal lobe
    axial magnetic resonance imaging of, 247, 247f
    fluid attenuation inversion recovery magnetic resonance imaging of, 244, 244f
    general images of, 205f, 235f
    magnetic resonance imaging of, 237-239, 237f-240f
Temporal process, 186f
Temporalis muscle, 196f
Tensor fasciae latae muscle, 154f, 156f
Tensor tympani muscle, 228, 228f
Tentorium cerebelli, 220, 220f-221f, 224f, 230f, 238f-240f, 252
Teres major muscle, 130f-131f
Teres minor tendon, 125f
Terminal ileum, 109f-110f, 113f
Testes, 91f, 114
Thalamoperforating artery, 250f
Thalamotuberal artery, 250f
Thalamus
    anatomy of, 230f-232f, 234f-235f, 237f, 241f, 255, 255f
    axial magnetic resonance imaging of, 252, 252f, 254, 254f, 259, 259f
Thigh. See also Leg
    arteries of, 166, 166f
    cross section of, 156, 156f
    extensor compartment of, 154
    lower, 159, 159f
    magnetic resonance angiography of, 167, 167f
    magnetic resonance imaging of, 157-159, 157f-159f
    middle, 158, 158f
    muscles of, 154-155, 154f-155f
    upper, 157, 157f
Third ventricle
    general images of, 230f, 232, 232f-234f, 255
    magnetic resonance imaging of
        axial, 252, 252f, 254f
        fluid attenuation inversion recovery, 242, 242f
Thoracic aorta, 40f, 49f, 84f, 86f
Thoracic duct, 40f, 49f, 58f, 60f-62f, 84f
Thoracic nerves, 25f

Thoracic spine
    metastatic disease in, 31, 31f
    osteoporosis of, 30, 30f
    scoliosis of, 68f
    T3 cross section, 59, 59f
    T7 cross section, 62, 62f
    T8 cross section, 49, 49f
    T10 cross section, 84, 84f
    T12 cross section, 85-86, 85f-86f
    T12-L1 cross section, 87, 87f
    T3-T4 cross section, 60, 60f
    T4-T5 cross section, 61, 61f
    x-rays of, 19f
Thoracic vertebrae, 18-19, 18f-19f, 23f
Thoracic wall
    bones of, 68, 69f
    soft tissues of, 67, 67f
Thoracoacromial artery, 128f
Thoracodorsal artery, 128f
Thorax
    anterior axillary coronal section of, 38f
    computed tomography of, 43
        anterior axillary, 39, 39f
        sagittal, 43
    imaging of
        lines, 66, 66f
        support devices, 66, 66f
        technical quality, 64f-65f, 65
        tubes, 66, 66f
        views, 64, 64f
    lateral chest x-ray, 42, 42f
    lateral view of, 58f
    magnetic resonance imaging of, 43
        anterior axillary, 39, 39f
        sagittal, 43
    midaxillary coronal section of, 37, 37f
    posterior view of, 58f
    posteroanterior x-ray of, 36, 36f, 68f
    topography of, 35, 35f
    vertebral levels in, 58, 58f
Thymus, 40f-41f, 60f
Thyrocervical trunk, 201f, 225f
Thyrohyoid membrane, 203f, 218f
Thyrohyoid muscle, 200, 200f
Thyroid artery, 200f-201f, 225f
Thyroid cartilage, 58f, 200f, 203f, 205f, 219f
Thyroid gland
    axial computed tomography of, 202, 202f
    general images of, 38f, 200f, 203f, 218f
Thyroid vein, 200f
Tibia, 162f-163f, 165f, 168, 168f, 173f, 178f
Tibial artery, 166, 166f, 169-170, 169f-170f
Tibial collateral ligament, 160, 161f-162f, 169f
Tibial nerve, 156f, 159f, 170f
Tibial plateau, 163, 163f
Tibial recurrent artery, 166f
Tibial tuberosity, 160f, 162f-164f, 169f, 171f
Tibial vein, 170f
Tibialis anterior muscle, 160f, 171f, 173f
Tibialis anterior tendon, 169f

Tibialis posterior muscle, 173f
Tibialis posterior tendon, 170f
Tongue
  anatomy of, 203f, 206, 206f-207f, 217f-218f, 245f
  mass in, 208, 208f
Torcular herophili, 248
Torus tubarius, 209f
Trachea
  bifurcation of, 37f
  computed tomography of, 37f, 46f, 60f
  general images of, 35f-36f, 58f, 199f, 202f, 218f-219f
  lateral chest x-ray of, 42f
Transversalis fascia, 85f, 89f-90f, 113f
Transverse cervical nerves, 200f
Transverse colon, 83f, 86f-88f, 91f, 95f, 101f
Transverse costal facet, 19f
Transverse facial artery, 201f
Transverse mesocolon, 91f, 98f
Transverse process, 19, 19f-20f, 24f, 78f, 198f
Transverse sinus, 190f, 220f-221f, 221, 239f
Transversus abdominis muscle, 90f
Trapezium, 141, 141f-144f, 143
Trapezius muscle, 37f, 200, 200f, 202f-203f, 203
Trapezoid, 141f-142f, 144f
Triangle of auscultation, 62f
Triangular fibrocartilage, 144, 144f
Triceps brachii muscle
  general images of, 130f-131f, 136f, 138f
  magnetic resonance imaging of, 132f
Triceps brachii tendon, 134f, 136f
Tricuspid valve, 38f, 49f-50f, 54f
Trigeminal ganglion, 221f, 238
Trigeminal nerve, 235f, 238, 242f-243f
Trigeminal tubercle, 234f
Trigone
  habenular, 234f, 255f
  hypoglossal, 234f
  lateral ventricle, 252f, 254f
  urinary bladder, 117, 117f
  vagal, 234f
Triquetrum, 141f-144f
Trochanteric fossa, 153
Trochlea, 122f, 133f, 135f-136f
Trochlear groove, 135f
Trochlear nerve, 221f-222f, 234f-235f
Trochlear notch, 133f
True pelvis, 104f
True vocal fold, 203f
Tuber cinereum, 230f, 235f
Tubercle of scaphoid, 143f, 145f
Tuberculum sellae, 194f
T1-weighted magnetic resonance imaging
  abdominal studies, 80f
  ankle, 179-180, 179f-180f
  brain, 231, 231f
  cerebral hemispheres, 258, 258f
  description of, 9
  distal radioulnar joint, 145f

T1-weighted magnetic resonance imaging
    (Continued)
  forearm, 140, 140f
  head, 219, 219f
  herniated disk, 29f
  hip joint, 152f
  illustration of, 7f, 9f
  lateral ventricle, 257, 257f, 259, 259f
  medulla, 246, 246f
  neck, 219, 219f
  optic chiasm, 251, 251f
  temporal lobe, 237-238, 237f-238f
  thalamus, 259, 259f
  thigh, 157-159, 157f-159f
  thoracic spine metastases, 31f
  uses of, 8
  vertebral column, 26f
  wrist joint, 144, 144f
T2-weighted magnetic resonance imaging
  abdominal studies, 80f
  ankle, 179-180, 179f-180f
  biliary duct system, 96, 96f
  cerebral hemispheres, 258, 258f
  description of, 9
  elbow, 136f
  female pelvis, 111f
  head, 219, 219f
  hip joint, 152f
  illustration of, 7f, 9f
  knee joint, 164-165, 164f-165f
  lateral ventricle, 257, 257f, 259, 259f
  medulla, 246, 246f
  neck, 219, 219f
  optic chiasm, 251, 251f
  prostate gland, 115, 115f
  shoulder joint, 126, 126f
  thalamus, 259, 259f
  thoracic spine metastases, 31f
  uses of, 8
  vertebral column, 27f
  wrist joint, 144, 144f
Twelfth rib, 35f, 89f
Tympanic canaliculus, 193f
Tympanic cavity, 227-229, 227f
Tympanic membrane, 195f, 209, 227f-228f

U
Ulna, 142f-143f, 145f
Ulnar artery, 128f, 137f, 139f-140f, 145f
Ulnar collateral artery, 128f, 130f, 138f
Ulnar collateral ligament, 134, 134f
Ulnar nerve, 130f-131f, 133, 137f, 139f, 145f
Ulnar recurrent artery, 128f
Ultrasound, 12
  applications of, 12f
  color Doppler, 12f
  pregnancy uses of, 12f
  principles of, 12
  pulse-echo concept in, 12, 12f
Umbilical fold, 109f
Umbilical ligament, 109f

Uncinate process, 83f, 87f-88f, 88, 91f
Upper abdomen, 71, 71f
Upper extremity vascular studies, 129, 129f. *See also* Arm; Hand
Upper gastrointestinal computed tomography studies, 93, 93f
Urachus, 114f
Ureter, 90f, 107f, 109f-110f
Ureteric fold, 113f
Ureteric orifice, 117f
Ureteropelvic junction, 88f
Urethra
  anatomy of, 107f, 116f
  female, 117, 117f
  male, 117, 117f
  prostatic, 117f
Urethral sphincter, 117f
Urinary bladder
  computed tomography of, 114f, 116, 116f, 118, 118f
    axial, 118, 118f
    coronal, 118, 118f
  coronal section of, 117, 117f
  cross section of, 116, 116f
  cystogram of, 119, 119f
  female, 117, 117f-118f
  general images of, 91f, 107f, 109f, 114f
  magnetic resonance imaging of, 115, 115f
  male, 117, 117f-118f
  neck of, 117f
  trigone of, 117, 117f
Uterine tubes, 107f, 109f, 112, 112f
Uterosacral ligament, 112f
Uterus
  anatomy of, 112, 112f
  body of, 107f, 112f
  cervix of, 107f, 111f-112f, 112
  computed tomography of, 118f
  fundus of, 107f, 112f
  general images of, 111f
Utricle, 227, 227f-228f

V
Vagal trigone, 234f
Vagina
  computed tomography of, 118f
  fornix of, 107f
  general images of, 107f, 117f
Vagus nerve, 40f-41f, 59f-60f, 202f, 210f, 221f, 235f
Vallecula, 204f
Vasa recta, 98, 99f
Vastus intermedius muscle, 156f-160f, 159
Vastus lateralis muscle, 154f, 156f-160f, 159, 169f, 171f
Vastus medialis muscle, 154f, 156f-160f, 159, 169f
Vein. *See specific vein*
Vena cava. *See* Inferior vena cava; Superior vena cava
Ventricle. *See specific ventricle*

Vermis, 236f, 240f, 247f-248f
Vertebra prominens, 197f, 199f
Vertebrae
    cervical. *See* Cervical vertebrae
    lumbar. *See* Lumbar vertebrae
    thoracic, 18-19, 18f-19f, 23f
Vertebral artery, 37f, 207f-208f, 225,
    225f-226f, 246f, 249, 249f-250f
Vertebral body, 42f, 218f
Vertebral canal, 19f, 23
Vertebral column
    imaging of, 18, 18f
    magnetic resonance imaging of, 26,
    26f-27f
Vertebral foramen, 19f-20f
Vertebral venous plexus, 23f, 220f
Vertebrobasilar circulation, 249
Vertebrocostal ribs, 68, 68f
Vertebrosternal ribs, 68, 68f
Vesical fascia, 117f
Vesicouterine pouch, 107f
Vesicular appendix, 112f
Vestibulocochlear nerve, 221f, 227-228,
    227f-228f, 235f
Visceral pleura, 69
Viscerocranium, 189-190
Vitreous body, 214f
Vocal folds, 203f, 218f

Volume rendering, 13
Vomer, 186, 186f, 190f, 193f, 210f

W
White matter, 8f, 240f
White rami communicantes, 22f-23f
Whole-body scans, 10, 10f
Window width, 5, 39
Wing of ilium, 78f, 104f, 149f
Wormian bone, 189f, 192f
Wrist
    anteroposterior x-ray of, 142, 142f
    bones of, 141, 141f
    joint anatomy, 143-144, 143f-144f
    magnetic resonance imaging of, 144,
    144f-145f
    osteonecrosis of, 144
    tendons of, 145, 145f

X
Xiphoid process, 35f, 68f, 84f
X-ray(s)
    ankle, 178, 178f
    anteroposterior. *See* Anteroposterior
    view
    chest. *See* Chest x-ray
    concept map of, 2f
    elbow, 135, 135f

X-ray(s) *(Continued)*
    foot, 181, 181f
    hand, 142, 142f
    hip joint, 151, 151f
    knee joint, 163, 163f
    lateral. *See* Lateral x-ray
    lumbar vertebrae, 21f
    overview of, 2
    posteroanterior. *See* Posteroanterior
    x-ray
    thoracic vertebrae, 19f
    wrist, 142, 142f
X-ray densities
    comparisons of, 2f
    interpretation of, 3, 3f

Y
Y ligament, 150

Z
Zona orbicularis, 150f
Zygapophyseal joints, 197f
Zygomatic arch, 189f
Zygomatic bone, 186, 186f, 188f-189f,
    193f, 195f
Zygomatic process, 186f, 189f, 193f
Zygomaticofacial foramen, 186f,
    188f-189f

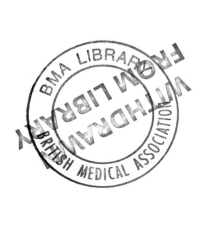